A Sceptical GP

A Sceptical GP

Elen Samuel

A Sceptical GP

Second edition (first print edition)

Published by Rheafield Publishing

Names and identifying details have been changed to protect the privacy of individuals.

This book presents memoirs and opinions and is not intended to be used to provide medical advice. The reader should consult a physician in matters relating to health and particularly with respect to any symptoms that may require diagnosis or medical attention.

ISBN 978-0-9576291-0-3

Research presented in Chapter 35 courtesy of Alison Hughes

Cover illustration by Teresa Jenellen

Designed and typeset by Rhiannon Miller

Printed in the UK by Cambrian Printers
http://www.cambrian-printers.co.uk/

Acknowledgements

With thanks to my long-suffering husband for his support and help throughout the writing of this book.

Also to Jane, Rhiannon, Marijke and Harry for their help and encouragement.

Dedication

This book is dedicated to the memory of our darling granddaughter Faith, who died in December 2009, aged two.

Author details

Elen Samuel is the pen name of a recently retired GP with many years of experience of the ups and downs of life in general practice in a rural practice in Wales. The patient anecdotes and stories in this book are based on real life, but in the interests of confidentiality all details have been changed and scrambled.

She still lives in Wales and enjoys playing music in chamber groups and orchestras, walking and travelling abroad, often getting as lost in other countries as she does at home!

Contents

Introduction

Healthcare in the developed world is a wonderful success story. Just think of the average healthy lifespan, the conquering of infectious diseases, the great advances in cancer treatment, and even the effective long-term treatment of chronic diseases. No wonder the media love a good positive success story, be it the heartwarming story of a young person battling bravely against serious illness, a new treatment available now, such as Lucentis, a new treatment for age-related macular degeneration which causes blindness in the elderly, or, more likely, a treatment that works in mice and might work in people in twenty years time. They also of course love a good health horror story, the dreadful misdiagnosis, the uncaring nurse, the long waiting lists or targets missed yet again. It all sells newspapers and magazines, and the money spent on health by both governments and patients, including on private health care, make the economy go round, as well as (mostly) helping patients.

What do patients make of it all? The wonderful explosion of information out there now makes for an extremely well educated population, at least for those who are interested in health matters. Medical information obtained over a lifetime quickly becomes out of date, and my knowledge of new developments in subjects that were once my field, such as diabetes, will become less relevant, so that before long there will be a time when my knowledge is not much better than the next person's. But what I have, and most non-doctors do not have, is a sense of perspective. I have been fortunate enough over the years to share with patients their concerns and hopes, and I have seen so many different sorts of treatment come and go. This is really what I would like to write about.

I was a GP for thirty-five years, and I firmly believe in a strong primary care system. A GP is usually trusted to act as the patient's advocate and can help and encourage people through their journey to get the most effective treatment. Patients fall into several groups when they start to need healthcare advice. There are those that have busy lifestyles and not a lot of interest in the hows and whys – they just want a quick and easy fix and to get on with their lives. There are the chronically worried and pessimistic who haunt the doctors' surgery but again have not

1

much interest in the details of how to get better. There are the deniers who hate anything to do with doctors and health and only access health care when they are forced to because of pain or disability. There are those who perhaps could have become doctors themselves, with a wide and balanced perspective on health care. And then there are the ones who frankly just like the attention of doctors, the more eminent the better, and those who will consume any healthcare option if offered in a persuasive way – or even if not!

This last group isn't going to like what I have to say, and so almost certainly aren't going to read it; if they do, they are likely to dismiss it. They are likely to feel that they know what needs to be done and it is only a matter of finding someone who will do what they think they need. This book isn't for them. It is for those, probably most of us at one time or another, who really would like to know what is likely to be effective, and who would like a bit more balance in their reading about health matters than they will get in the popular press, or on the internet. It is written to give a different perspective on the healthcare industry and how it affects us all.

Part 1

The GP's role in the developing NHS

Chapter 1
Primary care

The history of the gatekeeper role and how it affects GPs as gatekeepers to hospital care in the UK – Comparisons with other countries– The NHS and how it developed for GPs and hospital specialists

The extent to which the problems with recent underfunding in the NHS have affected patients and their GPs is illustrated well by the diagnosis of brain tumours. They are not common, but are common enough for many people to know of someone who has had one; they occur in all ages from children to octogenarians; and they often kill, sometimes quickly. It is well known that headache can, rarely, be a sign of a brain tumour and of course headaches are very common. So persistent headaches worry people a lot, and the first port of call is the GP. Like any other conditions, there are guidelines for the diagnosis of the various causes of headaches, and most people will have a simple condition such as tension headaches, migraine or neck problems. But even when these conditions have been diagnosed, headaches may not get better with treatment and many patients will have a nagging worry that they really have a brain tumour that their doctor is not picking up.

At one time in our locality when funding for the NHS was at an all-time low compared with other countries, we had diagnosed six brain tumours in people within three years, and these cases all clustered under a set of power lines that ran over our town. One in particular was a 16-year-old girl who developed a pituitary tumour, others were a mixed bag of brain tumours such as astrocytomas, a very aggressive and malignant type, and meningiomas, which are not so deadly but can recur after treatment.

The parents of the 16-year-old started a campaign to find out if the power lines were causing these brain tumours, and indeed there did seem some cause for concern. We reported the findings to the local public health team, and they investigated it as fully as they were able. Eventually they convinced the GPs (but probably not the patients' group) that power lines were not to blame, but even so there was a heightened awareness of brain tumours in the town. GPs of course had no access to magnetic resonance imaging (MRI) scans, which might diagnose these tumours early. There was an acute shortage of scanners and personnel to use them, and when they were available they were often not used to capacity, only between 9 a.m. and 3:30 p.m. for example. Even consultants could not get scans done. Computed tomography (CT) scans were more available but could give false negative results. One of my patients was reassured that he did not have a brain tumour on the basis of a negative CT scan, but his headaches persisted and eventually when he did get a MRI scan the tumour was found, but too late. The waiting lists to see a consultant neurologist were also very long, as our local neurologist had left and it was many months before a replacement was found. So GPs and their patients were in a very unenviable position. The likelihood of a patient with persistent headaches, dizzy spells or other vague symptoms having a brain tumour was very low, but it was impossible to reassure people without either a consultant opinion or a MRI scan, both of which took months to organise. After another of our young patients was found to have a brain tumour after nine months of headaches, we were all very anxious to make sure this did not happen again, and many of us were sending more and more people to see a neurologist even when the likelihood of anything serious going on was extremely small, thus putting even more pressure on waiting times.

Another case was that of a pharmacist who while on holiday suddenly developed a painful and uncomfortable sensation all down the left side of his body. He was a fairly stoical sort and preferred to finish his holiday rather than seek medical help in Thailand. When he came back I found his blood pressure was high and diagnosed a thalamic stroke. He was unwilling to be admitted to hospital and indeed he was not otherwise unwell and had gone back to work, so we treated his blood pressure and investigated him in the surgery. But it proved impossible to get him a quick neurological opinion either on the NHS or privately. It was two weeks before Christmas and no neurologist could see him privately until the middle of January.

What were we to do? If we (GPs) ring up the on-call doctor in this situation we will be advised to send the patient into hospital as an emergency. The patient will then get a good examination by the resident junior doctor and then sit on the wards while waiting for a consultant opinion and a MRI scan. Never mind that as hospital stays are the most expensive part of health care, this is very wasteful, it is also unpleasant for a busy professional, and in this case the patient really did not want to go. However at that time the Health Authority allowed us to do a limited number of MRI scans at a private hospital locally but paid for by the NHS. This was a system left over from fund holding days, which had been jealously guarded by our local GP groups which had followed fund holding. We could do 25 per year in our practice and they could be in any speciality.

So I was able to order a MRI scan, which confirmed that the man had suffered a stroke, and reassured the patient and the doctors in our practice, who could carry on treating him for his blood pressure in every way possible, secure in the knowledge that the diagnosis was right and he didn't have a brain tumour. Subsequently the local neurologist saw him as soon as he could. We were very lucky to have this facility as in most areas GPs could not order MRI scans directly. In his cases we had treated his blood pressure, and he did well, but it was an example of how difficult it was to work in the NHS at that time and how it affected patients.

Since 2001, millions of pounds have been poured into the NHS but I am not sure that such cases cannot still happen. The issue of GP access to specialised radiological tests is still with us. Now with an adequate neurology service, local GPs have agreed that only a neurologist can order these MRI scans but patients are sometimes very annoyed about this. After all, any episode of a TV medical drama, whether from the USA or the UK, will include patients getting MRI scans at a drop of a hat, and people do not understand why they are so difficult to access here.

The fact is that the amount different countries spend on MRI scanners is incredibly variable. In the UK the number of imaging examinations performed increased from 0.6 million in 2001 to 2 million in 2010.[1] But its total MRI capacity is still low compared to other countries – only 6 units per million people. In that time Austria has increased its spending on MRI units from 12 per million of population to 18.[2] The USA started with 20 units per million in 2001 and now has a capacity of over 30. Australia spends the same as the UK on MRI scanners and France only slightly more. I am sure that the optimum must be in the middle of these two figures. The USA spends far more than is needed whereas the UK could even now do with more.

Recently I went to a conference of GPs from all over the world. As with all conferences, it was an opportunity for time out to discuss, reflect and ponder upon the situation of GPs in health care in many different settings. I was amazed to discover the variation in systems of delivery of health in Europe, let alone in the rest of the world.

The conference was held in Austria, which has a very successful insurance based system, so GPs are working in a system with excellent secondary care, with low waiting lists and very efficient technology. But I was surprised to discover that they are restricted to single-handed practice – the system gives financial penalties for group practice. It meant that they could not provide many interventions themselves and had to refer everything to hospital. Austrian GPs only had one year of training and were not considered to be specialists in the same way as GPs in most other countries, where GPs usually have had at least three years and sometimes four of training, and have their own speciality organisation, such as the Royal College of General Practitioners in the UK. The Austrians were puzzled when I asked them about access to MRI scans and said that as patients would only have to wait a few weeks for a neurologist why would they need to ask for an MRI scan themselves? Australian GPs however could ask for MRI scans despite their availability not being much better than that in the UK. The federal government had introduced this specifically to improve childhood cancer detection rate. The Australian GPs were very satisfied.

Austrian GPs told us that the lack of specialist accreditation meant low status, and although their pay wasn't bad, it was hard being on your own. The discouragement of group practices made it especially hard for female GPs, who are now in the majority (as in most other countries) when they wanted to start their families. It also means patients have to go to hospital for almost every aspect of their care. It is just about the most expensive way to run a health service. Given that GPs usually deliver about 95% of care in a community, are often highly appreciated by patients, and a good system of primary care can make a health care system more effective, why do some countries like Austria fail to develop their primary care? In times of austerity one would think that this would be a no-brainer. But there are other factors at work.

The delivery of health care in most countries of the world (with the possible exception of Cuba) is not a Universal Good, acting in some mysterious way to enable us all to live healthier and more fulfilling lives. It is an industry that needs to make a profit and, like economies, always needs to grow. A good-enough drug, an adequate operation that does what says on the tin, may be what the patient needs, but that is not necessarily what the healthcare industry, insurance companies, pharmaceutical companies, specialists' leaders and the media want. They want new exciting developments that may indeed improve some people's lives but also makes them a profit. GPs are in the way here. If they are effective gatekeepers they will prevent many patients going forward to sample these new goodies, and may well give advice to the effect that there is a simple treatment available locally without the fuss and risk of more interventionist therapy.

The public loves to hear about new stories of breakthroughs and the media will cash in on this and provide them. They are fed by big expensive campaigns funded by all these health industries, which would dearly like to be able to advertise directly to the public, as they do in the US. When a patient actually talks to a GP she may realise that there is more to it than going straight for the wonderful new advance. So a really effective GP system is a barrier to profits. It can also undermine super-specialists' ability to promote their new operation, their new guideline, their influence and their power. As the prestige and the power usually resides in the super-specialists organisations, busily promoted and helped by the health care lobby, they are not keen to cede power to GPs. Hence in some countries there is a desire to keep GP practices separated from secondary care, keep them small, restricted in what they can do such as order modern up to date investigations, and keep them at the mercy of patients' wants rather than their needs – which may not be the same thing.

Of course, in the UK GPs may not be able easily to order MRI scans, but they can do a lot of other things. They are organised into groups of GPs with a lot of help from nurses and other ancillary staff. They also have, or will have, a lot of influence on what is provided by the National Health Service (NHS) with the new reforms in England. Countries without well-developed systems of primary care usually spend much more on health than those that do have such systems. The US is the prime example of this, and its health care system is the most expensive by far in the world. Quality does not necessarily improve either, as I will detail later.

The GP's role in the developing NHS

The reason why British GPs have a central role in patient care goes back a long way. The NHS was founded in 1948 with a commitment to health care for all, free at the point of delivery, and this has been kept by and large ever since. But all the money came from the Government, paid out of general taxation, so of course was cash-limited from the start. Governments have many competing calls on their purse. Not so in Austria and other countries with an insurance-based system. They have a two-tier system with all residents being entitled to free care but it is routinely topped up by many patients who pay into an insurance scheme, to get extra care, so the amount of money available is just much larger. New services in hospitals can be developed much more readily and the GPs can refer direct to these services with their patients being seen quickly. Thus there has not been a need to develop primary care, or at least not up to now.

In the early sixties, when the UK was still chronically short of money after the war, GPs were still mostly in single-handed practice working out of very shoddy premises, and not only had huge surgeries of people in real need, but also could not easily access good hospitals. The hospitals just hadn't been built, and there was a real shortage of doctors too. So in 1964, young doctors weren't becoming GPs, and GPs' morale was very low. Enough was enough. The British Medical Association (BMA), then as now a powerful trade union for doctors, told the government of the day that GPs wanted a new deal, which included incentives for group practice, a better contract in which the money they got did not depend so much on having a very large list of patients which they then had difficulty servicing, better premises, a less onerous method of dealing with on–call (it was 24 hours a day 365 days a year and the only break was when you employed a locum). Of course the Government refused to countenance any such changes, saying they were too expensive. But the GPs had something up their sleeve. The BMA threatened the government of the time with GPs leaving the NHS en masse, giving post dated resignations to be implemented if the government did not agree to their demands. As a result, 18,000 of the then 22,000 GPs signed letters of resignation letter from the NHS to be implemented if the Government did not agree. On 2nd July 1964 there would be no primary care health service, as 82% of GPs would have gone.

I remember that time well. I had wanted to become a doctor from a very early age. When we were three, my twin brother and I were hauling some books on a towel up the stairs. What we were doing it for I have no idea, but near the top the inevitable happened and my brother lost his footing and fell down the stairs, He broke his leg and was admitted to hospital where he stayed for six weeks in traction. When he came out I was apparently very solicitous and fussed over him constantly and as we were only three, must have been an awful nuisance. (Maybe I thought it was my fault as it probably was my idea to go upstairs with the books.) Anyway I decided then that I wanted to be a nurse, but when I was about five I heard that there were such things as lady doctors and I determined to be one of those.

When I was about fifteen I had quite bad acne, and went several times to see my GP, in a dreadful lock up surgery where the method used was to advertise the surgery hours from 9 am to 10 am. Everybody used to come in and crowd into the small waiting room. At a quarter to ten the doctor would arrive and at ten the surgery doors were shut. The doctor then proceeded to go through the patients in order of arrival, so of course the minimum wait was three quarters of an hour and the maximum probably two and a half hours. What a system! But patients were grateful – many still remembered the times when they couldn't afford to go to the doctor at all. I remember telling my GP that I was going to be a doctor, and I was surprised by his vehemence – 'whatever you do, don't do medicine. It is a terrible life. Do something else.' Of course I took absolutely no notice and by the time I qualified the battle had long been won.

The Government bowed to the inevitable. The Family Doctors Charter of 1964 secured a number of 'wins' for GPs, including improvements to premises, proper remuneration for out-of-hours work, and the ability to develop a really good standard of family practice.

It did take time for the low morale not only in general practice but also for doctors in hospitals to improve, and even when I qualified, 4 years after the new contract was implemented, almost 20% of the newly qualified doctors in my year left the UK, most never to return. Those were the heady days of wonder at a medical degree that would be accepted anywhere in the world. As conditions improved for UK doctors, the worldwide shortage of doctors began to abate and most countries slapped on restrictions for entry for doctors, and that combined with the improving conditions at home stopped the brain drain in its tracks.

Interestingly, by the late 70s and 80s, general practice was the career of choice for doctors in the UK. It was quite difficult to get training posts and jobs when you finished training. That was very clearly a result of how general practice had been able to develop.

In Austria it seems none of that happened. Austria has a very good standard of health care and came 9th in the World Health Organisation (WHO) health care rankings in its 2000 World Health Report, while the UK was 18th and the USA was 37th. This listing has not been updated since but Austrian indicators of good quality health care are still high. Patients can have free care as public patients, but have to wait for hospital appointments and tests. However the care is excellent when they get it. Most people pay for insurance and then get a better service with less waiting and some people choose to pay for all their care privately. GPs are used as personal mentors to guide patients through the system, and must have been satisfied in the past, but now it appears they are beginning to want a more important role. It seems that many doctors, certainly GPs, would like to work in the public system and there is a waiting list for doctors to join. Presumably therefore there are too many doctors trying to make a living in the private sector and this will reduce their bargaining power to get a better deal. It would certainly make for a more efficient service if they did.

Their healthcare system is expensive though: total health expenditure was 22% more than the UK in 2009.[2] Would the British public like to pay the difference out of its own pocket? I don't think so.

But after 1990 the British system was going to get much worse before it got better.

Chapter 2
Continued history of the NHS: waiting lists and healthcare rationing

History of the NHS (continued) – Acceleration of process of underinvestment in health care – Effect of long waiting times on diagnosis – Comparison with other countries – A new world of increasing funding – Austerity again and current cost pressures

So the golden age of general practice in the UK was from 1964 to 1990. During that time GPs were rewarded for grouping together (there was a 'group practice allowance' which you could claim if there were three or more partners), practices could employ nurses and ancillary staff such as receptionists, with a partial re-imbursement of the cost from the Government. The cost–rent scheme allowed GPs to design and fund their own premises using public money (this was in fact an embryonic PFI – Private Funding Initiative – scheme but it was much better run and didn't bankrupt the community as recent PFI schemes have tended to do), therefore many other health care professionals such as midwives, district nurses and community psychiatric workers were 'attached' – that is, they worked from the same premises, thus helping patients to get all the care they needed form one building. It certainly was great for me. I began a child health clinic, a well-woman clinic, and also started off the computerisation of the practice as early as 1983. It was very satisfying, and I could do it because we weren't over-worked. We even had a reasonable on call overnight commitment as we took part in a rota with other local practices.

After 1990, when a new contract was imposed upon GPs (they did not agree to it) a lot of the development of new services stopped. The contract linked GP's pay more strongly to performance. The terms and conditions of primary medical service delivery were closely specified and there was much less freedom within practices to change things. But it did start off a new development which put GPs in the forefront of commissioning service outside the practice, a system known as fund-holding, which I shall discuss in detail later on.

Meanwhile things were not going so well in the hospital sector. The UK has always been at the bottom of the OECD (Organisation for Economic Co-operation and Development) list of countries in spending in terms of health care costs as a percentage of GDP. In 1970 the UK spent 4.2%, while Austria (as an example) spent 5%,[3] and the USA, which has always been top, spent 7%. Then the gap widened so that by 1992 the UK was spending 6.8 % while Austria was spending 9.8% and the USA 13.6%. By 1996 the UK's costs had actually gone down to 6.5%, Austria's was 10% and the USA was still 13.6%. By 1997, it had fallen yet again to 6.3%, at which time there was a change of government in the UK. This puts it into context, and it is a wonder the NHS was functioning at all. We at the coalface could see what was happening very clearly.

Very little money was being made available for improvements in services and waiting times for hospital treatments were beginning to get longer and longer especially for surgical specialities. There were three main issues here. One was the lack of money for new operating theatres and intensive care facilities, causing waits for operations once it had been decided that an operation was needed, and another was a shortage of staff (mainly doctors) in out-patients departments which caused queues for people waiting to be seen by a specialist for their first appointment. These two problems were separate but obviously the total time a patient had to wait for definitive treatment was the sum of the two difficulties. Then, as a third problem, in between seeing the specialist and having the operation there was a lack of facilities for complex investigations such as scans, which prolonged the wait between seeing the specialist and getting listed for an operation, and also prevented GPs from investigating their patients properly before referral.

This lack of money therefore affected all patient care in hospitals in the UK, from diagnosis, procedures such as investigation to treatment for serious diseases and operations. Probably the most serious impact though was on cancer. To some extent the actual treatment of cancer was protected in that radiotherapy and other specific therapies were developed, mostly because of the efforts of the specialists working in the field. I am no expert on that. But the diagnosis of cancer in primary care was very difficult, and I certainly did know about that. I have mentioned the problem of diagnosis of brain tumours in Chapter 1, but probably the most difficult to diagnose were the ones in the stomach and bowel.

Diagnosing cancer early and reliably is not easy whatever health care system you are in. To some extent it has to be a trade off – investigating everyone who has a common symptom with complex tests to identify very early the few that have cancer may not be the best way to go, as many people will be harmed, by the tests, by the worry or by the treatment with false positive diagnoses. People say you can't be too careful and everyone should have these tests, but this is only true for some cancers. Stomach, pancreatic and lung cancers are often diagnosed as soon as symptoms appear, but treatment is not usually successful, as symptoms appear only when the cancer is already quite advanced. Often treatment in these cancers is not effective and it would have made no difference if the diagnosis could have been made earlier.

However for those cancers for which treatment is usually successful, such as breast, skin, and colorectal cancer, it is important that the diagnosis is made early and in the UK we have never been very good at doing this.

As an example there was one patient that really stuck in my mind from that time. She was in her late fifties, and it had to be said that she was a very frequent attender, both to her GP and to hospitals. Her husband had worked in the local pharmacy as an assistant and often helped with making up some of the prescriptions, so was quite knowledgeable about some medical matters. She came about general aches and pains, stomach aches and mild blood pressure problems, and had been investigated several times for unexplained stomach pains. I saw her early one year with more complaints about pain in her stomach. I did some more tests, which came back negative, but felt there wasn't much more we could do, but after the third visit I did refer her to the local consultant. Six weeks later she came back with her daughter (which was unusual), a very sensible lady, and asked for the appointment to be expedited and I agreed. The procedure was that you write another polite letter to the consultant saying that the symptoms were worse (or no better), and could she be put up the waiting list? However the consultant, who had after all seen this lady twice before, did not do this, and three weeks later she was back again. I was at a loss – I realised that the consultant did not think she needed to be seen any sooner, and to be honest she wasn't complaining any more than she had before. When I said that I would do my best, the daughter looked me in the eye and said, 'Can you guarantee that this isn't cancer, doctor?' That shook me and I said that no I couldn't. No one can until full investigations had been done. This time I rang up the hospital and she was seen within a few weeks. She was put on the end of a session with a junior registrar (doctor in training), and he couldn't find anything, the tests had been negative, and it wasn't until she had a laparotomy in due course that an inoperable cancer was found. She died a few weeks later. Even back then, in other countries she would have had her investigations much earlier, though whether she would have lived any longer can never be known.

Waiting lists are of course de facto rationing, and many countries do it. They can be effective for operations which have an element of desirability, such as cosmetic operations, and they may not cause too much harm for operations like joint replacement as a moderate wait does ensure that people are not offered an operation before they are really ready for it. But cancer is different. Cancer is an active process and kills, so diagnosing it early can be lifesaving. But all through this time when other countries were steaming ahead with new developments in diagnosis with more and more sophisticated scans and endoscopies, the UK was standing still. GPs obviously could diagnose the classical signs of cancer such as in the breast or skin very easily and did so, but lots of cancers did not present nearly so obviously. Many cancers such as colorectal cancer or womb cancer present with bleeding, and this is easily referred, but unfortunately this sort of bleeding can also be caused by common benign conditions like piles and hormonal problems. It is usually quite impossible to differentiate between these things in the early stages of cancer, and so referring all of them as 'urgent' does not help the hospital at all. They will still have to do a definitive investigation on everyone and when there is a bottleneck because the facilities have not been properly resourced then diagnosis will be delayed. The fact is that even nowadays waiting lists have to be short for everyone in these specialities in order to diagnose cancer early.

Countries such as the USA of course do it differently. There primary care is not well developed and most insurance companies will fund a patient to go direct to the specialist they think they need to go to, without seeing a GP first. The specialists are then funded on an item-for-service basis so that they will bill for each procedure they do rather than being paid a salary, therefore the market will ensure that there are always enough specialists with good facilities for investigation and treatment, so there are no waits longer than a few weeks. The patient of course (or their employer) is paying through their insurance payments, and this is one of the reasons the USA spends so much on healthcare.

Other countries in the OECD have developed their GP system as a gatekeeper because this is an excellent was of keeping costs down and avoiding some of the extreme waste and inequality the American system produces. Today GPs in such countries as Spain, Portugal, and Croatia and of course Greece report terrible problems with long waits and inability to get patients who really need treatment seen at the hospital because of lack of funding, because waiting times are the first thing to suffer when money is tight, and GPs refer more patients to hospital than the available funding can stand. In the UK in the nineties the specialities particularly affected were surgical specialities such as orthopaedics and oph-thalmology, although the problem can affect most specialities including medical specialities. Locally they got very much worse from about 1990 when there was a re-organisation of hospitals in our area, and over the next 14 years waiting times sky-rocketed. The system was failing to keep up with the demand from patients to get hospital treatment.

The fact is that it is necessary to control waiting lists to a reasonable level if patients are to be treated safely, and what happened over the years from 1984 to 1998 was tragic. No wonder the UK slipped down in the league of good health-care on many measures. Of course people could argue that it wasn't realised how fast medical care had been developing in other countries over this time, but the doctors in hospital and most GPs were well aware of what should have been provided.

It was certainly obvious that referrals had been increasing year on year in many areas and specialities. There were good reasons why this might be happening. There had been major new developments in many surgical specialities, such as joint replacement in orthopaedics and cataract surgery in ophthalmology. The population was getting older and more educated and people were increasingly asking for these treatments.

Far from being the envy of the world, the NHS was now a laughing-stock, and in America was held up as an example of the horrors of 'socialized medicine'. In a way they were right, as in a market economy you could never under-invest to this degree. Firms would always take advantage of gaps in the market, and indeed this was happening in the UK with more and more private work being done. NHS rankings for treatment of cancer got lower and lower compared to European countries that had insurance based systems. I have tried to detail the cost to patient health in my vignettes of the patients I treated, and the sense of impotence amongst NHS staff was pervasive. There was under-investment in new technology, in staff and in expertise compared to other countries, and of course for the patient the waiting times for treatment were horrendous. Though there were costs associated with repeated letters, rescheduling of clinics and of missed appointments as patients moved away, got better or died while waiting, they were nothing compared to the costs of putting more resources into the system, and politicians refused to do this.

At that time no one 'owned' the problem of waiting lists, as Health Authorities who were ultimately responsible had no power over the hospital waiting list system. They were supposed to regulate waiting lists by allocating more money to the departments most under pressure. But they never had any money to allocate and in any case had no levers to ensure that any extra money given was used for this purpose. The hospitals and specialist departments washed their hands of the growing waiting lists, as there was nothing in their contract to say that they should see patients in any given period of time. There were no sanctions on the hospital or Health Authority for keeping people waiting, and a culture developed where it was accepted as inevitable.

The system was kept frugal because each year an inadequate budget was set by the overall authority and hospitals had great difficulty keeping to it, so each year the managers overran their budget. Then there would be negotiation and the overspend was finally agreed and paid (or put forward to the next year). So the NHS got the worst of all worlds, there was never any money for new investment in a planned and orderly matter but when costs spiralled out of control because of inflation, inefficiency or sometimes bad management, the hospital would be sure that in the end they would be bailed out. There were no rewards for success, and nothing ever happened to the managers or clinicians who had presided over overspend so there was no incentive to improve.

Patients made angry telephone calls to the hospitals about the long waits and GPs and their secretaries made endless calls trying to negotiate urgent appointments, and they sometimes thought that the specialities were not trying to help, but in reality there wasn't a lot they could do. Individual consultants may have hated it that so many of their patients had to wait so long, but the solution was very complex. Some hospital consultants and other staff became very demoralized. Those that tried to see people quickly had a terrible load while some gave up even trying. Some indeed, though irritated no doubt, had a vested interest in not shortening the waiting times very much in the short term as they were about the only lever consultants had to protect their department from cuts and further under–investment. It might give them more power to demand more staff and increase in facilities. No doubt in some areas and specialities, some were not displeased that private work could take some of the load.

A new world

Eventually even politicians realised that this was a terrible situation for patients and doctors alike, and gave the NHS a very bad name all over the world. After a change of government in 2004 it was announced that they were going to invest in the NHS to bring the money spent up to the European levels. We GPs were very sceptical but indeed the government was as good as its word and soon doctors and managers in the Health Service could try to do something positive.

Resources began to trickle through in terms of staffing levels and technology. Cancer, its diagnosis and treatment, for so long an absolute disgrace, was now given priority for funding. Much needed investment in scanners and other equipment made a huge difference. For GPs on the ground though, it was the huge drive to bring the waiting times down that had the biggest impact. The governments of the time had a penchant for targets and in England that was to be 18 weeks from referral by a GP to treatment – not for first appointment but for actual treatment (in Wales it was put at 26 weeks, slightly more realistically).

So Primary Care Trusts in England and Health Boards in the devolved administrations were charged with the responsibility of implementing the targets of the Patient Waiting Time Initiatives. In Wales it was called T2T, Time to Treat. What a challenge when previously the waiting time from referral to first appointment could be up to 3 years and the waiting time for operation once on the list could be more than a year!

More money was now pumped into the system, and the amount of managerial energy used up in this process was phenomenal. Many new administrative jobs were created to try to ensure that each step on the pathway was scrutinised for ways in which efficiencies could be made. Of course they could and should easily reduce the figures by getting rid of the large number of 'ghost' patients on the list, patients who had died, moved away or had got better (there were plenty of those). I did wonder why this had never been done before. I suppose only in a system that was totally top down could this situation have arisen in the first place. It was certainly long overdue. After all, the first thing to do if treatment is in short supply is to make sure that the waiting list was accurate, as appointing all these 'ghost' patients meant that there were frequent 'Did Not Attend' patients (DNAs) – patients who did not keep their appointment. Of course what actually happened was that managers then overbooked patients to avoid the inevitable waste of time when an appointment was not kept. But that in turn meant very long waits in clinic when all the patients booked in did turn up.

What it did highlight was that previously waiting lists were not at all high up in Health Service priorities, so no one cared about them. This was brought home to me when I was talking to some Norwegian GPs recently. Now Norway is a very rich country – there is no lack of money to spend – but these GPs told me that currently patients can easily wait a year for an Orthopaedic appointment. They also told me that GPs in Norway do not have much 'clout' – they aren't involved in commissioning services as GPs in the UK are. So in Norway, despite the fact that there would undoubtedly be money to improve the system, no-one, apart from the patients and the GPs, thinks it is important to manage the waiting list and make sure that there are enough resources to ensure patients do not have to wait a long time. It isn't always a lack of money in the system, although for some reason spending on the health service in Norway overall has gone down in the last year we have records for.

So in the UK, after culling the lists of ghost patients, the new managers got more creative and took people off the waiting list if they missed appointments, or had other medical problems so that they were considered unfit for operation. In our area a lot of this was happening rather than investing in new clinics so not many new outpatient appointments were created at first. Eventually managers realised that it would not be possible to reduce the waiting times without creating more capacity so they started to do 'waiting list initiatives'. These were extra clinics, with the consultants paid extra on top of their normal commitments, in the evenings and at weekends, to come in and see patients to prevent them waiting too long. This continues today although it is a very expensive way of doing it. Some surgeons quite liked the extra money though others found it a lot of hard work. It was certainly very convenient for some patients to come in after work and have their appointments and sometimes tests as well. It suited the specialists who had never done private work as they could get extra money for doing something that was really worthwhile, though I do remember some doctors saying, as they treated those patients who had been waiting years, that there was really very little pathology there and not a lot of patients actually needed much done. This was because of course the waiting process had streamed out those with real problems and their GPs had usually managed to get them pushed up the waiting lists. Or sometimes they had died. But there were undoubtedly patients who needed treatment, and the others definitely needed answers to their problems.

Was the NHS system so short of staff that Diagnostic and Treatment Centres (DTCs) had to be set up to free the system? Probably the answer was yes. Years of underfunding had left the NHS acutely short of manpower. DTCs are run by private companies for profit, and are contracted by the Government to take the load off the NHS, with straightforward operations such joint replacements and hernias, and may also provide more scanners and other diagnostic equipment. They were staffed by surgeons outside the NHS at first, and they undoubtedly got waiting times down in many areas, sometimes to the NHS surgeons' displeasure, as of course it had a potential to reduce the private work these surgeons could do. DTCs are, of course, private initiatives and there were many problems with these, discussed in detail in Chapter 34.

So gradually there was increasing capacity in the system. All these new initiatives really made a difference and waiting times were coming down rapidly. It was relatively easy to make sure that patients coming through the system could have their surgery or definitive treatment soon after the decision was made to have the treatment as there were now enough theatre sessions, if you included the extra 'waiting list initiative' sessions outside normal hours, and hospitals achieved their targets. However they then found it was very difficult to keep the waits for the first appointment down as referrals from GPs kept increasing.

Of course if you can't improve the flow any further everyone realised that it was necessary to turn off the tap, or at least reduce the flow considerably and that meant looking at GP referrals as they were almost the only source of requests for consultant first appointments.

It was clear there was a rising demand from patients through their GPs. Was it just a reflection of the pent up demand that had built up while resources were scarce? Or was the system grossly inefficient and people were referred unnecessarily? If so, were there methods that could be used to improve it? No-one really knew the answer, but certainly for cancer there must have been a big rise in referrals – correctly, as this was the only way to ensure patient safety. The general public was getting more aware of the sort of symptoms that they needed to see their doctor about, and the concept of 'red flag' symptoms was. Patients with such synptoms had to be seen within two weeks, and this started to improve early detection of cancer. There is a lot more about red flags throughout the book as I think this is the key to ensuring good cancer outcomes.

But for other specialities the referral rates were rising without such good reasons. Orthopaedic referrals had risen almost exponentially over this same period, and so managers were finding that it was very hard indeed to keep to the 18-week target.

When I was still working in general practice I looked at what was happening to the patients whom we had referred to Orthopaedic surgeons in our practice, to discover how many of our patients got surgery and how many were treated in other ways. This was when waiting times were probably the longest they had ever been, and patients were definitely being denied the operations they would have benefited from, especially hip replacements. Of the 163 patients we referred to orthopaedic surgeons during 2003–4, 20 were referred to NHS consultant clinics for back problems. Of the 14 who were seen in the first 6 months, presumably those with the severest symptoms, only two were recommended for further investigation. The others were discharged immediately or were seen repeatedly in the back clinic and given physio (which they could have had anyway) or corsets, or referred to the pain clinic. Indeed some got better with no particular treatment, although many continued to have low-grade back problems. None of these patients were considered for back operations. I found it that hard to understand because I had heard that operations on the discs in the back were the answer. But our local surgeons did not do many of them on our patients and in retrospect they were right. I have given the evidence for this elsewhere but in many cases good active rehabilitation is a better way forward. If operations aren't very effective, then this raises the question of why we GPs were referring so many patients to hospital. In fact the reason was that we did not know the evidence. Indeed there was not a lot of evidence available at that time, but everyone hoped that there was a treatment that would reliably get rid of back pain and therefore we overloaded the clinics.

When I looked at what had happened to our 54 patients with knee problems, I found a similar pattern. Thirteen NHS patients were still waiting after 18 months to be seen for a first appointment. When I looked at their notes I found that some had had physiotherapy in the meantime (referred by the GP) and got better, but the hospital had not been told that they were better; and a few had had an MRI arranged by the GPs under a scheme left over from fundholding days, and found not to need referral. But eight patients were still waiting in a lot of pain over these 18 months, and as treatment of knee problems is now very successful it was most unfortunate that they had to wait so long. It looked as though we really should have been referring many people for exercises and physiotherapy first instead of to outpatient Orthopaedic services, but at that time physiotherapy also had long waiting lists. Some patients sensibly saw the physiotherapists privately. Then the few patients who really did need an intervention would have been seen quickly.

The fact is that GPs could be more careful about whom they referred to hospital and who could be treated just as effectively in community clinics, and this is a theme I come back to later in the book. Just as with waiting lists being allowed to build up with no effort being made to validate the lists or make the most of the appointments available, GPs always assumed that they had a right to refer to whatever specialist they felt would give the patient the best service. Consultants encouraged them in this because success is associated with having a lot of patients referred to them, and that meant more influence over managers who were getting far more important in running the hospitals. It was a right GPs felt was essential to their being able to do the best for their patient. But did GPs really know *what* was best for their patients? It was soon realised that there was no standardisation of referrals and GPs were unaware of how many referrals they made compared with their colleagues. It was found that all over the country that

GPs in the same sort of practice and seeing the same sort of patients were referring up to 15 times more than their colleagues. They can't all be right and maybe GPs did not really know the evidence behind their decisions. There has to be some evidence base behind what GP refer and this is again something that is explored later in the book.

It was beginning to be understood that perhaps the bonanza of burgeoning hospital care was being overdone, and patients would benefit from more local services, less high tech, which would give at least as good an outcome. But to set them up needed more money and it has always been difficult, if not impossible, to transfer money from hospitals to community services. When waiting times go up, the first priority is always to get the patients who have already been referred seen in hospital. It was considered unethical to take people off the waiting list to see health professionals other than the doctors to whom they have been referred. So any available money tended to go to the hospital for more consultants, more diagnostics and more operating theatre time (all also needed of course) and not to setting up services in the community, in health centres or in local hospitals where the full range of services was not needed. What was needed was cash to 'pump prime' the system, putting in more local services so that the patients wouldn't get on to the waiting lists to start with. This finally came about in many areas when NHS funding soared from 2004 on. Altogether the drive to reduce waiting times was a big success, waiting times did come down rapidly and was a big factor in the sudden huge rise in satisfaction with the NHS that occurred at this time.

Now however there is again a big squeeze on money for the NHS and attention is again being paid to GPs referrals. Commissioning groups, which had antedated the new NHS, and now have control over the system, had started to look in detail at evidence-based pathways and most GPs now find their referrals under scrutiny.

In 2004 the GPs had yet another new contract. This contract again changed the way GPs are paid, but paradoxically took away some of the aspects of general practice that we thought patients most appreciated. Previously a partner in a GP practice had his or her own list of patients registered with them and patients considered that doctor 'their' doctor. To some extent this had been eroded by the advent of very large group practice, but it was still an idea both patients and doctors liked. This was done away with, and all patients are now registered with a practice, and may not have a one-to-one relationship with any doctor. The practice is paid through a 'global sum' depending on the list size and other factors. Another big change was that GPs no longer had to commit to on call outside the hours of 8 and 6.30 and were no longer obliged to do Saturday morning surgeries. This was a big step and many patients are still not satisfied that their GP is giving as good a service as before. GPs work is now much more focused on management of chronic diseases in the surgery, and there is much less emergency work. The work is also more tightly regulated and is incentivised by a system of extra payment for meeting quality targets – the Quality and Outcomes Framework, (QOF) which has been copied by many other countries.

General practice in the UK is changing in other ways too. It is no longer a popular speciality as it had been and many training schemes struggle to find young doctors willing to train as general practitioners. Young doctors, who are trained in the hospital setting apart from a few weeks, are exposed to the highly sophisticated world of the hospital specialist and are choosing paths towards the really interesting work there. (Many are rapidly disillusioned however as the hospital ladder itself is changing, not always in the way these young doctors would like).

More GPs are part-time with both male and female doctors finding full-time practice too hard, and many do other things, both medical and non-medical in the times they are not in the surgery. The new contract enables experienced partners to employ salaried assistants who don't have the commitment to a lifetime in the same practice. Sometimes this is because they don't want it, but more often they can't get partnerships, as the senior partners will earn more when they don't share the global sum with other partners, because they earn more than the salaried assistants. This is likely to destabilize practices in the future.

These are all fairly abstruse points which don't directly impinge on patients now. But it is odd that primary care is under threat at the very time that it is most needed, to ensure that medical care is given to patients as near to their homes as possible and to avoid unnecessary and harmful treatments.

Where does all this leave the concept of Patient Choice, I wonder?

Patient Choice has been a mantra in England for over 6 years now. However it seems to refer only to patient choice of hospital – that is, once the decision to refer you to hospital for a specialist consultant appointment has been made you are supposed to be offered a choice of hospital. In fact if you don't remember about being asked later whether your GP did or did not offer you a choice, and say so in a later questionnaire, your GP will lose pay. Most GPs say however that outside London there is no appetite for choice. In general patients want their local hospital to be good enough. Patients usually ask 'what do you think'? And many GPs do not know enough about the consultants in other areas so won't be able to advise them. Some consultants do support patient choice and believe that it would stimulate them to improve services. However in a cash-strapped environment this isn't likely.

Patient choice of treatment other than hospitals would only work if there were really accurate data. I believe patients should have much more knowledge of what works and what does not, so that they can make realistic choices. But in my experience a choice of hospital has never been a high priority for people.

There is no doubt that as waiting times plummeted at last patients were getting a comparable service to most other European countries which had had much more money spent on them for years. By 2010 the waiting lists had all but gone, and patients were being seen within a reasonable time scale for the first time for decades. The overall number of referrals to hospital was also falling – by quite small amounts but it did seem as though the push for more effective treatment was having its effect.

Satisfaction with the NHS has also risen to a high level. A recent report by the Commonwealth Fund showed that when 9000 randomly chosen adults from 11 countries, were asked about their health care, the UK came top in measures such as: confidence that users would get the most effective treatment and lowest rate of errors, and second in fewer problems in getting care after hours.[4] Overall the levels of public confidence were higher than in any other country. When similar questions were asked of people with poor health who were actually using the service, confidence was even higher. And this is despite the fact that the NHS is still cost-effective; in 2010, it cost £2220 per person per year compared with an average of £2767 in the other OECD countries (an average of 20% cheaper, after adjustment for cost of living). The NHS in 2010 scored 4th out of 11 countries for waiting more than two months to see a specialist and 8th for waiting more than 4 months for elective surgery. It was 7th in breast cancer 5-year survival rates and in avoidable death rates, so no doubt more money targeted at diagnosis and high tech treatment in some areas would help, but by no means is the NHS now a laughing-stock, and much is good about the care people get.

Having done a whistle-stop tour through the ups and downs of Health Service functioning in the last 60 years, I now want to look at the really interesting side of life in general practice – patients and their problems. That treatments have changed, and patients have changed, over those years is not in doubt. The extent of those changes, and what is good and bad about them, makes an interesting story.

Part 2

Public health

Present-day challenges and vested interests

Chapter 3
Obesity

Demand for healthcare – health effects of obesity – evolution – food and nutrition – modifying market forces – bariatric surgery.

The UK health service has recently enjoyed a period of unprecedented increase in funding which has made a world of difference to patients, and by extension to their doctors. But now we are in 'austerity', and the Health Service will not see such increases again for the foreseeable future.

The problem is that demand for healthcare is on an upward escalator. The aging population, the increase in chronic diseases, the demand for more and more procedures, the epidemic of obesity are well known to cause increased costs at a time when there is no more money available. So what can be done about these?

Well, we can't say that either the aging of the population or the increase in chronic diseases is a bad thing. Both are due to lots of diseases not killing you off much earlier, such as infections, or heart attacks, and people with chronic diseases such as diabetes not dying well before their time. We can and should make sure these conditions are treated as effectively as possible. However the epidemic of obesity, like the epidemic of smoking before it, is something that has causes and solutions. We have to do something about it.

Obesity is an intractable problem for many people, as most people I saw hated being fat. If it were easy for them to lose weight they would but it isn't. We know that the body somehow regulates itself so the one's weight tends to stay at a constant level which is extremely difficult to alter by dieting. Unfortunately if we eat more, the 'standard' seems to set itself at a higher level each time. Some people do put on weight more easily than others but many just do like their food. There is no doubt of course that if you do eat less you will lose weight. I saw this time and time again when people got ill, usually with cancer.

There was one very nice lady who cheerfully admitted to liking her food, but who unfortunately also had valvular heart disease from rheumatic fever in childhood (very rare these days). As a result the extra load on her heart through being obese (and she was very obese) put her into heart failure, and for years she was blue, and very breathless with swollen feet, despite all the efforts of the cardiologists of the time. She also developed diabetes with all the consequent problems. Then she developed a slow growing cancer of the oesophagus, and could not eat. She lost weight very quickly and for about 9 months she was fitter than she had ever been. Her diabetes was cured, and her heart problem also got better so that she could go out shopping again for the first time in years. Of course she died of the cancer, but before she did she managed to get a lot more out of life.

But it has always been difficult to prevent obesity by just eating less. There have always been grossly obese people. In my early days in practice some were just as fat as people are now, but there were far fewer of them. I had a patient once, a lady in her early forties who could only be described as round. She was short, and very wide. She was very upset about her weight and came back to see me time after time. There were no dieticians then for GPs to refer to, so I found a diet sheet and encouraged her to stick to it, and to exercise. However she didn't lose any weight, in fact she kept on putting more weight on. Finally I put her on a diet of 500 calories one day and 1000 the next, and when that did not work, she persuaded me to admit her to our 10-bedded cottage hospital. Just think of that – she had no complications, not even diabetes, and she was in hospital for 3 weeks, on this very low diet. She was supposed to be supervised by the nurses to make sure she stuck to her diet. After 3 weeks she had lost 1 lb. I couldn't believe it and I honestly thought she had some sort of physiological problem. We discharged her from hospital, and it was only later that I realised that she had been cheating the whole time – going out and eating her favourite snacks.

Afterwards I didn't try nearly so hard, although GPs are exhorted to give advice and help people to lose weight, as they are expected to police many other behaviours. I felt obliged to give anti-obesity drugs but every drug that we have ever tried on obese patients has been a disaster, for example Fenfluramine, Tenuate Dospan and more recently Sibutramine. All were launched with high hopes of being the magic bullet, and each one turned out to have really serious side effects. None of them allowed people to lose more than a few pounds in weight anyway. Most have a run of a few years only before the problems appear and I was always relieved when each of them was withdrawn. While obesity can kill it is certainly not justifiable to give people tablets that would make them ill in other ways.

Well, how does obesity kill you? In my experience in general practice, some fat people were perfectly healthy. There did not seem to be a rule that if you saw an obese person in their fifties or sixties that they would die sooner than thin people. What did kill were two associated diseases – diabetes and hypertension, and those people were definitely likely to die earlier. But if you were fat, but didn't have either of these diseases, your blood pressure was normal and your blood sugar well in the normal limits, then what were your risks of dying earlier than thin people?

There has been a study recently in the US, which dealt with this question, looking at population-based data between 2000 and 2006.[5] The results were that for those people with severe obesity, meaning a body mass index (BMI) over 35, there was an association with mortality (due to diabetes and hypertension). But for those with milder obesity (BMI 30 to 35) there was a decreased association with mortality, in other words these people lived longer than their thin counterparts. And what was more, the mortality in diabetes was lower among obese versus normal weight individuals, so that you are worse off if you are a diabetic with normal weight. For those people in the study who were underweight, the associated mortality was definitely greater, something that does sound right. Underweight people are not often healthier, often because the reason they are underweight is that they are ill in some way.

I am not one of those people who think that the normal state of humankind is thin. The present tendency to aim for everyone to be within the magic BMI Body mass index of 20 to 25 is definitely a cosmetic thing, not a true health indicator. As people age they usually put on weight, but in moderation this is normal. BMI together with waist circumference is a better guide than BMI, as it is central obesity that is harder on the system. So again you need to eat sensibly in order to prevent diabetes, but not in order to get really thin.

What evolutionary advantage is there in being fat? I don't think that any one would quarrel with the idea that fat people are going to survive longer in a prolonged period of shortage of food. However the way this works isn't only to do with occasional famine. This works on a more everyday basis – having children. Babies have fat at birth unlike baby chimpanzees, which are skinny and look wizened compared to a human baby. The human foetus first starts to lay down subcutaneous fat in the third trimester, and then if all goes well will continue to become fatter during the first six months of life. This all comes from the mother when breast feeding, so it is not surprising that the mother too has to build up reserves of fat. There must indeed be an evolutionary advantage for babies to have this store of energy, and this may be the reason that women are more likely to put on weight all over their bodies rather than round their middles as men do. The skin is very elastic and can cover as much fat as needed to ensure enough food for the next generation. Babies then start to lose their fat as they go on to an adult diet, and normal diet and activity keeps most children slim – or used to. So fat is definitely normal. It is just unfortunate that there seems to be no upper limit.

The amount that has been written about why people are fat, and what diets to follow, is incredible. I don't intend to write much more about the subject as it is complicated and confusing and changes from month to month.

As for 'glands' causing overweight –a long time ago this was commonly thought to be the problem with those relatively few people who were overweight, and I wondered as I started my medical course what glands these could be. It seems that they were actually talking about the thyroid gland and under-production of thyroid hormone. This is dealt with fully in Chapter 10. Sadly you still see advertisements telling people they can lose weight if they take thyroid supplements, and several of my patients over the years went to private slimming clinics to get thyroid tablets despite not having a thyroid deficiency. As too much thyroid is extremely dangerous, having nasty effects on the heart such as arrhythmias and atrial fibrillation (see Cardiology) and heart failure, these practices are totally unethical and should never be part of medical practice.

But of course obesity never was primarily a medical problem. It is a social problem, a food problem and specifically a food industry problem, although a very complex one. Food products and the amount of processing of basic foodstuffs into palatable and tasty meals have increased hugely over the last twenty years. People in the post war era weren't generally overweight, but they weren't undernourished either. Their diet was similar to their parents, fairly basic meat and vegetables, and the consumption of processed foods has rocketed since then. It has been a market-driven process because women are no longer in the home with time to spend on shopping and cooking, but are out in the workforce, and they don't want to spend hours cooking for the family when they get home. So we can't blame the market – it has just responded to needs. But in order to make processed foods really tasty the manufacturers have to be very innovative in what they add to the food. The products of food manufacturers are regulated for safety but not for their effect on long-term health.

Now, I don't know what exactly it is in processed food that causes the rise in obesity, specifically in the last twenty years or so. Some people blame trans-fats, or any of the other sorts of manufactured fats which have been developed over the last hundred years, some the wrong sort of sugar, especially in processed and 'sports' drinks, others say it is just too much of everything. So it is imperative that we now look at the evidence and do more clinical trials to see exactly what the culprits are. Then, as the market has caused this problem the market will need to stop it. The answer is to tax everything containing foods that are proved to cause obesity very highly.

That sounds easy, but I am sure it isn't going to happen for a very long time. First you have to get the evidence. This would have to be done by very large clinical trials over many years, each one isolating a particular food which is thought to cause the trouble. They would have to be funded by governments or universities. The evidence would have to be compelling because food companies would argue against the evidence, and might try to 'bury' trials that don't go their way, as a the tobacco industry did for years. Once you have the evidence you would need to get governments to agree to tax the offending substances in order to get the companies to remove them from food and drinks. As this would almost certainly remove some of the 'tastiness' and palatability – after all this is what the food industry has worked on very hard over the years to appeal to people – the food companies would object and fight it all the way. The food lobby is likely to be as powerful as the tobacco companies were and fight just as strongly.

Then what would be the ultimate effect? The theory is that foods that are un-healthy would be very expensive, but basic foodstuffs like fruit and vegetables would continue to be untaxed so that poor people especially would be forced to eat more healthily. (The rich could still afford to eat badly, but of course they usually don't.) But would that happen? Smoking, despite being incredibly highly taxed, is still much commoner amongst poorer people than amongst the wealthy. People whose lives are harder, who have more of a struggle to keep things going, tend to hang on to what they see as the real pleasures of life, in this case eating tasty food (and smoking), sometimes at the expense of other more important things like paying the rent. The public would not really want this sort of 'nanny-ing', as it would be seen. So expect a long and rough ride.

It might be a self-limiting problem of course. By mid-century, on present trends, there will be 2.3 billion more people on the planet, and they will need 70% more food.[6] Food uses up large amounts of fresh water and energy, and though it has been projected that these extra people can be fed, big changes would have to be made in the way we eat in the developed world. The main problem seems to be eating meat, which though very good for you, has ecological, social and health consequences that are not sustainable.[7] Meat production uses more fresh water, uses up far more energy than food derived directly from plants and has a disproportionate impact on the ecological system, increasing global warming as the tremendous energy input involved in nitrogen fertiliser production causes significant climate change. Continuing to eat meat at the rate we have been in the developed world is not sustainable, and it will start to have a big impact on us in the next twenty years. Starvation in parts of the world has always been a fact of life due to crop failure and drought and will undoubtedly get worse with climate change, but there will be shortages of some foods in the developed world soon. There is no doubt that cultural influences are crucial here, with some societies eating far more meat than others – I can think of Argentina as an example where a meal out might consist of not just beef but four other types of meat as well – pork, lamb, rabbit and goat, all piled up in a pyramid on your plate! A vegetarian option is not usually on the menu! We need solutions that tackle our current obsession with food head on and which can stimulate consumption patterns featuring higher quality meat, smaller portions and more vegetarian meals. This will be a big challenge but can be usefully combined with a drive to get everyone to eat more healthily and reduce obesity.

Because the alternative of doing nothing at the moment is also extremely bad for the next generation's health, as well as being expensive and likely to bankrupt health services around the world. Children are most at risk. The combination of less exercise as they play games on their electronic devices and watch TV rather than playing outside with their friends, and unhealthy food, has already caused type 2 diabetes in adolescents and this is likely to rise so that, according to one view, the next generation is likely to be the first whose life span, on average, is going to be less than the one before. Diabetes is a real problem, and though once you have it you deserve the very best treatment, the best solution by far is prevention. Certainly I would suggest more education in schools and more public health advertisements as to what a healthy diet should consist of rather than taking the medical route.

Now, bariatric surgery has been hailed as the wonder treatment for obesity, and indeed it does work – a bit like having cancer, but not so deadly. I have seen people get their lives back after losing a third of their bodyweight, and able to discard all their pills for diabetes and blood pressure. It has been shown to be safe and very beneficial over six years,[8] although it is not a procedure entirely without risk, and people have died from short-term complications. A recent study in Sweden of twenty years' worth of healthcare use indicated that it was not possible to make a compelling case that it saved money in the long term by preventing diabetes,[9] as people who had had the operation used more hospital services than those obese people who hadn't had it, for the first six years at least. So one can understand the reluctance of society to roll out the intervention to all who might benefit in the short term. One common problem is depression after the operation, and I really wonder what is going on here and what is the relationship between overeating and brain chemistry. So many of the people I saw (unlike the lady above with heart failure) were fat because of comfort eating, which they did because they were depressed, or at least had nothing else in their lives which was really fulfilling. So were those people the ones that became depressed after stomach stapling? Or is there really a link between overeating and depression?

Apart from severe obesity and lack of exercise, and the people who still smoke, our health is generally improving. Present day lifestyle in the Western world is incomparably easier, more interesting and rewarding for many people than in previous generations. We expect the future to continue to improve and especially in the healthcare field. We expect there to be many more centenarians and for us all to have a long and hopefully well-funded retirement. But it is increasingly being understood that these are not givens and it may be that we are on a downward slope because of lifestyles. And more medical care is not the answer.

For the rest of the book I am going to have a lot to say about the effects on the world economy of the huge expansion of medical care. I am going to preach that there is too much healthcare, too many prescriptions written and it is really time we stepped back and looked in detail at what we are doing, what developments in medicine are really helpful and which are just expensive and misleading blind alleys. We all know that the present good state of our health owes far more to freedom from want, good sanitation and good preventative measures than from medical care. We, the public and its advisors, really need to cultivate 'the art of doing nothing.'[10]

Chapter 4
Alcohol and other abuses of the body's physiology

Effects of alcohol in the body – alcoholism – addiction to opioids – overdosage and suicide

It never ceases to amaze me at what we can do to our bodies and still stand upright. We are so much in control of our environment that we can overindulge in alcohol, drugs, smoking and eating, and mostly we still keep going, and only a few suffer really serious effects. Our bodies have a certain tolerance for changes from the 'normal' way of life – eating and drinking, eating 'natural' foods only when needed and not to excess, but there comes a point when the normal physiology of our bodies is overcome by deviations from this imagined perfect lifestyle. Yet we have a remarkable tolerance for some 'additions' to our environment, through our increasing sophistication in manipulating foodstuffs, because at certain times in history they have been beneficial to us, and our metabolism has adapted accordingly.

At medical school we studied biochemistry, the science of what goes on within our cells, and it absolutely fascinated me. The idea of all these tiny molecules rushing round inside our cells, interacting with each other, breaking down other molecules and in so doing producing energy and electric currents, building up complex proteins which were then used to make and repair the cell structures, then storing energy in the form of fats, and finally sending waste substances to the liver and kidney for elimination, was quite wonderful. What you learn about biochemistry and physiology is that everything is about balance and feedback. Too much of an end product in biological systems always produces a signal to some other part of the body to switch off whatever process it is that is producing the excess, for example if blood sugar levels rise you will produce more insulin to use it up but if your blood sugar falls too low insulin is switched off and a process will start in the liver to produce more sugar. Wonderful. And the tolerance limits are quite wide so that you can eat too much, drink too much for years and never suffer really bad effects.

But of course you can take this process too far. Over the years alcohol has probably been the most damaging self-inflicted poisoning of the system for some individuals, and yet it probably saved many lives in the past. Beer making has been around since 10,000 BC, and in times when water sources were not safe, because of infections like typhoid, people who drank beer rather than water did not get infected, not of course because of the alcohol content but because the water had to be boiled during the beer making process. Children drank beer. European populations have a high alcohol tolerance because their bodies have been exposed to regular use of alcohol over so many millennia.

Alcohol can be metabolised in two ways. In the usual way the end product is acetic acid, (vinegar) and this is quite well tolerated by the body. The other way is to metabolise it to acetaldehyde, another small molecule containing the basic atoms of carbon, oxygen and hydrogen, but this has quite unpleasant effects when in high concentration in the blood, causing the symptoms you get in a hangover, such as feeling sick, and generally unwell, and a thumping headache. The enzyme that influences the reaction when alcohol is metabolised to acetaldehyde is called alcohol dehydrogenase (ADH2) and if you have a lot of it you will metabolise alcohol to acetic acid and have fewer side effects if you drink a lot. However if you have a lower level of this enzyme in your liver, you will get a hangover easily. Your genes govern the amount of alcohol dehydrogenase you produce in your liver and so there is a strong hereditary component here. People who become alcoholics have a lot of this enzyme, so have a bigger tolerance from the start. Most of us have a natural toleration limit for alcohol and will vomit or get too drunk too carry on drinking, but people who become alcoholics don't have this natural feedback system and so are very vulnerable to alcoholism.

This is especially true of Australian aborigines whose bodies have not been exposed to alcohol over millennia,[11] and explains why they and their society have been so much destroyed by it. Another metabolic variation affects about one in three East Asians who lack another enzyme, acetaldehyde dehydrogenase, ALDH-2, one that helps to break down acetaldehyde itself, and so they suffer unpleasant facial flushing after drinking even small amounts of alcohol. This is again inherited and is known colloquially as 'Asian Glow'. An ALDH2-deficient drinker who drinks two beers per day has six to ten times the risk of developing oesophageal cancer[12] as a drinker not deficient in the enzyme. So Europeans have on the whole developed a way of living with alcohol that is not too destructive, but even so, for those affected individuals who are at risk from alcoholism sometimes the only answer is complete abstinence.

Lots of my patients asked me whether resveratol in wine really protects against heart attacks. We all know that despite the French drinking large amounts of red wine, their rate of heart attacks is low, and it has been said that this is because the resveratol in the red wine have a protective effect. This is supported by research on animals and in vitro which indicated the possible pathway by which this might happen, but there have been no studies in people that prove it. Other scientists deny that there is much resveratol in red wine anyway. I have always felt that the differing methods of death certification in the two countries might have something to do with the differing rates, as in France it is possible to put old age as the main cause of death on a certificate, whereas in the UK you can't – it can only be a contributing cause. Therefore when an elderly person in the UK dies suddenly, the cause of death is often put as a heart attack without a post mortem examination, while in France certainly in the older age group, old age, probably a more sensible cause of death, can be put down legitimately, thus reducing the cardiac element in the rate of death at a stroke in France. It is certainly true that differences of coding can account for about 20% of the difference.[13] I suppose it would be correct to compare the two in younger age groups, but if you are over 70 you might well want an excuse to enjoy your red wine! And why not, whether or not it does help your heart. Of course the J shaped curve for blood pressure[14] against alcohol consumption generally does show that 1 or 2 units of alcohol a day are good for your blood pressure and actually lower it slightly, the only trouble is the very steep rise in BP as the amount of alcohol you consume increases! So moderation is everything here.

I looked after many alcoholics in my time as a GP. I really felt sorry for these people, whose lives were often completely ruined by alcohol. One man in his twenties came to see me weekly for a very long time, and he begged me to try something new. I had often prescribed 'Antabuse', which is a substance that if you take regularly will give you a very nasty reaction to alcohol because it blocks the enzyme alcohol dehydrogenase and produces the dreaded acetaldehyde, giving you a very nasty hangover in 20 mins or so. So every morning you can make the decision whether to drink or not, and take the tablet at a time other than when you are already in the social circumstances when it is almost impossible to refuse a drink. Of course it does require a lasting commitment not to drink, and this chap didn't have it. He would come back and say that he had forgotten to take the tablet on just one occasion and that was when he had got drunk yet again. So I tried a newer tablet called acamprosate, which is thought to act to protect the brain from effects of alcohol. Regular excessive drinking will cause a reduction in the activity of some biochemical receptors in the brain, and as is the way with feedback systems in our bodies, the body attempts to compensate for the loss of activity by producing more receptors in people who drink too much. That is fine as long as you keep drinking but if you suddenly stop there are far too many of the receptors. Stopping alcohol produces glutamate, an excitatory transmitter that then floods these receptors. The result is symptoms of the DTs – delirium tremens, a most unpleasant experience. Acamprosate reduces the glutamate surge and therefore can help people come off alcohol and stay off it by stabilizing the chemical balance in the brain. So I read up about it and though it is usually prescribed by psychiatrists in hospital, I discussed it with the patient and he agreed to try it. I saw him weekly and he was doing very well, was back to work as a gardener and was even getting back with his wife. He developed some diarrhoea, a well-known side effect, but continued with the medication for about 4 months. Then he lost his job – nothing to do with his drinking, but the work he was doing came to an end – and that was it. Within days he had stopped taking the medication and was back where he started.

My impression was always that drinking alcohol is really not an unpleasant way out of any of life's problems. People with a high tolerance for alcohol don't experience the nasty effects and they aren't easily made sick or get hungover. Their families and work mates might suffer the nasty effects but they don't, and this means that they so often resort to alcohol when anything goes wrong.

Another patient, a woman in her mid sixties, had always enjoyed alcohol and probably had always drunk too much but she was a very sociable individual with lots of friends. I never suspected she drank too much. However she went through a painful divorce and both her offspring were messing up their lives. One son was a professional rugby player who made some money out of it but couldn't live on the money he earned and bizarrely then went on incapacity allowance (while still playing rugby) to make ends meet. The reason for incapacity allowance was binge drinking! He and his mother just drank all the time. Eventually the mother developed jaundice and I realised what was going on. She was detoxified in hospital and saw psychiatrists who told her she would need a liver transplant but must give up alcohol completely. She must have made a decision then that she would not stop drinking. Her son (she reasoned) needed the money that was tied up in her flat and she had lost most of her friends – this was an easier option than trying to give up the one thing that she enjoyed. A year later she was dead of liver failure. It didn't help the son of course despite the money he inherited; he still drank and his rugby deteriorated (he was getting older anyway) and presumably is still on benefits. It seemed such a shame.

And the first chap? He did come back to see me later wanting more of the tablets but this time I persuaded him to go to AA (he had been before but dropped out). I think that really AA has much more to offer alcoholics than a GP. It requires far more time and understanding than I had to give.

So addiction to alcohol is a great social problem. Acute alcohol overdose is a big problem for the health service, and is common, forming a sizable part of the average A&E attendance. In the past we often found ourselves visiting such people at home, and one man in his fifties sticks in my mind. He had taken some sleeping tablets and a large amount of alcohol, and had then called his estranged wife, who came to see him and then called me. Unfortunately by the time I got there he was deeply unconscious, and I immediately called an ambulance. The ambulance took a long time to arrive, and I found myself desperately trying to keep his airway going – he was an obese man and he was in real danger of respiratory obstruction. His wife refused to help in any way and went upstairs so I found myself having to phone the ambulance with one hand while keeping his airway clear with the other. He was whisked off to hospital and recovered, but he had a long-term alcohol problem and his life was a mess.

In contrast, I did not see much acute overdosage of heroin and other street drugs. Mostly they went straight to hospital and got treated there. When I first started in practice there were very few addicts and up to a few years earlier family doctors had been able to prescribe it legally for the few that were addicted. The Home Office kept a careful check on known addicts, and most addicts were wealthy, used it at home, and many were doctors. Heroin is a powerful painkiller prescribed regularly (and quite cheaply) for cancer and other very painful conditions, and many people who use it for pain can easily stop it if they no longer have a need for it. Its use as a recreational drug though is quite different and the dangers are well known, from the risk of spreading HIV and Hepatitis C through contaminated needles to the risks due to the fact that addicts never know what dose they taking – a dealer does not 'cut' heroin with Health and Safety considerations in mind. The risk to life of heroin comes directly from the fact that it is illegal. Logically, if it were legal, taxed (like alcohol and tobacco) most of the health problems would disappear. But too many powerful people make too much money from the illegal drug trade that any attempt at reform is unlikely to get anywhere. The lesson that prohibition of a substance just leads to big profits and crime should have been learned from prohibition of alcohol by the USA in the twenties.

Opioids have in fact been around for thousands of years and were commonly smoked, usually for the pain killing effect, and they were one of the first herbal medicines that really worked. Many people before the advent of modern medicine would have been extremely grateful for its ability to reduce the terrible pains people used to suffer from. It was the synthesis of heroin from the raw opioids in poppy seeds that became the problem, as instead of a painkiller it now became a mind-enhancing drug with the ability to cause addiction.

Of course people will overdose on many things – almost anything that comes at hand. Aspirin and paracetamol, barbiturates and Valium were the usual ones in the seventies, and then came antidepressants, and a mixture of new drugs, some of which were very toxic in overdosage.

The most memorable patient I saw was a young woman, whose partner called me at 2 am one night. 'Can you come quickly?', he said. 'My partner is breathing very heavily.' In my sleepy state I thought she must have been hyperventilating and said, 'Have you tried asking her to rebreathe into a paper bag?' That was the sensible thing to do when someone is really hyperventilating as the bad effect of over breathing comes from the fact that the patient has blown off most of the carbon dioxide in the blood causing the blood to become too acid. Rebreathing your own carbon dioxide will replenish the supply in the blood and relieve the symptoms. 'No, No,' he said, 'she really is ill!' So I got up and went. Again the call was in the country and it was difficult to find, but when I got there I realised that things were really serious. She wasn't rousable and was panting very hard indeed. Immediately I thought of an overdose and eventually we found an empty bottle of aspirin. Now aspirin is really dangerous in overdosage and causes respiratory stimulation by affecting the respiratory centre of the brain. So I called an ambulance, but gave her an intravenous injection of Valium, which worked very well on the breathing and she became more manageable though of course even more drowsy. I went with her in the ambulance and she was quite easily sorted out in hospital. The reason for the overdose was a quarrel with her partner, but what a drama that was.

It may seem that I was always getting called out to emergencies in the countryside and always getting lost. Maybe I am somewhat geographically challenged, but I can't emphasis enough how difficult it was to find farms or isolated cottages in those days especially in the dark. Peoples' ideas of directions vary a lot and they often confuse left with right, and often there is no idea of distance – is the green barn you are supposed to turn left at 500 yards away or 4 miles away? Farm or house names are never prominently displayed if they are there at all. Sometimes people would put the light on and wait at a gate but that was very rare. It wasn't only me – ambulances also got lost. As most calls were not real emergencies it was usually only a nuisance and an awful waste of time, but in an emergency it was a real problem. Phone boxes sometimes didn't work and you had to remember to carry a lot of change, as well as all the other paraphernalia that you might need. It was a problem for the patients too – I remember one man who had to walk three-quarters of a mile to a phone box to call me about his wife, and did it twice as she didn't respond to the treatment that I gave the first time. The advent of mobile phones was a godsend. After that when we were asked what vital bit of equipment we would need in our resuscitation sessions we always answered – mobile phones. Some areas though still don't have any reception and you are back to square one. Satnavs aren't so much use as they are not accurate in the countryside to the extent they are in the town, although they do get you in the general direction of where you want to go.

Of course it was often the same people who overdosed time after time, sometimes as a call for help. Psychiatric teams now roam the hospitals to see these people and try to sort their problems out but often the patients don't keep follow-up appointments and do the same thing again a few weeks later.

Other methods of killing oneself can be by road accidents, which are otherwise unexplained. Once I was called in the middle of the night to a layby on a major road. A car had run into a stationary lorry in the layby at full speed and it had run underneath the back of the lorry, cleanly decapitating the top part of the driver's head. When we looked at it objectively the only possible scenario was that he had done it deliberately. How else could we explain the fact that the trajectory of the car was almost straight so he would have had to turn into the layby (which was a fair length) and then accelerate?

In the country farmers use guns and I was once called to a farmer who had almost certainly killed himself by using his legally held gun. But a few weeks later I got a call from the police querying the time of death. It was then felt it could have been murder. But there wasn't enough evidence one way or the other and the case was never solved. Another time I was called to a farm early on the morning where not the farmer but his 20-year-old son had shot himself. He had been seeing my partner with depression and there wasn't much doubt he had killed himself. I was very upset and could not really relate well to his mother. The last thing you want in that situation is for the doctor to start crying but that was what I nearly did. In the end the only thing I could do was to certify that he was dead (not difficult as he had shot himself at close range) and ask my partner whom the mother knew well to call as soon as possible.

Chapter 5
Water consumption and dehydration: inconsistent health advice

Clinical dehydration in babies – the bottled water industry – sports drinks – salts and ions in the blood – over-hydration – potassium levels – sodium levels and need for salt – intravenous hydration – diuretics – chronic kidney disease – referral to nephrologists – transplants – shortages of donors.

When I was newly qualified as a doctor, I did a job in Paediatrics in a district general hospital. There were only six doctors in the team serving a population of more than 200,000, but we weren't overworked. What we did see though was a steady stream of tiny patients coming in dreadfully dehydrated – dry. They had suffered from infections such as D&V (diarrhoea and vomiting) or vomiting from other causes, but their mothers hadn't realized the importance of keeping their fluid intake up. This was before even the salt and sugar method of rehydrating kids in the developing world where dehydration was even more of a killer. Anyway, it was my job to insert drips into tiny veins in the scalps of these infants. First we shaved their heads, then sterilized the skin and inserted the needle into the veins that happened to be easier to see and manipulate because of the lack of subcutaneous tissue on the scalp. Then we immobilized the needle with cotton wool and sprayed ordinary glue on to it to fix it. It was wonderful to see how quickly these babies picked up with the life giving water, from being half dead scraps to being howling normal infants. None died while I was there but it seemed so sad that they should have to suffer this. I felt then that surely mothers should be told how important it was to keep their infants well hydrated.

I didn't of course do anything about it then, as I went on from Paediatrics to Obstetrics and Gynaecology, Anaesthetics and then to become a GP. Then I realized there was a complete change. Every one knew about dehydration, every health visitor in the land had drummed it into families and now there were no more infants being admitted to hospital with near terminal dehydration. We GPs played our part giving out endless sachets of Rehidrat and Dioralyte to mothers on out of hours calls. What happened about the simple one teaspoon of salt and one of sugar that was used routinely in Africa? Dioralyte and Rehidrat were 40 times the cost but they were well packaged and palatable for the kids so let's not quibble. It was a wonderful result from very simple advice efficiently given. Then I saw things almost going the other way. Mothers were terrified their seven year olds were going to die after vomiting twice, and I saw my job as trying to make sure these children didn't have to be admitted to hospital – the mothers just needed to wait until the fluids worked, because the fact that a child often had diarrhoea straight after drinking did not mean that the fluids were going straight through them. The very act of drinking started a reflex, which would make the bowels open with whatever was in the lower bowel at the time, and the fluid that went into the stomach would get absorbed and immediately help to rehydrate the child.

Then suddenly there were advertisements everywhere about how wonderful water is and the health benefits of drinking more of it. I saw advertisements in public toilets claiming that drinking water was good for your skin and your body and that tap water had lots of impurities that would do harm to our bodies. Who had put them there? People were to be seen everywhere with bottles of spring water, expensively obtained from supermarkets and bearing provenance of some extra special spring water usually from miles away, drinking from them every few minutes as though they would die of dehydration if they left it an hour. One doctor I knew began to advise patients with various illnesses to drink at least 3 litres of (tap) water a day.

I really could not understand this. I had been taught that adult kidneys were excellent at maintaining a good fluid balance in the body. If you were deprived of water for any length of time your kidneys would in effect shut down and conserve the fluids in your blood and body fluids. Your urine would become very dark reflecting how concentrated it was. If you drank a lot your kidneys would respond very quickly and you would find yourself running to the toilet every few minutes, passing very dilute light coloured water. If you really were in the desert without any water, you would by these means manage to live for at least 48 hours and sometimes up to 7 days. It is only in children and especially the under twos that water balance is critical and you have to avoid dehydration at all costs. And what was wrong with tap water anyway?

What was going on here?

Of course people need to drink fluids, and water is a lot better than soft drinks with high sugar content. But bottled water isn't any better than tap water in most areas. Tap water in the UK is of very high quality, and this is monitored regularly. In fact both sorts of water may contain bacteria or carcinogens and the more you drink the more of these impurities you will ingest. It is of course a market ploy to persuade people that bottled water is better, but this hides the real downsides of bottled water. Bottles made from certain plastics contain oestrogen-mimicking chemicals which can leach into the drinking water (and other beverages) they contain,[15] and these oestrogens can depress men's sperm count. The manufacture of plastic bottles also uses up a lot of environmental resources, and their disposal uses up landfill sites and often disfigures beautifully scenic countryside and threatens marine wildlife. Why not re-fill your bottle with tap water?

Your total fluid requirement (i.e. all fluids not just water) depends on the weather, your level of activity (both these will govern the amount of fluid you lose by sweating) and the amount of food you eat. So although many official bodies recommended drinking eight glasses of water of water a day, or 1 millilitre for each calorie of food, and this would seem to be a reasonable amount, you don't have to drink this amount if you are not exercising and are in a cool environment.

There may be some situations where drinking more than usual is good for you, for instance if you have stones in the kidney or polycystic disease (a quite rare condition), and it may help to prevent young women having repeated bladder infections, but it can make kidney infections worse as it reduce the concentration of inhibitory factors which would otherwise help with infections. So it is a complicated situation.

A view strongly promoted by the manufacturers of so-called 'sports drinks', is that drinking more water than you need to replace lost fluids will improve your performance. So sports participants were encouraged to drink for 'performance' rather than thirst, but the studies that seemed to show this were performed under conditions which did not reflect what normally happens.[16] The 'less well hydrated' sportsmen started the exercise not with normal hydration but with artificially induced hypovolaemia (a low total amount of fluids) sometimes by using diuretics. This immediately puts the body at a disadvantage and their performance is going to be lower. More water than you need to replace your greater fluid loss during exercise will not improve your performance. Other studies[17] that purport to show this are very small, of poor quality and usually use surrogate endpoints (see later) such as rehydration rates, and none used the performance of actual athletes in a race as an end point.

Many websites promoting the good effects of drinking water say still state 'you can never drink too much'. This is definitely wrong. You can die of over hydration because this dilutes the amount of sodium in the body, a condition called 'hyponatraemia', both during exercise and when users of ecstasy have followed advice and drunk excess water. It causes brain damage and occasionally death, when severe.

The evidence for this water bonanza has been well reviewed in the British Medical Journal.[18] Suffice to say that there is no really good quality evidence that we need to drink so much water or that it has any properties other than to keep a normal balance of fluids in your body.

Some friends of mine had had a very hard life – they had tried one business venture after another and nothing seemed to go right, they had been made bankrupt once and had failed at most things they tried. When they came to our town the husband tried running a small computer outfit and his wife made and sold fresh sandwiches. They didn't last long; her sandwich business dried up when a nearby supermarket started selling them and his computer business never prospered, as there was a lot of competition. So they sold up and bought a derelict farm in the country and started selling spring water that they claimed came from a pure spring on their land. I saw them a short time later and they were over the moon. They had struck the beginning of this craze and their bottled spring water was selling like hot cakes and for the first time for years they were actually making money. I felt pleased for them, but it underlined that there were lots of money-making opportunities here, so there was lots of advertising, and that was why water drinking became so popular. Sports drinks are particularly well promoted without any good evidence, but it makes lots of money for big business.

Of course this has no knock-on effect for the NHS. People are free to spend their money on whatever they want and such water is certainly harmless. But it does show how we are all susceptible to advertising and how our habits in any sphere but especially our health can be changed quite quickly. It all makes the markets go round. However, certainly in the US, gallon for gallon, bottled water is more expensive than oil, and people on low incomes could spend their money in ways which would be much better for their health, for instance buying more fruit and vegetables.

Personally, although I do a lot of walking on holiday, I don't usually carry much water – it is heavy stuff! If I am going for a morning walk I drink plenty of water at breakfast and then rely on the fact that there will be a nice cold drink at the hostelry at the end. But the attitudes of my fellow walkers are sometimes quite hysterical, offering me their water at every stop and being quite worried if I say I am quite all right thank you. Some people of course should be careful – although adults usually have excellent kidney function, mild kidney failure gets quite common as we age. It is much commoner in people with high blood pressure, and those on diuretic and other drugs for hypertension do have to watch their water consumption, and similarly diabetics.

I don't think that up to now anyone has disproved the hypotheses that if you drink when you are thirsty,[19] enough to quench your thirst, you will be fine. Health food shops are full of information about the various salts in your body and what you need to take in your diet, but some of this is very misleading, so here is some more information and evidence.

The balance of fluid on the body is regulated by the distribution of sodium and chloride (as common salt), potassium and bicarbonate. It is a very complex subject, and very interesting.

The most important ions (charged atoms or molecules in dissolved salts) in the body are sodium, potassium, chloride, and bicarbonate. Sodium is the commonest, and of course is ubiquitous mostly occurring in common salt (sodium chloride) and sodium carbonate. It is the main positive ion in the blood and tissue fluids, while potassium ions, (occurring naturally as potash), are the main constituents within cells. I laughed when I saw one of the adverts for potassium on a website when I was looking up this subject. The website says potassium is good for muscle weakness, confusion, irritability, fatigue, heart problems, chronic diarrhea, and is needed with regular, intense exercise and with the use of certain diuretics.

That is true, though I would substitute 'potassium deficiency can cause' for 'potassium is good for', but I can tell you that if you have these symptoms, the cause is most unlikely to be potassium deficiency. If you do have potassium deficiency and have any of these symptoms then you will be very near death. Potassium levels in the blood have to be kept within very tight limits and low potassium below 1.8 or above 7 millimoles per litre may cause your heart to stop. Period.

I have only seen potassium deficiency, not due to prescribed medication, twice in my career. The first was a lady in her fifties who called me out one morning because her legs were weak. Not a very unusual symptom, but when I got there I found that one of her legs was actually paralysed – weak and floppy, with no reflexes and very low tone. She wasn't otherwise very ill, but I thought she must have a rare form of a virus infection (Guillaime-Barré) so I admitted her to hospital. I heard later that her symptoms were due to potassium deficiency. She had been very constipated and had taken an over-the-counter laxative, which could leach potassium out of the bowel. She had taken far too much of it, and if she hadn't gone into hospital then she would have died. Fortunately, measurement of serum potassium (together with sodium chloride and bicarbonate) is one of the first tests done after admission to hospital for most conditions. The test is called 'serum urea and electrolytes,' measuring urea, the main nitrogenous waste product, and four ions, sodium, potassium, chloride and bicarbonate, so the diagnosis wasn't difficult. That particular laxative was subsequently removed from the market.

The second case was a young child who had quite bad diarrhoea & vomiting, and was admitted to hospital, as she seemed very floppy. She had very low potassium – much lower than you would get with normal virus diarrhoea and vomiting, and turned out to have a rare congenital syndrome causing leakage of potassium from the kidneys. It is extremely rare, and with proper potassium supplementation she grew into a healthy adolescent who excelled at sports. However her mother told me that she had to take over a hundred tablets a day. Potassium tablets are unpleasant to take in any sort of dose and it was amazing how little she complained. But her parents were warned that if she got any sort of infection especially a bowel infection they were to watch her potassium very carefully. It could easily slip below a critical level and then her heart would stop. It was often difficult to persuade doctors who didn't know her of this too, which made travelling with her sporting activities very difficult. She carried a letter from her consultant at all times explaining the need for immediate potassium supplementation if she was ill in any way.

The usual need for potassium supplementation arises from medication, prescribed correctly by doctors. All diuretics, which get rid of excess water fro the body and help reduce blood pressure, work by getting rid of more sodium than usual, and in many cases this means they cause the kidneys to let through more potassium as well. So serum electrolytes are measured regularly in people on these medications and either potassium itself or another diuretic that works by the kidneys preferentially saving potassium, is given concurrently. It is a delicate balance and all doctors will do this every day for their patients by measuring the potassium level in the blood and seeing whether it is in the normal range or not. You can certainly have too much potassium as well – too much in the blood and the heart may go into an arrhythmia (beat very irregularly) and cause heart failure. It is difficult to raise your potassium too high by taking potassium, but if you are in kidney failure and didn't know it (the symptoms can be very vague and make you feel just not very well) then as the kidneys fail they no longer can excrete potassium and the level in the blood rises. If you then take potassium it can push your levels up above the safe level.

So potassium is not something you should mess around with. Otherwise healthy people do not have to worry about potassium and your doctor will diagnose its deficiency or excess correctly in the rare occasions where there is a problem. If your doctor tells you your potassium is a bit low and you need supplementation, because of medication you are taking, you can always eat plenty of bananas as well as, or instead of, potassium tablets – they are a very good source.

The level of sodium ions in the blood is also very important but not so critical as there is a wide range of tolerable levels in the blood. It is very difficult to get sodium depletion even if you are on a salt free diet – there is plenty of salt in most naturally occurring foods, let alone the supplementation in so many processed foods that you don't know about, but you can get a sodium dilution by drinking too much water. This dilutes the salt in the blood and causes the level to drop. It causes weakness and tiredness but is not life threatening except in extremes. If the levels fall too low there is a risk of fits, and one woman following a special diet recommended by a so-called nutritionist, which involved drinking huge amounts of water, suffered brain damage. I also heard of a case once where a man was admitted to a hospital after suffering a road traffic accident, who had two broken bones and severe bruising but not much else. However he was put on a drip (almost everybody admitted to hospital as an emergency these days seems to get one) but this wasn't monitored properly and far too much fluid was pushed into him. He died, but the hospital did not admit the mistake until months afterwards. Fluid overload can be serious.

Interestingly, we don't have any sense that our bodies might be lacking in salt, unlike animals. Many animals in low salt areas will actively seek out salt by eating earth if necessary, but we don't. It may well be that our bodies have evolved in areas where there is plenty of salt, near the sea, and so we have lost some of our sensitivity either to the lack of salt or to excess. In the past stokers and miners used to get severe cramps when working in hot environments when they were sweating a lot, but never thought to take extra salt, though presumably they could have. The scientist JBS Haldane advised adding 10% seawater to the drinking supply, and solved their problem.[20] Nowadays we don't have problems like this – Health and Safety will see to that!

Low sodium, or hyponatraemia, can also be due to diuretic treatment and sometimes it does not respond to just eating more salt. At all times you should be in touch with your doctor. The electrolyte balance in the blood is very delicate and these salts should be used judiciously.

The main organs in your body that regulate these ions in your blood are your kidneys. There are many diseases of the kidneys but most are quite rare in young people. However in older people, their kidneys can wear out like every other organ and this is an insidious problem that affects a high proportion of the over seventy fives.

Chronic Kidney Disease (CKD), or early kidney failure is almost a 'new' disease. We GPs did not usually test for it until recently, and it is symptomless unless the body is stressed with water deprivation or overload. In my practice the people with kidney problems were those who had specific kidney diseases such as recurrent kidney infections, diabetes or polycystic disease, and of course we measured their kidney function regularly. Only a very few people have bad enough kidney function to interfere with their lifestyle. However, as people age their kidney function does deteriorate and there was evidence that treatment of early kidney disease (with expensive drugs) could benefit people's health, because it was thought that if CKD could be identified early and managed well, the number of people needing expensive dialysis would fall, quality of life and longevity would improve, and the cost to the NHS would diminish. So as part of the drive to increase the quality of GPs work, CKD had been identified as one of the targets of good practice (the QOF, Quality and Outcomes framework, discussed in Chapter 8), so now GPs have to measure the kidney function annually of all patients who might be at risk for CKD, with a simple blood test. Then if a certain threshold is reached people have to be referred to hospital to see a specialist.

It is interesting to look at the effects of this on referral rates to hospital over time. Inevitably referrals to hospital rose exponentially. Nephrology departments were overwhelmed, and it was felt that now too many people were being referred, because the guidance was not clear enough. So new guidelines were created in our area, making it clear at what stage people were to be referred, and these were published on a particular web site, the 'Map of Medicine'. It was hoped that a decrease would now occur. So GPs looked at their referrals over the next year – and found that there were only a few referrals in the whole year from the four practices looking at nephrology, so indeed there must have been a huge drop. Was the guidance reducing the number of referrals? Well, no. The fact was that the new contract guidelines had been well publicized to GPs in 2005, and they had been actively encouraged to refer all patients with stage 3 kidney problems, so there had been a huge surge of referrals in 2005 and 2006. In the second year many of those patients had already been referred so it was only a question of referring the newly identified. And there weren't very many of them.

In fact it is now realised that the new guidance was making more than 1 out of 10 elderly people suffer from a symptomless and probably harmless disease, and there are moves afoot to remove it. This illustrates a problem that has resulted in overdiagnosis in many areas. The main beneficiaries of lowering the thresholds for kidney disease are the pharmaceutical companies, as people with mild kidney failure were now to be required to take even more expensive tablets (ACE inhibitors and others). You can see how this happens as many of the experts sitting on the panels of experts that decide on the guidelines have links to the drug companies which make the tablets, and though they may genuinely believe that these drugs will do good it is hard to be completely unbiased. Such experts should declare their interests and if possible should not sit on such panels, but that is very hard to implement. In this case the experts are looking at the guidelines again with a view to changing them.

When kidneys have completely failed, transplanted kidneys can be very successful, and this is now the standard way to treat patients rather than by dialysis using artificial kidney machines. The lack of donors is a real problem – when asked, 90% of people say they support organ donation but less than 25% have registered their wishes.[21] Even when donors are available the problem of tissue matching can mean that a person cannot find a kidney. The Human Tissue Authority regulates this process in the UK, and in England, Wales, and Northern Ireland last year more than 1200 organs from live donors were transplanted, but this is not enough.

Recently a trend has started to use social media sites as a means of finding an altruistic donor – a live donor who can donate a kidney and to widen the number by connecting families and friends of people who need a kidney. This can then form a chain connecting people who had wanted to donate a kidney to a family member or friend, but were incompatible, with a suitable stranger. Their loved one then received a kidney from someone else along the chain. The world's longest chain of organ donations was completed in the US, in 2011, with 30 patients receiving a kidney from 30 living donors.[22] The complicated process lasted for four months and involved 17 hospitals across 11 states. There is a worry that some people can be coerced into donating a kidney, and that relationships formed through Facebook aren't so enduring as the more usual local relationships, but so far everything has gone well and this seems to be an excellent way of ensuring that people get the kidney they need.

Water is of course the most basic and crucial requirement for life. We in the developed world really don't have to worry about it unless we are already ill. It is amazing how much is talked about it here, where good water is on tap, when there are vast areas of the world which suffer form that most damaging of conditions – lack of water. If some of the verbiage could be directed to raising awareness of the importance of a clean water supply for every one, the world would definitely be the better for it.

Part 3

The evidence base
for treatments

Risks, benefits and vested interests

Chapter 6
Hormone replacement therapy: development of an evidence base

Supposed benefits of HRT – side effects – marketing to GPs – results of Women's Health Initiative Study – current recommendations – continuing effects of HRT – PMT

At the beginning of my time in general practice most treatments were 'custom and practice' taught from one generation of doctors to another, as there was good evidence only for the big advances, such as penicillin and other antibiotics, insulin and so on. The change in emphasis to what truly works and what does not has come in gradually. To illustrate it I will talk about hormone replacement therapy (HRT), as a salutary tale. My experience of prescribing HRT was one of the biggest influences on my thinking about how important it is to be sure treatments actually do work. For about 20 of the 34 years I spent as a GP, many postmenopausal women consulted me about the menopause, and the use of HRT as treatment for relief of symptoms and to prevent the effects of aging, including preventing heart attacks, strokes and even cancer. I was for most of this time the only woman GP in a four-partner practice, and the men in the practice were very pleased to see me take up this workload, so I became almost a single-issue doctor.

The bandwagon began slowly, as my first years in the practice coincided with the rapid expansion of use of the contraceptive pill and so my work was dominated by contraception for young women. I went on courses to improve my knowledge of the pill, learnt how to fit coils and generally was pretty knowledgeable about female hormones and contraception. While oestrogens are the primary female hormones produced by the ovaries, progesterones, also produced by the ovary, are important in the menstrual cycle. To some extent they act against the effects of oestrogen and even on their own are capable of acting as contraceptives. There was considerable discussion at that time about the best form of progesterone to use in the pill, as it was known that some progesterones could actually promote atheroma – the plaques in your arteries which can build up to block arteries and cause heart attacks. So it was essential to develop new progestins (synthetic progesterones) with fewer side effects. Over the next few years this was done, and doctors (and of course the drug companies) began to consider whether these improved progestins might actually benefit women after the menopause.

The theory went roughly like this. It is well known that the rate of heart attacks in women both before and for a time after the menopause is a lot less than men's, and it was thought that oestrogens were preventing these heart attacks.[23] So, the theory went, the menopause was a bad thing for women as it caused the risk of heart attacks for women to increase. Also this theory chimed in with women's need to keep looking young, and it was assumed (without evidence) that there would be beneficial effects on the skin, for example. However there were also very well known side effects with giving more oestrogen than a woman normally produced, such as blood clots (deep vein thrombosis and pulmonary embolus), which could be fatal. Also it was known that oestrogens affect cancer in some cases, for instance it will definitely cause endometrial (uterine) cancer unless given with progesterones, and can make breast cancer worse. Of course there was also the obvious disadvantage that a woman's periods came back – just as she had been enjoying freedom from that annoying problem every month for the first time for 30 odd years. You couldn't give oestrogens alone if a woman still had a uterus as this would affect the lining of the womb and cause endometrial cancer, so progestins had to be given to counteract this, and so the menstrual cycle had to continue. This of course was not a problem with women who had had a hysterectomy; they could be given oestrogen alone.

It all sounds very convoluted and complicated now, but because of the big profits in it, there was an all out push by Big Pharma to come up with safer and more convenient forms of HRT. The basic oestrogens and progesterones were now quite cheap, and initially all the companies did was to agree the exact formulations of oestrogens and progesterones in each packet, rather than have to develop more drugs. Now the menopause had to be made into an illness, and many everyday problems such as lack of libido, lack of sleep, and tiredness were put down to the menopause, to be cured by HRT of course.

Soon pharmaceutical representatives were besieging me as more and more companies waded in each with their own combination of oestrogens and improved progesterones. At the time I was arranging evening meetings for our Female

Medics Forum and so offers to pay for our food in return for the ability to put up a stand came in thick and fast. Was I popular!

In time I put more and more women on HRT and this was a big part of my work. There is always a tendency in a general practice for patients to choose their doctor deliberately because of what is known about their competences and of course this is to be welcomed. I saw the menopausal ladies, the men saw heart problems – that was just how it was.

The claims at that time therefore were that HRT

- Prevents hot flushes – there was good evidence of this
- Improved your skin – there was no evidence at all that this was so
- Regularized periods – correct if you were still having periods, but brought them back if you weren't
- Prevents heart attacks – there were some longitudinal studies indicating it might be so
- Combined therapy (oestrogen and progesterones) prevents some cancers e.g. cancer of the colon, cancer of the uterus (endometrial cancer) – there was some evidence of this
- Prevents osteoporosis (thinning of the bones) – good evidence that this is so.

It was also postulated that it would reduce the incidence of Alzheimer's disease – there was no evidence at that time, and the theory has since been disproved.

The known side effects were:

- Periods continue or return and sometimes are troublesome
- Makes established breast cancer worse
- Increased rate of thrombosis (blood clots).

But the side effects were downplayed, and eventually it got to the point where it was being advocated that every woman should have HRT after the menopause whether they were having symptoms or not, because it would be good for their health. We all had algorithms of the risk/benefit which we were to explain to each woman who came in so that they could decide whether to take it, but the pressure by the media – women's magazines, TV programmes, newspapers was intense, even though all the publicity was well in line with advertising standards.

Fortunately many women were quite sensible about all this, and many resisted their doctors' desire to put them on the drug, but by the early 2000's it was being noted that only 37% of post menopausal women were actually taking it and shouldn't we be doing more to persuade the rest?

Then in 2002 came the results of the Women's Health Initiative study.[24] This was a randomized placebo-controlled clinical trial of therapeutic and dietary interventions influencing postmenopausal women's health. Initial publication of the preliminary results suggested overall harm from hormone replacement therapy, leading to a dramatic worldwide decrease in its use. In detail, 8,506 women participants received standard HRT in 1 tablet, and 8,102 women received a placebo (an inactive tablet which looked the same). The results were that there were

- 7 more heart attacks (a 29 per cent increase),
- 8 more strokes (a 41 per cent increase),
- 8 more pulmonary embolisms (blood clot which went to the lungs),
- 8 more invasive breast cancers,

per 10,000 person years in the people taking HRT. As against that there were

- 6 fewer colorectal cancers
- 5 fewer hip fractures (due to the beneficial effect on osteoporosis).[25]

The absolute excess risk of events included in the global index was 19 per 10 000 person-years. There was no protection against mild cognitive impairment or dementia (the study included only women 65 and older).

Of course these differences either way are not big, but are very important when you are trying to improve everybody's health. If the trial had gone the other way, these small differences would have influenced everyone to make sure that all post menopausal women took these drugs, as this is what drug companies do. Marketing such huge numbers of pills will make them a lot of money.

For women who had had a hysterectomy and were taking only oestrogen the results were:

- No difference in risk for heart attack
- Increased risk of stroke
- Increased risk of blood clots

- Uncertain effect for breast cancer
- No difference in risk for colorectal cancer
- Reduced risk of fracture

So this, the first big randomised controlled trial of HRT ever done, comprehensively debunked most of the claims of benefit from HRT and proved that it did in fact increase the risks of cancer and heart disease rather than reducing them. So all those years I had been putting women at risk by peddling unsafe drugs.

So what went wrong? It seemed reasonable to suppose that HRT might work and it is true that a lot of women do develop heart disease after the menopause, although it has been found that the recent increase is actually down to more women smoking. I think there is no doubt that people, including GPs like me, had a very trusting attitude to the media stories of the benefits of HRT. We were just not aware of some of the tricks that were used to publicise these drugs. For instance, in 2009 it became clear that the makers of some of the HRT medicines might have regularly 'ghost-written' articles about the benefits. It was disclosed during a court trial in Arkansas in 2009,[26] where women who had developed breast cancer after taking their products were taking the company to court, that the company had prepared medical journal articles about HRT for general publication but failed to disclose its role. The problem was that there was a secrecy agreement whereby the company could withhold the evidence of what they had done from the court. The US federal court decision resulted in the release of approximately 1500 documents detailing how articles highlighting specific marketing messages written by unattributed writers, but 'authored' by academics, are strategically placed in the medical literature. I certainly was taken in. I had no reason to suppose that these articles, some of which I read, were not unbiased accounts of the importance of HRT to women's health, as I trusted the medical experts whom I thought had written them. Of course it raises the question of what those experts were doing – putting their name to papers that had been written by someone else.

In the 90s the emphasis was mostly on the possibility that HRT would protect against heart attacks and the results which indicated that the incidence of breast cancer had increased obscured the fact that heart attacks weren't prevented either. In 2003 the results of the 'million women study' in the UK (1.3 million women were followed up) were published and they confirmed the findings of an increased risk of breast cancer in the treated women.

But now the wheel is coming full circle again, and the bandwagon for HRT is starting to roll. In 2012, some scientists reworked the results of that trial[27] to say that in fact it is only older women (over 60) who have an increased risk and the younger ones (around 50) might benefit. However, the article's authors, from South Africa, Germany and the UK, admitted that they had all acted, or continue to act, as consultants for pharmaceutical companies that make HRT, and presumably this is the result they would like to see. And now there has been a more recent study in Denmark, which looked at women taking HRT in early menopause, rather than at older women, and this will reassure those women who really need HRT to see them through the worst symptoms of the menopause that taking HRT for a short time is safe.[28] (Some of the authors of this study have also disclosed ties to companies which make HRT.) I think we should all be very careful indeed this time. If we had just kept to the idea that HRT was for treating severe symptoms of the menopause, I would not have been misled into putting many women well past the menopause who had minimal or no symptoms on to HRT, in a misguided effort to improve their health.

The current recommendations are that hormone therapy should be used at the lowest doses for the shortest duration needed to achieve treatment goals. Postmenopausal women who use or are considering using hormone therapy should discuss the possible benefits and risks to them with their physicians.

Any individual GP is unlikely to have caused a death from HRT as the numbers are too small, but there were other problems with this excessive attention on HRT during those years, and that was that, because so many symptoms got drawn in to 'the menopause', many of us spent far too much time on discussing the details of hormone levels, and tended to ignore other possibilities. This could be serious if it meant that we missed other diagnoses that might have been serious – for instance one woman was eventually found to have a rare type of epilepsy which partly explained her symptoms, but she was convinced that her problem was with the menopause, so the diagnosis was delayed.

Quite apart from the human cost, just think of all that money wasted over 20 years. It is the way the system works in a market environment (in which of course

Big Pharma is a major player), but a system like the NHS has to look at every penny to make sure that taxpayers' money is spent effectively.

Nowadays many post-menopausal women use herbal remedies, up to 38% in a recent study.[29] St John's Wort is discussed fully in the appendix, and there is some evidence for its use, but this is likely to be due to its proven anti-depressant activity and it is not clear whether hot flushes are helped significantly. Black cohosh is also widely used, though the evidence is conflicting.

PMT or premenstrual syndrome (PMS) was also a very fashionable diagnosis at one time, being an explanation for all sorts of maladies affecting young ladies and even being held up in court as an excuse to get off with various episodes of bad behaviour. The recommended treatment was to suppress the ovulation cycle altogether, but you need very high doses of oestrogen to do that. Then for a long time we used Pyridoxine, vitamin B6, in very high doses. It never did a lot of good and it went out of fashion. Too much pyridoxine can cause tingling and neurological problems. A herb, Agnus castus, from extracts of the fruit of the chaste tree, *Vitex agnus-castus*, has been shown to have beneficial effects in two adequately powered placebo-controlled RCTs, and some people bought it. Since there is not a lot of evidence in favour of conventional treatments either, this may well be a better alternative.

So gradually PMT disappeared from diagnostic classifications. If there is no money in selling treatments then publicity soon goes away.

And indeed I got no more visits from reps about HRT.

Chapter 7
Evidence-based medicine: 'good' and 'bad' science

Concept of EBM – RCTs – outcomes and surrogate end-points – Lorenzo's oil – statistics – meta-analysis and systematic reviews – guidelines – validity of published trials – relative risk – NNT – fraud and mis-representation of studies – conflicts of interest

What is evidence-based medicine (EBM)? The debacle with HRT showed conclusively that treatments have to be based on evidence. It seems amazing now, but as late as the early 70's when I started working as a doctor, there was no recognition of any evidence behind what we had been taught and what we were doing in medicine. In other words, for most of the treatments we used in day-to-day practice there was no proof at all that they actually worked. In 1972 Archie Cochrane working in Cardiff published *Random Reflections on Health Services*[30] and after this people began to accept that treatments really did have to be proven to work, if at all possible, by trials which compare one treatments with another. The term 'evidence-based medicine' itself only came into existence in 1990.

It is unclear how much the general public knows about or understands the concept. My feeling is that people know that it is important but don't necessarily want it applied to their treatment. I recently was talking to an American mother who had purchased some unlicensed and expensive treatment for her son who had a genetic condition. When I asked her if there was any evidence behind it she said, 'we are trying to find out by using it'. It seemed there was no controlled trial at all and this was just a marketing ploy directed at someone with plenty of money, but despite being an intelligent lady it was not clear to her that using it on her son was not going to help her find out whether it worked or not. Her son might improve but that might or might not be due to the treatment. If he did not improve that did not mean that the treatment would never work in anyone. It was just a hope that something might work, which is understandable though not scientific. Medicine has to have more reasons for its use than that.

In general, patients put a big premium on trust in their medical advisor and also are strongly influenced by the wider community of friends, the internet, newspapers and so on. They rely on these sources for information on whether a treatment works and lack a perspective with which to understand what the difficulties are in choosing treatments.

It is worth re-iterating that many treatments may not do any good, and are used only because of custom and practice. Doctors themselves often need to be convinced of the need to change what they do – I certainly remember being amazed that Paroven, a treatment for restless legs, had been shown to have no effect. I had used it for over ten years – restless legs is a common complaint but usually not serious, and my patients did not come back after being prescribed a 3 month course, so I had presumed they had got better. Sometimes they reappeared after some time after the course of Paroven had finished saying that the restless legs had recurred and could they have some more, and this confirmed its effectiveness, in my view. When double-blind controlled trials were finally done it was clear that the tablets were useless. I can now think of many reasons why I had been misled, for instance by the usual placebo effect, possible misdiagnosis (restless legs is an odd condition to describe), and because it is often a self-limiting condition (doctor-speak for 'gets better on its own'). Also the tablets needed to be taken four times a day for six weeks and not many patients would take that many tablets for a relatively minor complaint, so I think they had assumed that if it hadn't worked it was their fault for missing out doses. Anyway I don't remember any patients coming back and saying that it didn't work, but nevertheless studies later showed that the tablets were completely ineffective.

The gold standard of evidence for whether something works or not is a randomized controlled trial (RCT). In these trials the study subjects are randomly allocated to receive one or other of the treatments before the trial starts. Then the two (or more) groups of subjects are followed up in exactly the same way, and the only differences between the care they receive, for example, in terms of procedures, tests, outpatient visits, follow-up calls etc. should be those intrinsic to the treatments being compared. In this way you can get a true reflection of the effectiveness of one treatment compared with another.

One of the fundamental rules about doing a clinical trial is that you decide what outcome you expect to get (from your hypothesis) before the trial is started and not afterwards. You should have a primary end point, which is the main point of the study, such as length of survival for instance when considering how long people will survive with or without treatment for cancer. In the HRT trial the primary efficacy outcome was a heart attack or death from a coronary heart problem (myocardial infarction or coronary death), and when the results came in showing that the results were worse in the treated group than in the placebo group the trial had to be stopped. The results should also be analysed statistically and only significant results publicised as such. There can be secondary outcomes, and subgroup analyses, but the main outcomes should be clear in the final report.

Ideally, a trial should have a single endpoint based on just one outcome measure. However, as the art of trial design has evolved, most large trials have a primary (composite) endpoint consisting of multiple outcome measures. An endpoint can also be the time taken for an event to occur. For such an endpoint, the events of interest for which a time is to be recorded—such as stroke or heart attack—must be predefined. Trial endpoints can also be a quantitative measurement of a biochemical or socioeconomic parameter such as cholesterol level or quality-of-life.

However, sometimes outcomes are combined which are not the same, such as sudden death from stroke and heart attack, as in the ACCORD trial published in 2010 on blood pressure in diabetics,[31] but these are caused by quite different things which are as different as oranges and apples. In some cases these different end points can be combined to increase the power to reach statistical significance in order to favour the interests of the industry (device and drugs). But in the ACCORD trial control in diabetics the results did not reach statistical significance and the conclusion was that intensive blood pressure control is not worth doing, neither for cardiovascular outcomes (a 'combined end-point'), nor for progression of diabetic eye disease. Intensive blood pressure control was good for fatal and non-fatal stroke prevention but this was only a 'secondary outcome'. In this way the interpretation of trial results can be misleading.

More importantly, we have come to realise that when collecting evidence that a treatment works, that you have to be sure you use an outcome that definitely improves people's health. An example of a useful outcome would be that more people live longer because they don't get the disease in question, or suffer fewer bad effects of a disease like diabetes such as less blindness, when they take the new treatment. It seems very obvious.

But what medics have tended to do until recently is to use a result of a blood test as a marker – such as HBA1c, which measures a substance in people's blood which shows how well their diabetes is controlled (it is based on overall results of blood sugar levels). Then the doctors will go further and assume that because their blood sugar is better controlled then the patients will have fewer complications. That again seems very likely but few trials have gone on for long enough to actually show this. Do patients care if their blood sugar is more normal? Well, not really if they still get the same complications such as kidney problems, blindness or amputations at the same rate as before. So there should be another step that correlates these improved measures of blood sugar control with a reduced complication rate, and this mostly has not been done.

Manufacturers of new diabetes drugs have always based their claims on improved performance of their new drugs on their effects on blood sugar alone, and often these new drugs do indeed show better control, but at the expense often of more severe side effects. It is much easier and quicker for doctors to show a change in a blood test result which favours their new treatment, than wait years for the real outcomes such as prevention of death or blindness, but this means that expensive new treatments now tend to be used far earlier and far more often, and patients may suffer more side effects and in the end may not get the benefits they were promised. Sometimes it would be better to wait for the results of trials in which the outcomes, which actually matter to patients, are measured.

This is a common problem, to use a surrogate end point such as the result of a test instead of whether the patient really gets better. An early example was Lorenzo's oil. A film was made of the heartbreaking story of a family's search to find a cure for their son Lorenzo who suffered from a rare metabolic disease called ALD, adrenoleucodystrophy, which caused paralysis and mental decline. The parents were upset when they found that no-one was doing any research into treatment (presumably because it was a rare disease and there would not be big profits in any new treatment) and so read up about the biochemistry and researched the known causation of the disease themselves, despite not being biochemists. Against all the odds, they found a treatment, a long-chain fatty acid, which when added to the diet appeared to overcome the abnormality. Laboratory test showed the blood marker for the disease was quickly normalized so that it appeared that the condition's terrible effects could be stopped. Tragically though this could not have been the whole story. The film ended with Lorenzo improving, but in reality the improvement stalled and though Lorenzo lived for many more years with the therapy, he never recovered enough to have a useful life. In addition when the oil was given to new sufferers of the disease before damage to the central nervous system had happened, it did not seem to stop the progress of the disease. The surrogate end point, the blood test, did not reflect what was really happening and Lorenzo's oil is not recommended for treatment by most health authorities, although people still buy it privately, in spite of controlled trials indicating that it does no long-term good.

All clinical trials of different forms of treatment should give results that are statistically valid, that is, the result could not have happened by chance, and statistics is a science in itself. A very useful tool in statistics is the ability to combine different studies on the same theme, to give statistical results that could not have been gained from any individual clinical trial, for instance because it was too small or too limited in scope. The method is called meta-analysis, and is defined as the statistical analysis of data from various sources for the purpose of integrating the findings. By combining studies, a meta-analysis increases the sample size and thus the power to study effects of interest. It is used a lot in medical research, although care has to be taken to ensure that the elements that are compared are in fact comparable. We have to take it on trust that these big meta-analyses are done correctly and are valid, as many of the important studies that change recommendations for treatments for patients are now derived from meta-analyses.

Systematic review is another major way in which treatments can be assessed – by combining trials and studies which are similar but where the statistics can't be done because the studies are too varied. Researchers therefore go through each trial reading them and combining the relevant results. As an example, when a friend of mine did research for an article on the early use of palliative care in cancer and whether this would be cost-effective, he found that very few of the articles he looked at said anything about the cost, so he could not combine them in a meta-analysis. Instead he did a systematic review which meant that he had to go through the articles one by one, taking out the results that he was interested in.

If there aren't any of those then we can look for other controlled clinical trials or observational studies. Less useful evidence is found with case studies and personal experience, but it can be valuable. Finally patient's views need to be taken into account, so evidence-based medicine is made up of the three pillars of (i) evidence, (ii) clinical expertise, and (iii) patients' views.

People may be convinced that certain treatments work for them, and in the busy world of general practice (and sometimes specialist practice too) it may be easier to agree with them and carry on prescribing. But in the modern era when costs are escalating it has become imperative to use only those treatments with good evidence behind them in publicly funded systems like the NHS. So recently, evidence-based medicine has been the rallying cry of clinicians and managers alike. Does physiotherapy work for this? Does acupuncture work for that? Does homeopathy work for anything? So it is said that no doctor or health professional should advocate any intervention that does not have evidence behind it, yet we know that people do so even when the evidence is clear that it is not effective. Did I look up every treatment I prescribed? No. I tried to do what was recommended in the medical press and what I knew my colleagues did, and I always did what consultants recommended even though in some cases I thought they may not be correct. Most doctors were the same.

When the vogue for evidence-based medicine first came in there was a rush to develop guidelines for doctors to help them follow the evidence. At first many doctors dismissed this approach as 'cook-book medicine' – follow the recipes in the cook book and you should get a perfect meal every time – but what happens if you haven't got the ingredients, the implements or even the skills? The problem has always been that only a few treatments even now have really reliable evidence. For other conditions the evidence is very limited or is conflicting. For instance it is not clear from existing studies whether vitamin D can prevent colon cancer. More studies will be needed and the doctor needs to use personal experience and give the patient the choice of the options available.

Can we be sure that the evidence that seems to say that something works, is reliable? Well, often the answer is 'no'. There are all sorts of ways in which poor evidence is used to persuade doctors that something works and the big pharmaceutical companies ('Big Pharma') are past masters at this. Research is expensive and so drug companies, rather than research labs, fund a big proportion, and they really want their drug or treatment to work. Scientists, including medical scientists, are pretty good at proving what they want to prove – they are only human after all – but if the evidence is wrong it will lead to patients not getting the best treatment, or even harmful treatment.

Most people know now that there is a bias towards only publishing trials with a positive result, usually one that would benefit the people who fund the trial, be it Big Pharma, or research groups. Therefore studies where the treatment did not work are buried. At the very least this will mean that researchers will repeat the study, wasting their time and the sponsors' money, and at its worst, trials with positive results will look too good when other trials on the same theme are not published. Even worse, when studies which show unacceptable side effects are not published, this can mean that patients are harmed.

Sometimes it is not clear from initial studies that there is a problem, and it only comes to light after many patients have taken the drug. One famous example was the Opren case when many people with arthritis who had taken this drug suffered kidney and liver failure.[32] More recently the drug Varenicline, marketed to help people give up smoking, was found after a few years use to cause psychiatric symptoms such as depression, suicidal thoughts, and erratic behaviour in some people. It is well known that tobacco firms have been guilty of denying the harmful effects of tobacco by not publishing material they have commissioned. They also were guilty of altering the evidence to make it look as though tobacco was not as dangerous as it is.

It is also important to look at how the evidence, which may be of excellent quality, is presented to and by the media. The most common way of doing so is by using relative percentages rather than absolute numbers, which always make the effect seem much larger. Consider this example – if the risk of getting breast cancer is 2% over ten years, so two out of a hundred women like you will develop cancer, then an increase of 50%, which seems a whopping increase that will make huge headlines, will increase your risk to 3% – so that one extra person in a hundred will now develop cancer – important, but not stuff you would think would make headlines. On the other hand if your baseline was 20% then an increase of 50% means that an extra 10 people will develop cancer. But very few people have risks as high as that for common conditions, at least in the younger age group, so the media are exaggerating the risk in order to sell their papers.

The fact is that a change in relative risk will matter much less when your absolute risk is small. Using NNT (number needed to treat – the number of patients you need to give the drug (or other intervention) to in order to prevent one instance) is a very useful way of presenting the evidence. For statins, used to prevent heart attacks and strokes in people who already have high blood pressure, you need to treat nearly a hundred people over three years to prevent one cardiovascular event. If you then expand your population to people with a 10% risk of a coronary event, the number will be much higher. When for a short time I presented these figures to my patients as part of a study, people really did question whether they ought to take the drug in question, and several said they just weren't going to take them. That wasn't the point of the exercise at all, and I soon stopped giving the figures (actually it was quite hard to get the up-to-date figures on most conditions, as NNT isn't often included in journal articles). In such cases, presentation of the evidence is all, and it can be difficult in everyday practice not to bias what you say to the outcome you want, when you know that whatever intervention it is, it will save some lives. (But of course probably not the person in front of you.)

These bad practices are now well discussed.[33] But there are other ways in which evidence is not what it appears to be.

Sometimes the design of clinical trials is very strange, for instance when patients who are less likely to do well in responding to a certain treatment strategy, or to a new drug, are just excluded. In the highly publicised ACCORD type 2 diabetes clinical trial for high cardiovascular risk diabetics, mentioned above, the following patients were excluded: people over 79, some people with kidney problems, people with high blood pressure and high levels of cholesterol. Excluding older people from clinical trials is commonplace, yet elderly people's bodies do not react the same way to diseases and treatments as younger people do, and this means that the findings in younger people do not apply to them. With more and more people living longer and being treated with these drugs it makes no sense to exclude them.

The other conditions excluded are all complications of having diabetes, and patients with them will need to be treated with something, so this is obviously selecting only the fittest and youngest patients who might be expected to respond the best. The most severely affected patients are excluded from the trials but these patients won't be excluded from the licence to treat and so GPs will use the new drug in these people – but with no evidence that they will work, nor knowledge of what harm may be caused. GPs always have patients with not just one disease but also several at the same time, and if such patients are excluded there aren't many who actually fit the criteria for entry to the trial. For GPs the problem is that patients are often elderly, and if they have diabetes a high proportion will have high blood pressure and kidney disease (because diabetes and high blood pressure damages the kidneys). If patients like this were excluded from the trials we are basing our evidence on, then the evidence may not contain enough information to tell you how to treat them in real life. Sometimes trials are so selective that very few of our actual patients will match the group that were actually studied.

I am not saying of course that the trials were useless – far from it. But it is necessary to be critical and to be cautious in making big changes to treatments in response to well publicised trials. My point is – and it is one repeatedly being made in the BMJ and other well-respected journals – that evidence does have to be looked at critically, as there will be a big bias towards a positive outcome that will lead to more treatments such as drugs, strategies or technologies, that will make money for the healthcare business.

Outright fraud in the scientific community is becoming more obvious. It certainly has always been there but in the past it has been difficult to prove because of the culture of deference to senior scientists, and, it has to be said, the bullying of junior scientists. Things are now changing and scientists are now facing trial for fraud in the US. At the moment some researchers into Alzheimer's disease are being prosecuted under the USA's False Claims Act of 1863,[34] which penalises people who defraud the Government. This is a new development, because previously people thought that researchers were always ethical. Now whistle-blowers are coming forward to publicise fraud (usually falsified data), because their jobs are being safeguarded. Even more than this, whistle-blowers in the US are now receiving large cash sums for giving evidence resulting in conviction. This turns the tables completely, and junior researchers who see something funny going on are no longer compelled to remain silent. The case of the MMR scare, where the researcher was convicted of fraud and struck off the British medical registrar, is one of the most famous examples of fraud, leading as it did to a falling-off of public trust in MMR vaccination, and subsequent rises in cases of measles, and consequent deaths.

Conflicts of interest can also occur, and researchers now have to be more transparent in declaring what links they have to profit making companies.

Research is done by Research Institutes, Hospitals, University Departments, and commercial companies; and increasingly academic institutions have entered into partnerships with drug companies to create research centres because of the enormous cost (US $100 million), lead time (10 years) and uncertainty of a successful profitable drug. While these collaborations may be essential to ensure that new developments are funded, they also create conflicts of interest and raise ethical concerns, particularly when research involves human subjects in clinical trials. Lapses in oversight of industry-sponsored clinical trials at universities, and especially patient deaths in a number of trials, have brought these issues into the public spotlight.

In the US potential conflicts of interest extend to government advisors. In 2005, an FDA advisory panel voted to allow the painkillers Celebrex, Bextra, and Vioxx to remain on the market, despite data showing that they increased the risk of heart attacks. A week later, the Center for Science in the Public Interest reported that 10 of the 32 panel members had recently provided consultations to the manufacturers of the drugs, leading to speculation that if these conflicted researchers had been left off the panel, the drugs would have been withdrawn from the market. Many scientific journals now expect every researcher to list all conflicts of interest with each paper published, so such ties to industry are being more obvious.

So more and more attention is now being given to every aspect of research to make absolutely sure that research which results in the spending of huge amounts of public money are being scrutinised in the interest of both public safety and effective health spending.

Chapter 8
Guidelines: paperwork, keeping track of the evidence, financial incentives and media misinformation

Best practice – GPs' use of guidelines – NICE – pressure to fund new drugs – QOF – patients' decision aids and the internet – treatments not funded

When the results of clinical trials stand the test of time there will develop a consensus amongst doctors about what is 'best practice'. In hospitals, clinical pathways have been developed to describe the best route the patient should follow through the system. Guidelines for GPs are then developed by specialists on how they should identify, diagnose refer and treat the patients that the specialists wish to be referred to them. They don't of course take into account whether the GPs or the patients see a need to do so. However GPs may be faced with literally hundreds of different guidelines from each speciality, being deluged with a new guidance document every 48 hours on average, all of which land on their desk. Sometimes they came in paper form, with detailed instructions on what the GP should do. Sometimes they are huge laminated posters you are supposed to put on your wall. Then of course GP's get emails and attachments from major interest groups –this society and that society each promoting their diseases and the latest evidence based pathway developed in the hospitals. With the best will in the world GPs cannot keep up with all this. You do not even know who actually made these up sometimes – they may be from a lone consultant with a bee in his bonnet about a condition.

When we asked our GPs in a recent study[35] whether they had followed any guidelines at the time they had referred patients to hospital, the results were so variable that it was impossible to say that the GPs took the question seriously at all. It may indeed have been a stupid question to ask – we probably needed to be more specific: which guideline? when? In one area 100% of the GPs said they had looked at a relevant guideline that other doctors thought likely to have been reliable, in another it was 4%. We were following these doctors' referrals for a year and the percentage did not even improve during the year. And when a group of doctors were asked in an online poll recently 'Are you able to keep up with the latest guidelines?' only 5% said yes, 74% said no and 21% weren't sure. So it seems that the production of all these guidelines have not been very successful at primary care level. (Of course on-line polls aren't firm evidence of anything. I tend to put the results in if they agree with what I think! But they mustn't be taken as gospel.)

Using evidence-based treatments is something, of course, that those GPs should do, but if they do not use the guidelines how do they keep up to date? Le May et al[36] have written an excellent book on mindlines – these are the patterns of thinking that they say GPs and other doctors often use in order to consolidate their learning. They say the process of learning how and when to use new treatments needs to be a collective social process, so that doctors can try to make sense of them and put them in context, rather than trying to learn guidelines, however attractively produced.

Most doctors learn about new treatment and what works and what doesn't from their training and then by further reading on their own, looking up the evidence as they go, and discussing any new treatments with their colleagues. Their own personal experience of treating their patients influences the consensus they come to about what pathways they would recommend. GPs take on new evidence and ideas better when recommended by well-trusted opinion leaders in general practice rather than of those of 'experts', who often don't know the context in which GPs are working. Web sites and forums for doctors are also very useful. So rather than just sending out guidelines it would be more helpful to facilitate meetings within and between practices, which are free from health care industry influence, for general discussion of real life cases and the evidence available. It is crucial to get GPs and consultants meeting together so that GPs can get the feedback that has so often been lacking. In this way they can strengthen the use of the most relevant guidelines (e.g. NICE) and try to stop the flow of confusing guidelines. When new evidence comes out it is important to get ordinary (i.e. not specialist or token) primary care referrers involved in the production of all directives/ guidelines from above.

However Medical Defence organisations, which of course are the organisations that pick up the pieces when a GP doesn't follow a guideline and a patient suffers as a result, have to be very keen on guidelines, and one of them has proposed that a monthly roundup of summaries of new guidelines should be sent to GPs, who could then electronically 'tick' it once read. The likely result would be that this sits on the shelf with all the other guidelines.

From a hospital standpoint it still would be helpful to develop an overall 'map' that summarises the evidence for each pathway that patients can take in their journey through the health system. The idea is good; obviously it is right that all patients should benefit from the right action at every stage in their journey from diagnosis to treatment and a cure.

One of the most successful attempts to codify what doctors should do in each stage for every condition is the Map of Medicine. Each pathway is supported by robust clinical evidence and so is authoritative. However we found in our area that it really wasn't much help for GPs. It was developed as a tool for hospitals, where usually the diagnosis, or at least the area of diagnosis, was already known. The tool did not take into account the huge breadth of types of presentations that face GPs. It had operational problems too; it did not integrate well with GPs own clinical systems, so it was not possible to use it in a consultation. Also it was not possible to customize it to local pathways. For instance, there was an excellent clinic that had been set up in one small local area for GPs to get a test to diagnose heart failure. It had been publicised to local GPs and they used it. However because it was a local initiative and wasn't available to all GPs everywhere it couldn't go on Map of Medicine.

So Map of Medicine remains a very useful tool for hospital staff and managers, but will need more tweaking before it can be really useful for generalists such as GPs. The fact is, as most GPs quickly realise, if you really need a guideline, there probably isn't one because if there were one, you would probably already have heard about it.

So where does this leave the patient? If doctors have to search and work to find out the evidence for a certain treatment, what hope is there for the patient?

With the availability of the good evidence on the Internet (along with a lot of frankly wrong and dangerous stuff) it is easier to look up the evidence base behind many, though not all, common treatments. Sites such as NICE, GP Notebook, NHS Choices, Wikipedia, NHS Direct and so on will help. There is a lot of information available specifically on evidence-based medicine. Certainly it is essential to use only evidence-based pathways for treatments that are funded from the public purse, as in the NHS, though I presume people who are paying themselves (as with the example of the American mother above) are entitled to do what they want with their money. Even they however should only be presented with treatments that are known to be free of any harmful effects.

Also recently there has been a lot of effort put in to Patient Decision Aids on many important topics and your doctor will certainly give you one of these if your condition is one where there is an informed choice to be made. In some cases they are available on line. If there isn't one for your condition or you don't know what you have because no diagnosis has been made, you are back to that tried and trusted decision aid – your GP. He or she should be able to give you the benefit of their knowledge and experience and give you tailor made advice for your particular needs – with or without Google!

NICE, the National Institute for Health and Clinical Excellence, was set up on 1 April 1999 to ensure everyone has equal access to medical treatments and high quality care from the NHS – regardless of where they live in England and Wales. NICE is an independent organisation responsible for providing national guidance on promoting good health and preventing and treating ill health. Its aim is to quantify health benefits for patients against cost so that only the most cost effective medicines and treatments are to be funded by the NHS. It works alongside the licensing system of drugs and treatments, which ensure that only drugs that, have passed rigorous safety and effectiveness tests can be sold in the UK.

NICE is in fact envied the world over, for its ability to put a brake on spending huge sums on very marginal treatments. But it is constantly under pressure in the UK and there have been many media stories about its effects on hard cases – patients who have been denied the chance of a few extra months at huge cost to the public purse. Behind these press stories is often intense pressure from powerful lobbies of drug companies that want the NHS to buy these new drugs. The usual ploy is for a drug company to fund patient pressure groups, without making it clear that they are doing so, and in turn these groups will lobby the media.

The other problem for the NHS is that sometimes the drug companies price the drugs extremely highly and often hold the health systems of the world to ransom when the drug really would be of value. They say the drugs have to be priced so highly because of development costs, but in fact the development costs are usually only a fraction of the total, the rest being marketing costs. NICE at present goes on a rule of thumb, which says that a drug should cost less than £30,000 per quality life year granted. But this has been raised to £40,000 for certain cancer drugs, which might prolong life for a few months.

Herceptin, a drug used to treat certain types of breast cancer, is an example of a very expensive drug. When first licensed in 2002 it appeared to offer a great deal of hope for patients with certain types of breast cancer, and NICE had to do an appraisal very quickly. This came out against using the drug routinely in cases where the cancer had spread, and the company quickly appealed. They won the appeal on a technicality, but in 2012 the committee ruled that it was not cost effective – it gave fewer than six months of extra life at a cost of £50,000 per patient.[37]

Another example was drugs for Alzheimer's disease, where it was first thought that they did slow the disease significantly, but soon it became clear the effect was fairly marginal. However even small reductions in the rate in which deterioration occurs is useful and will save money as well as give extra precious months of better functioning for the person with Alzheimer's. There is at present a big advertising campaign exhorting carers to take their family members to the doctor to make sure Alzheimer's is diagnosed early. I am sure that the makers of some of these drugs will be funding these adverts, and they do tend to raise the expectations of the general public that a lot more can be done than is the case. How early would you want to know if you are suffering from Alzheimer's disease?

There are often stories in the media about how terrible it is that patients are being denied treatment but never is there a mention of the alternatives if the country really cannot afford to pay the huge price – that the drug company should reduce its costs to what the market (i.e. the NHS) can afford. Otherwise if the high amount is paid out of the public purse there will be less for other deserving treatments. It is the unbalanced nature of these stories that betrays what they are – special interests backed by powerful drug companies that need to maximize their shareholders' profits and have very little real concern for patient care.

I have sat on many committees that decided whether the NHS should pay for drugs or interventions for certain patients. They were usually cases where a specialist had decided that a patient would benefit from an extra treatment which was either not available locally or considered too expensive. It was the job of the committee to look at all the available evidence and question the consultant, GP and patient. Though some of the members of the committees were well trained, they were still dealing with rare conditions with no medical knowledge and it was a struggle. In the end a decision would have to be made and there was always an awareness of what the local media might say. There were some people who had a sense of entitlement that was quite brazen and they would appeal and go to the newspapers each time. One man wanted specialist out-of-area treatment that had very little evidence behind it but he was a past master at using the local paper to publicise his case and in the end he got his referral – though not his treatment as the consultant at the other end thought it was not indicated. These are difficult decisions and people on these committees, including lay people, do their very best to be fair. I am not at all sure whether the patient will be able to appeal under the new system in England now.

For GPs, the Quality and Outcomes Framework (QOF), a voluntary incentive scheme for GP practices in the UK that was first implemented in 2004, has linked some evidence-based quality indicators to GP's pay, such as the measurement of the test for how well a patient's diabetes is controlled, to GPs' pay in an effort to improve standards. This is the reason why GPs will now 'chase' patients, sometimes mercilessly, to have some tests or treatment for which there has been enough evidence to put on the system. For instance one of the indicators is blood pressure measurement (not only for people with hypertension or diabetes, but also for most of the population), and so anyone going to their doctor is likely to get their blood pressure measured. Of course not everyone wants every test that is suggested, so there is a get-out clause – exception reporting – that means that if a patient has failed to come for a tests after 3 requests they can be 'excepted' i.e. excluded from the count (a doctor will have to get a threshold percentage such as 70% of patients to get the cash). This system, the first in the world, has been very successful in getting GPs to follow those guidelines to which the cash has been attached – in fact that was the reason why most GPs earned such huge pay rises in the 2004 contract. The DoH underestimated how successful the GPs would be, or perhaps the BMA was too good a negotiator for the civil servants. QOF NICE oversees the development of indicators used to show that GPs should be rewarded for providing good quality clinical care and for helping to improve people's health.

I am sure that it has brought up standards, but there are some people who will say that this does not translate into better outcomes for patients. This may be due to faults in the way the system is set up, 'gaming' by the GPs or the fact that the patients who are 'excepted' might be the very ones who really need to have the tests. Another problem with the system is that it only applies to certain conditions such as diabetes and hypertension, and although there are more than fifty of such conditions altogether there are an awful lot more that do not have a QOF target, and so these tend to get less attention. Every interest group now wants a target so that standards in their speciality will improve. Nevertheless the programme has been successful, and standards of patient management, though possibly not outcomes for patients, have improved. Each year the evidence for the various indicators is checked and the results looked at in depth so that indicators can be dropped changed or added.

Financial incentives are used at least in part because law courts are still not very likely to take evidence-based medicine into account.[38] Clinical practice guidelines in healthcare litigation involving quality-of-care and entitlement-to-benefits claims are sometimes not upheld. This may be due to the politics of the situation, and just as clinicians have been reluctant to use clinical practice guidelines in practice, courts have been, and likely will continue to be, slow to apply them in deciding cases.

Apart from looking up randomised controlled trials (RCTs) or systematic reviews (Wikipedia is very helpful here) to decide on whether a treatment will work, you can use the 'experts' – people who have specialised in this field, written books and papers and so on. Even NICE accepts expert opinion as a form of evidence. So long as the experts declare their interests, this can be OK. But often they don't, and this problem is considered in more detail in Chapter 17.

All GPs can do is to try to keep as up to date as possible but beware of big claims from drug reps and bandwagons in the media. As a patient I would want to know my doctor was up-to-date and careful, and that is the best you can do. Evidence-based medicine is great when it is there but it is still limited in its relevance and scope. However, who is going to say they practice non-evidence based medicine?

Many areas are developing lists of procedures for which there is good evidence of effectiveness, and others where there is evidence that they are not cost-effective.

The question is then, what should be done about the latter? Should they be available for patients even if a doctor thinks it might be inappropriate? Should a doctor be able to refuse a patient a remedy that has been around for some time but for which it is realised that the evidence is not there? What if the doctor does not believe in this evidence because the treatment seems to her to have worked in the past? Well, the answer is obvious in a publicly funded health service; the procedure should not be available. But it is difficult to change habits, of patients and doctors. In Wales there has been a document around for some time that has been produced using latest evidence, and lists procedures that should 'Not Normally be Funded'(NNF). It lists those procedures which are not considered cost-effective or clinically necessary and which the NHS could decline to perform.

GPs have been told about the list, and in some specialities there has been attempts to implement it, but politically there are difficulties as, if the local paper publicises a 'hard case' where some one has been denied treatment, there may be a complaint and the Health Board may have a lot of bad publicity. At bottom, the politicians have not been brave enough so far to give a lead and this causes uncertainty. So far not many NNF conditions have in fact been refused. Doctors at the front line cannot agree about many of them, though they have been informed of the evidence behind the decisions so that they could share it with their patients. But we know that any decision to refuse treatment should be clear, transparent and consistently applied by both primary and secondary care. It has been difficult to achieve clinical consensus so far.

Sometimes this list is in fact rationing. For instance cosmetic surgery on the face such as face-lifts or blepharoplasty (rather than cosmetic procedures necessary because of a disease process) has long been considered to be outside the NHS. For many years spots or blemishes that need a diagnosis to make sure they are not cancer have been removed through the NHS, but nowadays the cost of doing the ones that are definitely not cancer has been rising and so after diagnosis they now are left alone, unless the patient is very 'concerned' (which may be another term for 'likely to make a big fuss').

Most doctors agree that some conditions such as mild uncomplicated varicose veins should not be funded, as the symptoms are generally not worth the extensive surgery required and should respond to much simpler measures. Other conditions should be done under strict guidelines – e.g. tonsillectomy and Caesarean section, otherwise it seems there are always surgeons and patients who will get them done somehow, with little benefit to the patient. Recently it appears there has been a big increase on tonsillectomies in the USA.

The there are the procedures that have a bad outcome if the patient's lifestyle is not healthy, such as knee replacements for the overweight, lots of heart operations where the results are poor if the patient continues to smoke, or liver transplants where the patient does not stop drinking. Each case here has to be considered on its merits, but if there is clear evidence that a procedure does not work so well in these cases, it is going to be very tempting to stop funding them when money is tight.

If you want an excellent critique of how evidence is misused by the popular media in medicine then I would recommend a book – 'Bad Science' by Ben Goldacre, which comprehensively demolishes many fads in medicine, including homeopathy and the MMR scare, which are fuelled by media misinformation.

Chapter 9
Cancer: detection and treatment

Evidence about diagnosis and treatment of cancer – waiting lists and cancer survival – early diagnosis – health spending in different countries – access to investigations in primary care – end of life care – screening

So what is the evidence about diagnosis and treatment of cancer?

Cancer is, of course, a major killer disease in western society, and has become the most feared, as infections such as TB and pneumonia have been beaten and even heart attacks have effective prevention and treatment.

The term cancer covers a whole range of disorders of varying degrees of seriousness. Cancer is defined as any disease caused by cells that grow out of control, and ultimately will spread to other parts of the body – a process known as metastasis. Some locally growing tumours are not malignant, and once removed will not appear elsewhere (though they may recur). There are referred to as benign tumours. The real fear in any form of cancer is that the cells that are out of control will spread to other areas of the body. We can only understand the likelihood of this happening when the tumour cells are examined under the microscope. Cells that are out of control begin to look different and lose the normal cell structure. A well-differentiated cell (i.e. looking very like the normal ones from which they have arisen) is less likely to spread than one that is less well differentiated in which the structures of the cells begin to degenerate. It is the job of pathologists to decide by looking at the cells which type they are, and hence what is the likelihood of the cancer spreading.

However, even cancer is slowly becoming less of an immediate death sentence, as vast amounts of money have been poured into healthcare by governments and private finance, and many forms of cancer are now treatable and some even curable. Cancer pathways have been developed, research is now better funded and large multi-national trials are going on which give even peripheral areas access to the best treatment that money can buy in the NHS and other systems of healthcare. Breast cancer treatment now is so much better than it used to be, as is treatment for many types of leukaemia, some brain tumours, cancer of the womb, and even some cancers of the ovary, a notoriously difficult cancer to diagnose.

In my career I have looked after many people with cancer. The majority have been adults, some very old, but some have been children. The most upsetting case was a lad of 11 who developed osteosarcoma of the leg. He came in with his mother at the end of surgery one day and showed me a lump on his knee. I could see immediately that it was probably cancer, but they obviously were unaware of that. I sent them down for an X-ray straight away, and he was admitted to hospital. Over the next 6 months his leg was amputated and he received chemotherapy but it was to no avail. He soon developed secondary tumours in his lungs. The specialist hospital was many miles away and soon visits there became less and less frequent and I was visiting the house every day. They were a fantastic family and so brave. He died peacefully at home, but we all found it very hard. No wonder cancer is such a feared diagnosis. Treatment has improved since then and amputation can be avoided in most cases of osteosarcoma, but children still die from it.

There are two areas where there improvements in cancer care can still be made – diagnosis, and end of life care.

I have already mentioned the difficulty in diagnosing cancer early and reliably in whatever health care system you are. To some extent it has to be a trade off between under and overdiagnosis, both of which have their benefits and harms.

Recently it has been reported that despite all the money that has been poured into the Health Service, survival after diagnosis for patients with some cancers in 2010 were lower in the UK than in many continental countries.[39] The figures for this are difficult to interpret but it seems possible that part of the reasons is the in built delay in diagnosis in the NHS, because of the need for a local doctor to refer to a specialist. Specifically, in a paper from Denmark[40] it was noted that British and Danish citizens have a poorer cancer prognosis than citizens from other countries, and this study hypothesises that their low cancer survival could be partly rooted in the gatekeeper function undertaken by general practice in these two countries. They did an ecological study with data from EUROCARE-4 and primary care. It was found that healthcare systems with a gatekeeper system do have a significantly lower 1-year relative cancer survival than systems without such gatekeeper functions.

It is undoubtedly true that some cancers need to be diagnosed early and treatment started soon in order that survival from diagnosis times might be maximized. This holds for breast cancer, bowel cancer, and some cases of prostate cancer, testicular and ovarian cancer. These are all cancers in which treatment has improved immeasurably over the last 20 or so years. Regrettably this is not necessarily true of the difficult to treat cancers such as lung cancer, pancreatic cancer and stomach cancer. For these cancers treatment is rarely curative and people who contract them die almost regardless of treatment, although treatment may be palliative and prolong life to some extent. In these cases the time from diagnosis to death will be shorter if the person is diagnosed later but the overall length from the start of the cancer to death will be much the same. So although obviously it is right to make the diagnosis early, it does not influence the statistics.

In breast cancer, colon cancer and some others it is crucial to make the diagnosis early as it may make the difference between death in a few months and survival for 5 years or more. So why should survival in the UK be worse than in other countries? If we assume that GPs are to act as gatekeepers (because any other system is wasteful and probably unaffordable, see below), then from my experience part of the reason may be GP's lack of access to investigations together with long waiting lists. Consider bowel cancer for example.

Many people complain of abdominal problems, the causes of which vary from irritable bowel syndrome, diverticulitis, gallstones, or coeliac disease to cancers such as bowel cancer itself, ovarian cancer, pancreatic and liver cancers. The way GPs decide to investigate such problems depends very much on recognizing so called RED FLAG symptoms such as bleeding, loss of weight, persistent pain. These symptoms are referred very quickly by GPs and there is usually a maximum waiting time to see the consultant of two weeks. Only a small proportion of these people actually turn out to have cancer, fortunately. But unfortunately there are a sizable number of people who do not have these red flag symptoms who do in fact turn out to have cancer. In my experience it is impossible for GPs to be sure they are recognizing and referring these people, who may have very mild symptoms, and to refer them under the two-week rule. There just isn't enough to go on at first, and a GP may be following guidelines perfectly yet still not realise that there is something more serious going on until she has seen these people several times – sometimes months. In the meantime the GP may well have done tests, such as occult blood testing, abdominal scans, blood tests and so on which may have indicated that referral is necessary, or the tests may have not shown much but the patient's symptoms are getting worse.

But the alternative, that everyone is able to go direct to a specialist, will have its problems too. In the American system there is a fee-for-service system where doctors get paid for each procedure, and you can sometimes go direct to the specialist of your choice. You are likely to get investigations for cancer done very early, as each doctor has an incentive to investigate immediately, but this can mean a lot of over-investigation for the wealthy, which may cause harm, but poor people without health insurance are very likely to have a delay in diagnosis. Not only that but such people are systematically excluded from figures in the USA, so its high showing in survival rates for cancer is very suspect.[41] You have to look at international figures with great care.

The lower rates of survival for cancer in the UK may be also be due to the fact that some people will just not go to the doctor soon enough. This seems to be associated with inequalities of health in different areas, as it is known that in poor areas diagnosis is more likely to be delayed, regardless of the availability of medical care. People in these areas may not recognize the significance of 'red flag' symptoms such as coughing blood, lumps in the breast, or unintended loss of weight, and so may not consult until the symptoms are well established and it is too late. It is said that such delayed presentations account for half of avoidable deaths. This also shows up between countries because the distribution of income levels in the UK is much wider than in most continental countries especially the Scandinavian countries. There may be other factors though – in my experience people sometimes know that their symptom might be serious but don't go to the doctor out of pure fright. They don't tell anyone and hope it will go away. I think that only when people feel more comfortable about the possibility of cancer and the likelihood of its being cured will they see the doctor earlier.

However if one remembers the history of funding for the NHS in recent years it may be that investment in cancer services takes time to work through into people's consciousness. After all, investment was abysmally low before 2000. It was commonplace then for patients to wait months or years to be seen after referral for what would now be considered to be a 'red flag' symptom even when the GP put urgent on the referral letter and wrote several letters of expedition. When I first went into practice it was possible to phone up a consultant or their secretary and the patient would be seen very soon, but this changed in the late eighties and early nineties as the gap between what could be done and the funding to do it got ever wider. The problem with the system as I saw it was that there had been so little investment in cancer services, general surgeons were overworked, we GPs were getting to feel that whatever we did we could not get patients seen quickly, and there was absolutely no urgency felt about any of these cases. This situation went on and on well into the nineties. It is not surprising then the notion of 'red flags' and patients going to their doctor straight away and getting referred and seen within two weeks has taken a bit of time to get established in most people's minds, especially if you live in one of the poorer areas of society. It is also recognised that doctors and well-trained specialists are more available in richer areas.

The UK spent 3,445 US dollars per head of population on healthcare, public and private, in 2009,[42] while France spent 4,000 and Austria 4,200,[43] so there is still a gap of 20%. It is said that the French tend to over use their system, and there is now great pressure to reduce costs with direct payment by patients. The French system, like the British, has a well-developed system of primary care, and my argument would be that waiting lists to see a specialist should be shorter for everyone, not only for possible cancer patients, as sometimes there are no specific symptoms that might lead a doctor to think cancer is a possibility. Also the more investigations GPs can organise themselves, the better. It is certainly true that if any patient waits a long time before seeing a specialist for further investigation when cancer is not considered to be a strong possibility, then there will be delays in cancer treatment, as it is often impossible to pick out the patient with hidden cancer from those with similar symptoms who do not have cancer.

Not all cancers of course are easily treatable and so early diagnosis does not improve life expectancy anyway. Pancreatic cancer, lung cancer, stomach cancer – survival rates have not changed much. For lung cancer there have been slight improvement in 5-year survival, and more people are getting operations to surgically remove the tumour, which theoretically should increase survival rates. The big problem in treating lung cancer is again getting the patient diagnosed quickly, as almost three-quarters of patients present with advanced disease that can't be treated, and 38% of them are first diagnosed following an emergency admission.[44] As usual it is said to be the GPs responsibility to diagnose them earlier but there is no evidence that GPs delay referring patients. After all the main tool of diagnosis is a chest X-ray and all GPs have good access to this. That said there is indeed an enormous variation in rates of chest X-rays performed by various GP practices, but no one knows what the correct rate should be, as this would depend on the area, smoking prevalence and so on. Regular audits of X-rays by GPs shared amongst themselves would help in getting some sort of consensus on which patients need a chest X-ray.

But again, symptoms such as cough in lung cancer often do not appear until the cancer has been there for some time and also sometimes patients do present late. I certainly saw some who had delayed coming. I think part of the problem might be that most patients with lung cancer are smokers and by now after years of carrying on smoking regardless of the risk they almost feel that it is inevitable that they will get it, and the current survival figures are so low that patients feel there is no point in getting the diagnosis any sooner than they have to. It is a bit of a chicken and egg situation, and currently we are in the middle of a big public education campaign to get patients to go to their doctor if they have had a cough for more than three weeks. I dread to think what GPs are making of this, if patients expect to get a chest X-ray every time. There are indeed lots of things GPs can look at as mild asthma, allergies and even problems with the gullet can cause chronic cough, but X-rays may not often be necessary.

Of course cancer specialists obviously want to get patients early enough to treat them with more cutting edge treatments. As against that, the evidence for lung cancer in the USA shows higher death rates in those investigated early for cancer,[45] because almost all with 'suspicious' lesion underwent very risky surgery from which a number died. The problem is that some of these lesions may not have been, or developed into, cancer. The famous Mayo Lung Study showed a persisting long-term increase in deaths in the screened group,[46] and 25% or more screen-detected cancers in the lung may be over-diagnosed, according to another study.[47] It could even be as high as 50%![48] Of course smoking is not always the cause of lung cancer. My best friend, a lady in her late fifties, died of lung cancer within 8 months of diagnosis and more recently my (female) cousin in Australia died aged 67, again within months. Neither had ever smoked, and neither had any red flag symptoms. The first symptoms in my friend's case was pain in the neck, and in my cousin's case a slight cough for a few weeks only, while the cancer was already too advanced for treatment in both cases. It is said that HRT may have contributed to a higher rate of death from lung cancer in women,[49] although not to an increased occurrence of lung cancer. There is no doubt that it is a dreadful cancer to have.

Once cancer has been diagnosed there is also a big variation in how lung cancer is managed around the country, according to the National Lung Cancer Audit.[50] Measures such as the proportion of patients receiving an operation for their cancer ranged from 9.7% to 16.1% in different areas and the proportion of patients receiving anti-cancer treatment such as chemotherapy and radiotherapy varied from 54% to 66.5%.

Survival is also lower for late stage colorectal cancer in the UK than elsewhere in Europe,[51] and the number of people dying in the 30 days after an operation varies a lot between hospitals and is worse if the patient has to be admitted as emergency.[52] This variation is certainly not going to get any less with the dismantling of the 'National' in the Health Service in England.

Now we have a cancer plan with guaranteed funding, but it will take time to improve early diagnosis – it is likely that the NHS cancer plan needs to go on for over 7 years before you will see full benefits. So providing that overall funding is kept up to that of other countries then we will see improvements to the UK's cancer survival just because of the improvements in funding and equipment that have been made particularly in the last five years.

So to summarise, in order that cancer is diagnosed as early as possible you need two things most of all. Firstly that the waiting times for everyone, for all specialities, are kept as short as possible and certainly should never again be allowed to get back to the sorts of times people had to wait in the early 2000s. Otherwise those people without obvious symptoms of signs of cancer will wait too long. And secondly those GPs should have access to as many tests and radiological investigations as possible. Not withstanding the relative shortage of such equipment, a really good primary care system can improve on cancer diagnosis and in my opinion it is a false economy to restrict these.

If diagnosis of cancer is made late for whatever reason, when treatment is eventually given some patients will survive longer with the treatment, but some have a poor quality of life in their remaining months. As a doctor I saw many people going back and fore to hospital or trying treatments of last resort, which made their lives considerably more distressing than if they had had no treatment. I do remember people who made the other choice. Early on in my career I looked after a very cheerful fat man, who always came in with a joke and a smile. He developed gastric cancer, but this was in the time when you did not ever tell the person that they had cancer. You always told them they had an ulcer, giving hope that it would get better, but you always told a relative the true diagnosis if you could. It seems amazing and very patronizing now to do this, and of course most patients soon guessed what was happening. They had probably seen friends or heard of people who were never told, but I was never confronted with a person who asked me to tell the truth. Anyway this man must have realised what was going on and he point blank refused to have any treatment for his 'ulcer'. He lost weight rapidly but still kept cracking jokes when I visited him at home. He had a good quality of life to the end, and never had much pain. I admired him greatly and often wondered later on when patients went for extensive surgery and chemotherapy then still died quickly, whether they had made the right choice – or whether we had even given them any choice.

Doctors themselves don't often go for the last ditch treatments. According to one medical blogger, what's unusual about them is not how much treatment they get compared to most Americans, but how little. For all the time they spend fending off the deaths of others, they tend to be fairly serene when faced with death themselves. They know exactly what is going to happen, they know the choices, and they generally have access to any sort of medical care they could want. But they go gently. There is a tale (possibly apocryphal) of a doctor who had won acclaim for developing a new treatment for a difficult to cure cancer that could increase a patient's life for 6 months although not with a high quality of life. While still working he developed this cancer himself. He did not use his new treatment: he retired from practice and spent the next eight months doing all the things he had wanted to do for years, then died peacefully at home.

So a question a patient might ask is, 'What would you do, doctor?' And the onus should be on the doctor to be absolutely honest.

One way to get cancers diagnosed very early, it is thought, is by screening the whole population for specific cancers. Successive UK governments have set up the breast and cervical cancer programmes, and the cervical cancer screening has undoubtedly saved many lives. Bowel cancer screening is now being funded but so far in the UK there has been no prostate cancer screening. Screening is not the answer to everything – you will never get a system when say, you reach 40 and then are screened every few years for a whole range of cancers, as it is not always clear whether any given cancer type will cause problems in a person's lifetime.

For breast cancer it now seems that the type of cancer picked up at mammography screening is sometimes just not the sort of cancer that will eventually cause you trouble; at least not when prognosis is estimated using a proprietary test, the Netherlands Cancer Institute's 70-gene breast cancer prognosis test.[53] This test has been proven to be predictive of overall survival and the development of distant metastases.[54] A recent study in women 49 to 60 years of age, has shown that more cancers, 58%, were considered low risk in a cohort of women diagnosed with breast cancer during the era when mammography was routinely done (2004–2006), compared with 40.6% considered low risk in 1984–1992 when screening was not offered,[55] so that we are diagnosing more cancers through screening which carry a low risk. Many women may be treated with chemotherapy or radiotherapy who really wouldn't ever need it. Their cancers, which showed up on the mammogram, were small and may never have grown into a lump you could feel. This shows how difficult it is to get screening right. It's fair to say that mammography screening per se has failed to demonstrate a significant impact on reducing deaths from breast cancer, as opposed to the benefits of newer treatments, and the latest study from Sweden showed limited or no impact of screening on mortality from breast cancer.[56] The number of new diagnosis between 1975 and 1995 in the USA rose by nearly 70%[57] but the death rate was largely unaltered. This could indicate considerable over-diagnosis – up to a third of all screen detected breast cancers. The latest recommendation is for women to be very carefully counselled as to whether they should go for breast screening, and I am not sure how long the breast screening programme will continue in its present form.

And of course this is even more true of prostate cancer, where it is well known that as men age their likelihood of having cancer cells in their prostate gland rises so that in men over 90 nearly all of them will have some. Yet in older men prostate cancer is not a very virulent cancer and most men will die of something else. This is why prostate cancer screening has never been recommended in the UK. In the USA, where men were exhorted by advertisements to have their PSA done yearly from the age of forty, evidence shows that the number of diagnoses rose exponentially between 1975 and 1995 and, although the numbers have fallen since then, they are still 50% more than in 1975.[59] Yet the death rate from prostate cancer has remained essentially static with only a slight fall in the last decade, well after the rise in diagnoses began – indeed after it had started to decline again – and probably due to newer treatments.

However in both these cancers the death toll is much bigger in younger people. Women developing breast cancer under 40 have a very poor prognosis, but mammography is not very accurate because younger women have thicker breasts and cancers may be missed. We know that older women (past the menopause when diagnosed) can live for years with breast cancer, having treatment to stop the spread, and surgical treatment for breast cancer is now very specific with only the lump, not the whole breast, being removed. In younger men too, cancer of the prostate can be much more aggressive, but is much, much rarer so it wouldn't be cost effective to set up a screening programme. So screening programmes have their limitations, and a great deal of care should be put into the decision to start them.

If we look harder for cancer we will, of course, find more cancer but we have no way of knowing which lesions would have caused harm if left undiscovered. But having found it we are compelled to act thus exposing our patients to all the physical and psychological traumas of unnecessary investigations and treatment. It has been argued that prostate screening isn't just about mortality; it's about improving length of survival. But, of course, if you find something earlier which is still going to kill you in the end your perceived 'survival with cancer' will be longer.

What is really needed is some sort of understanding as to which screening-detected lesion, which is likely to be much smaller than the usual symptomatic one, is likely to go on getting bigger, and eventually reach the stage when it will cause symptoms. We know now that some cancers can regress (get smaller), fail to progress, or grow slowly while never causing any symptoms or contributing to death. There must be something different about these small cancers that we are unaware of, and some mechanism within the body that can indeed fight off cancers – but it seems only when they are very small. This is what researchers need to concentrate on. Otherwise people are going to be put in an impossible position – hardly anyone I saw would refuse to have treatment once a cancer had been diagnosed.

Chapter 10
Hormonal disorders and autoimmune diseases: diabetes and thyroid disorders

Diabetes in different populations – insulin resistance – prevention of complications – new drugs and their problems – weight reduction – type 1 diabetes – hypoglycaemia – surrogate outcomes – thyroid disease

Diabetes is already a huge problem in every western country, and unfortunately is also increasing almost exponentially everywhere, because of the recent changes in diet in Western culture towards more sugar and fats. Other developing countries are also starting to change their diet and they too will see an increase in diabetes. Soon a big proportion of people in the world with diabetes will be Asian, as people from South Asia are six times more likely to develop Type 2 diabetes than Northern Europeans and they are likely to develop it ten years earlier.

Other groups of people are at risk as well. Diabetes in Aboriginal Australians is very common and this is considered to be because they were originally efficient hunter-gatherers in an environment where food was scarce. Therefore they have a very efficient metabolism, which made very good use of the food resources they had, and some had a mild glucose intolerance and high cholesterol so that they could put down stores of fat more easily when needed. When they lived a traditional lifestyle and ate high-fibre, low-fat meals such as wild animals, vegetables and fish, and keeping very active, they had a low body mass index, and a naturally light body type, and thus were protected from becoming obese or developing diabetes. Nowadays far fewer are living the traditional lifestyle and they are exposed to Western ideas of diet, so are eating foods rich in fat and sugar. Together with smoking and drinking alcohol this amounts to very bad news for their health, with obesity, diabetes, heart attacks and high blood pressure problems becoming much commoner. Like measles, TB and other scourges in the 16th, 17th, and 18th centuries, we Europeans have visited some dreadful problems on people in other parts of the world.

However we ourselves are far from immune, and each year the incidence of diabetes goes up. It can of course be treated but there is no cure and the complication rate is very high indeed, taking up a lot of the resources any country will spend on healthcare.

Type 2 diabetes is not of course primarily a deficiency of insulin. Insulin is required so that sugar (glucose) can pass into the cells from the blood and tissue fluids, and once inside the cells can be metabolised within the cell, thus releasing the energy that the cell needs to perform its functions. In type 2 diabetes the receptors on the membrane of the cell do not respond to insulin, preventing the carriage of sugar over the cell membrane. At first the pancreas stimulates the production of more insulin to try to overcome this block but it only helps for a while and soon the pancreas is unable to produce more insulin, and there then may be a deficiency of insulin. To complicate things further, insulin makes you put on weight so that, in the phase when you are insulin resistant (perhaps because of your genes) and your pancreas is producing more insulin on an attempt to reduce the blood sugar, you are going to put on weight, despite eating the same things. So weight gain at that point becomes a vicious circle, and very, very difficult for the patient to get out of.

There are other problems in that the cells are deprived of this source of energy so they switch to other pathways, and so lead to increased storage of fat, so people tend to put on weight (again). It seems to me that our physiology is marred in a way, which isn't the case in other mammals. Most mammals have a 'cut-off' point at which they do not gain any more weight (the exceptions are either hibernators such as bears, or domesticated animals bred for certain traits). They do not store much fat under their skin, and though they can get diabetes, as far as I am aware this is type 1, not type 2.

But dolphins are different. These are sea-going mammals that have subcutaneous fat for very good reasons – it is by far the best insulator in water. They can get insulin resistance but can also turn it on and off. When they are fasting, they make themselves insulin resistant. Glucose is not removed from the blood and their brains continue to be supplied with vital energy. When food is available, they switch off their insulin resistance and blood sugar levels are controlled again. Assuming that our relative fatness is a response to famines to ensure better survival of our offspring, and that diabetes is an unfortunate result in some people, the researchers say that diabetes may have evolved in our prehistoric ancestors to cope with famines in a similar way,[60] but the off switch has been lost over the millennia. Of course, dolphins store their fat under the skin, just as we do. Research is now going on to find out how dolphins turn the switch on and off, which would be a really incredibly neat solution to the problem.

The passage of glucose into the cells is a very fundamental pathway in physiology, and without it glucose builds up in the blood with bad effects on the very small blood vessels in the circulation and the back of the eye. These effects pile up so that years after people develop diabetes they will develop complications such as heart attacks and strokes, worsening kidney function, poor peripheral circulation leading to amputations, and blindness. This is where the disease changes from being something you can control and live with, to being something that really messes up your life, and is the cause of early death.

People rarely die of diabetes itself these days, as blood sugar can easily be controlled in all forms of diabetes, with modern treatment. But recent trials have shown that if you have type 2 diabetes you can try too hard to lower your blood glucose. One part of the recent ACCORD trial on people with diabetes for some years and at high risk of complications showed that there was a higher death rate from cardiovascular events in people who were treated to have their blood glucose right down to non-diabetic levels than in those who just had ordinary control. In addition, the intensive-therapy group had significantly higher rates of hypoglycemia, weight gain, and fluid retention. It wasn't clear why the extra people were dying, as it wasn't due to hypoglycaemia, but now patients are not advised to control blood sugar intensively. However moderate control is essential to prevent eye and kidney complications.

The most common cause of death in diabetes is due to cardiovascular complications, heart attacks and strokes, and these are about three times more common in people with diabetes than the rest of the population. High blood pressure alone can also cause these things so it is important to keep blood pressure low with drugs if necessary. But again the most recent trial showed that there was no advantage in lowering levels of blood pressure to normal or below normal levels in people with diabetes, as the number of strokes and heart attacks were the same in both groups. So moderation is important here.

What is absolutely clear is that smoking and diabetes is a terrible combination. I was always surprised at how many patients of mine did not stop smoking after they had been diagnosed with diabetes, even after they developed eye or circulatory complications. One man had to have both legs amputated, but carried on smoking. That shows either how addicting smoking is (and it certainly is very addicting) or that this man didn't really want to live.

A lot of work has been put into finding drugs that will reduce some of these problems and every year there are new expensive classes of drugs, which are supposed to help. However they don't tend to be tested against the old drugs that are now out of patent and have stood the test of time, but against other newer tablets. Some quite quickly turn out to be dangerous for some patients. For instance rosiglitazone was all the rage in my last years in practice and huge claims were made for its beneficial actions, but a warning was issued in 2010 when it was found that it actually increased the risk of heart attacks, when it was supposed to reduce them. Other drugs in this class also have proved to have big problems, so that the big breakthrough trumpeted with this new class of drugs has proved a blind alley.

Many other treatments for diabetes actually make people put on weight, when their excess weight is what has caused the problem in the first place. Even injecting insulin will make you put on weight by increasing appetite. (Indeed I remember injections of insulin being used to treat young girls who suffered from extreme anorexia nervosa in order to override their reluctance to eat, by making them extremely hungry, I'm not sure if this would be considered ethical now).

The latest drugs for diabetes do appear to allow those treated to lose weight, but this is in the context of many of the drugs that are currently used for diabetes making people put on even more weight, which is an extremely unhelpful side effect. They are known as gliptins and their structure is based on the hormone glucagon-like peptide 1 which is found in the small intestine and produced after stimulation by foods. There are several drugs in this class which have been licensed for use in the UK.

GLP-1 regulates glucose levels by stimulating insulin secretion and biosynthesis, and by suppressing glucagon secretion, (which is a hormone which can increase sugar levels by releasing sugar from glycogen in the liver), delaying the emptying of the stomach and making you feel full, and this can actually contribute to weight loss, the holy grail of treating diabetes. Doctors are even looking at whether it will be good to promote weight loss in non-diabetics as well. There is, one might think, only a fine line between treating people with diabetes with these drugs and people who are obese and in a pre-diabetic state, in other words people who are very likely to get diabetes soon if they go on as they have been doing. Then only a further small step before treating obese people who don't have diabetes with these drugs. They are relatively new, untried drugs with an unknown side effect profile and are very expensive. I don't think this is going to be the solution, though no doubt such drugs will be promoted as such.

So one future beckons in which people may think they can take a drug like this rather than eating less. But eventually we will find side effects for this magic bullet as well – so far pancreatitis and thyroid cancer have been found in patients taking it, and consumer groups in the US have now recommended that the drug should be pulled from the market. Other studies indicate that this class of drugs are generally safe.[61]

It may in fact be true that we already have enough antidiabetic drugs available and it will be very difficult to find drugs that are better and safer now. This is particularly applicable to developing countries. One would think that if money is short then every person with diabetes should be treated with the well tested and trusted, effective drugs for diabetes that we already have. But no, much more expensive drugs are heavily promoted in poor countries too so that precious resources are used in hospitals (which of course want to keep up to date with the most modern treatments) without any understanding that the new drugs may be 50 times more expensive and overall not really much better.

It is easy to medicalise this problem. The test used to diagnose diabetes traditionally has been the fasting sugar – how high the blood level of sugar is when you haven't eaten or drunk anything containing sugar. The fasting sugar level rises very gradually as people become more insulin resistant as they get older, fatter or for other reasons, and the old cut off level was 8mmol/l. Over that level you were considered to have diabetes (it was slightly more complicated than that as you also had to have a positive Glucose tolerance test) but in 2002 the cut off point was suddenly lowered to 7. This immediately identified many thousands more people as having diabetes and is one of the 'causes' of the increased numbers of cases of diabetes in the world, but very little mention seems to be made of this.

There is another test for diabetes called the glycosylated haemoglobin (HBA1c) test. Glucose in the blood makes a complex substance with haemoglobin, which is the oxygen-carrying molecule in the blood, so that as well as carrying oxygen it carries glucose to form glycolated Haemoglobin, HbA1c. The amount of this substance in the blood can be measured easily and accurately and the amount is proportional to the amount of glucose there has been in the blood over the previous three months or so. So each patient will have a range of level of HbA1c within which they should try to keep and it is one of the targets that GPs have to look at in the QOF.

NICE has now proposed asking GPs to test all their patents over the age of 25 for their risk of diabetes by doing the HBA1c test in order to identify people already in a pre-diabetic state (those whose fasting sugars are already higher than they should be). Those people would then need to be assessed and treated where necessary. It has been thought that doing this could prevent twice as many cases of diabetes, but you would have to give advice or treatment in up to five times as many people. Would it do any good? Well, probably not. Such screening has recently been shown to have no effect on death rates from problems relating to diabetes, cancer or cardiovascular conditions.[62] This is a lifestyle problem not a medical one.

At bottom the most realistic way of tacking diabetes is to help to stop us eating too many starchy and fatty foods. But these foods are easy to eat and pleasant tasting (the manufacturers take care to make them so) and so it is an uphill battle. The products of food manufacturers are regulated for safety but not for their effect on long-term health. Doing this test on so many people would enable doctors to target those at special risk, but really everyone needs to change their diet.

This is well illustrated by a recent trial, the Diabetes Prevention programme (DPP),[63] funded by the National Institute for Diabetes, Digestive, and Kidney Diseases. It randomly assigned roughly 3,500 adults on the brink of diabetes to one of three treatments: usual care, the drug Metformin (Glucophage), or a lifestyle intervention comprised of a prudent, healthful diet and moderate exercise. Dramatic results led to early termination of the trial at about the four-year mark.

Metformin, a very effective drug, reduced the incidence of diabetes by 30 percent -- meaning nearly one in three high-risk people who would have developed diabetes without the drug, did not. The lifestyle intervention, however, was twice as good, reducing the incidence of diabetes by 58 percent! The problem, as ever, is how to persuade people to do this.

So the debate goes on.

Type 1 diabetes is a completely different disease, although it too is increasing in incidence. It is an autoimmune disease, that is, the body for some reason unknown makes antibodies to its own tissue, in this case within the islets cells of the pancreas where insulin is made. Eventually the islets are destroyed and the patient becomes deficient in insulin. It occurs predominantly in young people and is a disease which kills very quickly without treatment. The patient first complains of passing too much urine, because the high amount of glucose in the blood and urine draws water with it into the urine, then the cells in the body start to use other pathways to get their energy and this leads to a condition known as ketoacidosis, which is caused by high concentrations of ketone bodies, formed by the breakdown of fatty acids. These molecules have a very characteristic smell and I was all too familiar with it while working in hospitals at the start of my career.

During that time diagnosis of diabetes by GPs in our area was, I have to say, very poor. In the course of my training and the first year while I was working in the medical and paediatric wards I saw at least four young people admitted in a coma, suffering from ketoacidosis, because doctors hadn't recognised the early symptoms and signs of diabetes. I remember being immediately able to make the diagnosis just by the smell of ketones, a rather sweet smell, in the room. Then we had to work very hard to correct the metabolic problems by giving insulin and fluids via a drip, and preventing the rise of potassium in the blood, which would be fatal very quickly. It usually took a day or so for the young person to wake up and take notice, and then they needed to be treated properly with insulin for the rest of their lives.

The differential diagnosis was with diabetic hypoglycaemia, which could also cause coma, due to too much insulin (by mistake or accidental overdose). The levels of glucose in the blood would get so low that that the body could not function. Subsequently in our area, doctors (especially those who had not been trained in the UK) rapidly learned about the presentation of diabetes and now everybody will have their diabetes diagnosed in the doctors in surgery and then stabilised by an out patient appointment.

However I saw a lot of hypoglycaemia from over-treatment of diabetes, (if you give too much insulin or other medication it will force more glucose into the cells and leave very little in the blood stream) until well into the nineties before easy methods of home monitoring of blood glucose became available. I remember on one occasion being called out to a woman in her 40's who was well known to us. She had had type 1 diabetes since her teens and unfortunately had become blind because of it. Her diabetes had always been difficult to control and on this occasion she had managed to phone to tell us that she thought she had had too much insulin. She lived on a farm in the country and I went there very quickly. She was still conscious but drowsy and also being very sick into a bucket. She was alone – her children were in school and her husband (a farmer) was at market, and the hospital was miles away. So I settled her down, and gave intravenous glucose slowly. You have to give a large volume of glucose into a vein and it takes some time, and it is also rather sticky stuff, but very quickly she came to, wondering where she was. There is always a lot of satisfaction in making a patient better so quickly.

Later we used glucagon, which could be given by intramuscular injection rather than IV, it works by stimulating the liver to break down its stores of glycogen into available sugar, which then floods into the blood stream. It s a much neater way of treating diabetic hypoglycaemia but it does take longer to work. I wanted to send this lady into hospital afterwards to improve her diabetic control but she wouldn't go. Nowadays there would have been a diabetes specialist nurse who would have probably prevented her getting into that state in the first place, and would certainly have come to give further advice afterwards but we didn't have such help then. So eventually I left, but to my chagrin on the way home I left open one of the three gates I had to open and close on the way to the farm and all the sheep got on to the road. The farmer rang me in high dudgeon later to complain!

Diabetes specialist nurses, home monitoring of blood glucose with acutest and other kits have revolutionised diabetic control since then, although in some people diabetes is still very difficult to manage ('brittle diabetes') and 'hypo's still occur. Now the tendency seems to be monitoring of blood glucose very often, as people think more is better. However it is important not to let diabetes completely run your life. Close monitoring of blood glucose is an unfortunate necessary in people with insulin dependent diabetes especially the young. But of course people with type 2 diabetes often use it as well. Close monitoring of blood glucose in type 2 diabetes is considered likely to prevent complications such as blindness and kidney problems, and so people with diabetes have often been taught to do home monitoring. But there has undoubtedly been a lot of hype here from drug companies. The way the pricing goes is that the machines which read the glucose level in the blood are very cheap, but the testing strips are very expensive, so advice form manufacturers and drug firms is often towards over measurement rather than the opposite, especially in the elderly. Now studies have been published that indicate that home monitoring may not be very effective anyway. A meta–analysis published in 2012 in the BMJ[64] showed that there was indeed a statistically significant reduction in HBA1c levels in those who regularly test their own glucose levels at home and use it to fine-tune the amount of medication they take, but it was very small. There is no evidence as to whether it actually does prevent complications, which is what patients really want to know. GPs have been asked recently to discourage its use unless it is really considered absolutely necessary to prevent hypos.

As I mentioned earlier, originally it was thought that the level of HbA1c would also correlate well with the number of patients getting complications of diabetes so that if you kept the level only slightly above normal levels you would get fewer complications and if you had high levels (i.e. poor control of your diabetes) you would get more complications. There has been a lot of recognition recently that these two outcomes may not correlate well with each other and that clinical trials should also continue to look at the complication rates. So far however this tends not to be done, as it takes too long, and is expensive. But it isn't really possible to gauge how effective treatment really is unless you do look at how many people get complications with a change of treatment rather than what their HbA1c or any other blood tests is.

Incidentally, many people without diabetes who have symptoms such as faintness or dizziness think that hypoglycaemia might be the cause and they then eat or drink sugary substances. However real symptomatic hypoglycaemia in people not on treatment for diabetes is extremely rare. The only causes are very rare tumours of the adrenal glands and other rare metabolic diseases. I often found myself having to prove to patients with funny turns who were convinced that lack of sugar was the problem by doing a blood sugar level when they had symptoms. The level was never in the range that might cause symptoms -usually the problem was due to anxiety.

Thyroid disease is the other major endocrine problem found in general practice. It can go different ways – people can have too much thyroid hormone or too little, and often the people who initially had too much (hyperthyroidism) run out and then have too little (hypothyroidism). Thyroid trouble can be due to a deficiency of iodine, and it is well known that in areas where there is only a small amount of iodine occurring naturally, young people can develop a swelling of the thyroid called goitre. This can be unsightly and people will have an operation to remove the swollen gland. However it is getting very rare now because of iodine supplementation.

Most thyroid trouble is caused by an autoimmune problem where the body makes antibodies to thyroid tissue. In younger people the antibodies, far from blocking the thyroid hormone, actually activate it. Normally the pituitary gland produces a substance called thyroid stimulating hormone (TSH), and the auto-antibodies produced abnormally in the body, called TSHR-AbT, also stimulate the thyroid. Thus the thyroid is forced to make much more thyroid than usual and this can have very severe effects. The effects tend to mimic those of adrenaline, so people feel very hot, develop a racing pulse, thyroid swelling, sometimes heart arrhythmias, and a tremor, and they can feel very ill. They can also develop thyroid eye disease which is a most unpleasant condition. It causes the extreme 'starey eyes' and squint seen in comedians such as Marty Feldman, as it affects the muscles and tissues in the orbit around the eyes. What is less well known is that it is a very unpleasant condition with affected people suffering dry irritable and often painful eyes, and the eyelids becoming puffy and red. The muscles of the eyelids contract, producing a staring appearance as the lid is retracted and the muscles and fat surrounding the eye swells, pushing the eyes forward so that they bulge out of the orbits (exophthalmos). Lid retraction and exophthalmos make the dry eye symptoms worse. The swelling of the muscles which move the eyes produces unequal movements and double vision (diplopia) and the orbits may become painful, particularly on eye movement. Unfortunately, treating the original problem, the over production of thyroid does not make the eye problems go away; in fact it sometimes make the eye problems worse and in severe cases the condition may require surgical decompression.

Graves disease is the acute form of an overactive thyroid, or thyrotoxicosis, usually seen in young women. It is a severe disease and can cause heart failure as well as making you feel ill, and it has to be treated. This is usually done by drugs and then radiotherapy, which shrinks the thyroid. In nearly all cases the patient will eventually become thyroid deficient either because the thyroid runs out of juice, so to speak, or because the drugs or the radiotherapy destroys the thyroid tissue. So the end point is that these patients will take replacement thyroid hormone – thyroxine, which is easy to take, the disease is easy to get right and the problem is solved as long as the patient goes on taking it.

There is a strong hereditary component of this sort of thyrotoxicosis and when I was in Labrador as a student I was told that in one particular coastal settlement there was a particularly high incidence of thyroid disease. This was probably because they had inter-married within this very isolated community over several generations. Most of the people had come from Ireland and the fens region of England originally and must have included some families that suffered from thyroid problems. There were no roads in Labrador at that time apart from one between the American Air base and North West River where the hospital was, and all transport was by small plane, which went out visiting the coastal communities twice a week. On one occasion I was on the plane with the public health nurse who was making routine visits to vaccinate the children. Suddenly the pilot of the plane got an emergency call to go to this village. We diverted and found that a 34-year-old woman was being loaded on to our plane to be taken to hospital. But I was shocked – she was in extremis with slow shallow breathing, an unrecordable pulse and she was cyanosed around the mouth. Neither of us really knew what to do except give immediate basic care and soon we were trying to assist her respiration by partial mouth to mouth. We also gave nikethamide which was a respiratory stimulant but which was pretty useless in these circumstances. It was all in vain though and she died on the way to the hospital. We got a debriefing shortly after from the superintendent of the hospital and it seemed that she was one of the people suffering from thyrotoxicosis. Whether she died from that or because she had also developed a chest infection, which is what the villagers said, I never did find out. It was a terrible tragedy though as she had young children. Back in the practice I saw several people with severe thyrotoxicosis and they recovered well after medication and radiotherapy.

Quite commonly the presentation of hypothyroidism (lack of thyroid hormone) was of a gradual onset of thyroid deficiency in more elderly folk and was known as Myxoedema. This causes people to feel tired and feel the cold a lot. Eventually the thyroid level could go so low that mental function was impaired and people could actually go mad with it, suffering loss of cognitive function and sometimes psychotic ideas – so called 'Myxoedema Madness'. One of my favourite detective stories was one by Dorothy Sayers involving thyroid disease. It centred upon a controlling villain who tracked down a lover who had spurned him and found her suffering from myxedoema. He then contrived to get control of this woman and deprived her of her thyroxine until she went mad, becoming ugly, slow and mentally retarded. It seemed this was for a purpose – to show to another ex-lover of the woman (who had been very beautiful) how powerful he was. A good story, but one in which the extreme forms of thyroid deficiency were portrayed, which are never seen nowadays.

Sometimes people with myxoedema put on excess weight, although weight gain solely due to 'glands' i.e. thyroid trouble is extremely rare.

When patients are diagnosed with an underactive thyroid they often give a history of a period when they had lost weight rather suddenly or had had thyroid swelling, and this presumably had been due to autoimmune thyroxicosis.

It was easy to diagnose hypothyroidism as thyroid function tests showed a low titre of thyroxine (T4) in the blood. Sometimes they also had a high thyroid-stimulating hormone (TSH), which meant that the pituitary was trying to make the thyroid work harder, and this meant that the level of active thyroid hormones in the blood would inevitably fall. We then started the patient on a very low dose of thyroxine and monitored the heart to make sure it wasn't being compromised. Once the dose had been stabilised the patient had to stay on it for the rest of their lives.

However there was a group of people in whom the tests were borderline. Should we treat them or not? The trouble was there were many people in that age group who felt tired all the time (TATT) and some of them had borderline thyroid test results. Some people were also overweight, and would like a quick fix, and many rather unscrupulous doctors at one time used to prescribe thyroid in 'slimming pills' to those with borderline thyroid tests and also some with entirely normal tests. This was a very dangerous practice indeed and usually offered by 'slimming clinics' but was difficult to detect unless patients complained or became suspicious. I remember people who were taken in by such clinics but were very reluctant to stop the treatment. Doctors have been struck off the medical register for doing this.

The patients that I treated with thyroxine in this category who had borderline results didn't seem to feel any better for it but it was always difficult to make the right decision. Now there is NICE guidance on the exact level of test results before a doctor should consider prescribing thyroxine, although it is not always followed. Incidentally, people tend to like a diagnosis of hypothyroidism as it means they can get all their prescriptions free! Perhaps because of this change of guidance from NICE or because the population is getting older, the number of people taking thyroid hormone has increased quite markedly recently. People taking it have to have their blood levels measured regularly to make sure that levels do not go too high but overall it is a very successful treatment and thyroid hormone is very cheap. It is nice to have a disease that responds so well to treatment with so few side effects!

Chapter 11
Heart disease: primary prevention, public education and treatment

Heart attacks – heart failure – treatment of angina – AF – statins

Heart problems – coronary heart disease, heart valve disease and heart failure represent the field in which a GP's role has changed the most during my working life. If a person develops sudden chest pain now, an ambulance will be called straight away using 999, and paramedics will attend with a full complement of equipment to diagnose and treat immediately, before transport to hospital and a coronary care unit if a heart attack is likely. If necessary, emergency investigation and sometimes an operation are performed within minutes. Local health services have to measure the pain to needle time (how soon the patient received the injection of clot busting drugs) because the speed at which a heart attack is treated makes a difference to the eventual outcome. In rural areas paramedics can do this. Even untrained observers can do resuscitation with a defibrillator and nowadays you don't even have to do mouth–to–mouth resuscitation, as it is only necessary to keep the circulation going by chest compression to ensure brain perfusion. Clot-busting drugs given by paramedics and on arrival at hospital have now been superseded by immediate transfer to a centre where facilities for reperfusion treatment such as angioplasty are available. This means that the blocked artery can immediately be unblocked before the heart muscle is damaged and improves survival. Hence the number of patients getting clot-busting drugs has been dropping as survival with these is not as good.

On a cruise recently a man had a heart attack, and as the leader of his group was trained in resuscitation he did so, using a defibrillator successfully, and a helicopter came to take him off to the local cardiac centre, where he was operated on and made a full recovery. There is no role at all for the GP except to route an urgent call through to the ambulance service if it comes initially to a practice or out-of -hours service. In my last years in practice any GP not specifically trained in BASICs (a scheme run by GPs to get themselves up to speed in the latest emergency medicine techniques) would be elbowed out of the way pretty quickly by paramedics, working to strict protocols, and even in nursing homes when we GPs did actually know the patients and had a better idea of what might really be required, our services were definitely not required if a paramedic team was there.

How different from when I started in practice when we had a crucial role in immediate emergency treatment. When we were on call for the practice outside normal hours we would be expected to visit a patient with chest pain to make sure the diagnosis of heart problems was correct and to give pain relief before ringing for an ambulance and sending to hospital. We could reassure those who were actually suffering from indigestion (the diagnosis of one versus the other was actually often not simple at all). Surprisingly though, we were not classified as emergency workers and therefore were not allowed to put a flashing light on our cars or even be excused from a summons if we were caught speeding on the way to hospital with a patient! Often at that time the ambulance would take hours rather than minutes to arrive. When patients arrived in hospital (if they did) they would be admitted to an ordinary ward and put on a monitor if they were lucky. The death toll was enormous, but the knowledge of how to treat just wasn't there, and even emergency resuscitation was usually unsuccessful.

There was so little you could do for an acute heart attack that an academic paper came out in the early 70's which indicated that patients who were sent to hospital with a heart attack were more likely to die than those kept at home (the stress of the heart monitors in hospital was supposed to cause their deaths) and we GPs were exhorted to look after such patients at home. That wasn't easy – I remember being on call one weekend and visiting a man three times whose crushing chest pain wasn't responding to pain killers including an injection of morphine – and at the third visit I sent him into hospital of course. He survived, remarkably. Subsequently of course coronary care units were set up where patients were monitored for ventricular fibrillation, which happened when the electrics of the heart were damaged and stopped the heart beating – the commonest cause of death with a heart attack. Then better drugs such as B blockers and ACE inhibitors were developed which could treat and prevent recurrences, and now of course, statins the wonder drugs of the nineties can prevent coronary heart disease in those at risk. Even the damaged coronary heart vessels can be unblocked using stents. The death rate has plummeted with the saving of countless lives of men in their prime.

People also were less aware of what chest pain meant. The first patient I saw with chest pain just after I had joined my practice was a man in his 50's who had chest pain all night, but was convinced he had indigestion. His blood pressure was low – a bad sign – and I wanted to call the ambulance straight away. But he refused – basically he didn't believe me because I appeared so inexperienced I suppose. I called the ambulance anyway once back in the surgery, but he died before the ambulance got there. Undoubtedly he would not have survived in those days anyway, but it was a lesson for me to try to inspire more confidence. Actually indigestion and heart pain are very similar and it has taken many campaigns and advertisements to convince people that they should call an ambulance with any sort of chest pain. It shows again that it isn't only resources and money that a health service needs – the general public has to be educated as well, before outcomes will improve.

Another sad story from the 70's was the patient who suffered very badly from gastritis and indigestion after most meals, and found out for himself that milk was a very good way of ameliorating the symptoms. So he drank over 2 pints of milk a day as a minimum. Milk of course would indeed neutralize the acid and therefore help the symptoms, though it did not cure the problem. And the large amounts of milk, plus a family tendency to high cholesterol gave him coronary artery disease, and he died suddenly in his late forties of a heart attack.

Heart failure was the commonest reason for necessary call-outs in the small hours (usually 2 am), when a person would awake acutely short of breath, gasping, and would try to get to a window to get some air. This was due to the diseased heart failing to pump properly. During the day the circulation just about managed to keep going (though the patient would be breathless), but at night in the horizontal position there is redistribution of blood volume from the lower extremities to the heart and big vessels so there is an increased load of fluid backed up in the lungs, which are then fuller of fluid than they should be, leading to breathlessness. This was a medical emergency and we GPs used to go out from our beds and visit the patient to give an intravenous injection – usually morphine and a diuretic. The treatment worked quite quickly, although if truth were told it is likely that the very fact that the patient was now sitting upright would have relieved the symptoms in milder cases anyway. This would happen perhaps once or twice a month to every GP. I remember one lady in her 80s came in the morning describing just such an experience but had not called the doctor. When I asked why she hadn't she said, 'Well it has happened several times and I expect quite soon this will carry me off. It is not such a bad way to go'. That was the level of acceptance that was quite usual only 35 years ago. You can't imagine that nowadays!

Now the GPs job is much more effective and doesn't get him up in the night either. A GP needs to refer to hospital patients with chest pain who haven't already got there by themselves, and then after discharge to monitor the effects of all the drugs given, firstly to prevent, and then to manage the symptoms of heart problems after investigation by the hospital. High blood pressure, high cholesterol, often exacerbated by smoking and a poor diet, are the causes of preventable heart problems and so the incidence of heart attacks and severe angina has plummeted as these factors are got under control.

That said, that is not quite the whole story, 'heartening' as it is to think of this improvement as being solely due to better diagnosis and treatment. The fact is that deaths from coronary heart disease (CHD) started to fall before all the big breakthroughs in treatment,[65] and we don't know why there was such an epidemic of CHD in the fifties sixties and seventies. It is said from a study looking at midwives' records early in the twentieth century, that poor nutrition in the womb may have contributed, but that surely wasn't a factor that had just suddenly arisen then as poverty was widespread at that time and earlier. Nevertheless modern prevention and treatment does save lives.

One big problem for GPs has always been the early diagnosis of heart failure. A heart attack does not necessarily lead to heart failure because the muscles which do the pumping can recover if they have not been damaged too much from the sudden lack of oxygen when the blood clot stops the circulation. The patient may get angina when the blood supply isn't enough, and then the blood vessels can be opened with anti-anginal drugs. But congestive heart failure, when the muscles of the heart can no longer pump blood round the body, can result from long-term damage to the heart muscle in several ways. It can result from damage to the muscle due to heart attacks and severe angina, but also from infections such as myocarditis and pericarditis, and from cardiomyopathies, when the muscle itself is diseased. It can also be due to damage to the valves of the heart, but the epidemic of valvular heart disease that resulted from streptococcal infections such as scarlet fever and rheumatic fever is again a thing of the past. Either the streptococcus has got less virulent or the rising level of overall health has put it out of business. The main cause of valve problems now is sclerosis of the valve due to calcium deposits on the valve, often due to aging.

However as people age the heart muscles can just wear out. So an elderly patient might come to the surgery complaining of shortness of breath and swollen ankles, due to the excess backpressure on the lungs and high pressure transmitted from the heart down to the circulation of the legs and the rest of the body. When these symptoms are together and there are signs of poor heart function then the diagnosis is easy. But shortness of breath is common in the elderly and is more often due to lung problems rather than heart problems, and of course some patients have both. Swollen ankles are often due to poor circulation and lack of exercise as blood only gets back to the heart from the feet and legs as a result of the action of the muscle pump of the legs squeezing the blood upwards. If you don't take any exercise and sit around all day the blood can tend to pool in your legs, and if elderly people have problems with their mobility, from arthritis, say, then they tend not to exercise. The high backpressure of the blood that hasn't been pumped upwards now causes fluids to leak out of the veins. Varicose veins where the valves in the veins become incompetent (often a hereditary problem) make things worse. So swollen legs aren't necessarily a sign of heart failure.

Sometimes there are obvious signs of poor heart function such as abnormalities in the heart rate and often there are signs on the ECG, and if so then we start treatment with important classes of drugs developed recently such as ACE inhibitors, beta-blockers, calcium channel blockers as well as diuretics. Early on in my career we only had diuretics, which work on the kidney, to get rid of the excess fluid in the circulation that has built up due to the heart failure, and digoxin, which as every one knows was developed from digitalis found in foxgloves. We prescribed an awful lot of digoxin in those days. We were told it increased the force of contraction of the heart muscle, and so improved the pumping ability of the heart. The dose was difficult to get right and digoxin is toxic to the heart in high doses so we had to measure the levels of digoxin in the blood and adjust the dose carefully on each patient. Yet when controlled trials were done it was found that patients with normal heart rhythms who took it regularly did not live any longer, though they did get fewer stays in hospital. Presumably the symptoms were relieved but digoxin in this case did not solve the basic problem. Nowadays digoxin is only used where there is an abnormality of the heart rate such as atrial fibrillation, a common problem of the electrical conduction of the impulse through the heart. Even in these cases now there are better drugs.

So GPs had to quickly learn alternative treatments as they were developed, but the guidance from above often seemed to be by trial and error, and beta blockers for instance were first thought to be bad for heart failure and then good, and then bad again. Treatment of blood pressure can again be very tricky as results of new trials lead to further refinements of the correct treatment.

Now cardiologists are very confident that they have got really effective medical treatments for heart failure, and it is important to diagnose it early. In general practice it is common to see an elderly patient with shortness of breath which could easily be due to heart failure or COPD (chronic bronchitis and emphysema) and if the ECG and Chest X-ray don't show very much it is difficult to be sure what is going on. The best test at the moment is an echocardiogram (ECHO) that gives a moving picture of how the heart is functioning. This is an expensive test however and there can be long waiting times for a patient to get one. A quicker and cheaper solution would be to do a simple blood test that has recently been developed called the Brain Natriuretic Peptide (BNP). This is secreted by the heart in response to excessive stretching of heart muscle cells (the brain bit comes from the fact that it was first identified in pigs' brains). In many areas there has been a dispute whether GPs should be able to do this. The BNP test costs roughly a tenth of the cost of an ECHO and could easily be done in primary care in those cases where the diagnosis is not certain, but where a lot of effort and money has been put in to developing ECHO services, many organisations still don't allow GPs to use the BNP, even when patients are clearly not getting ECHOs quickly enough. In the USA at present BNP is not advised in the initial evaluation of typical heart failure findings. However many GPs think it would be ideal in finding out whether these patients with mild shortness of breath are actually suffering from heart problems rather than lung problems. It would definitely at the very least make it more likely that the patient ends up in the right hospital department first time, which must be a cost effective thing to do. We will have to wait to see whether this test does eventually trickle down. As far as I know no one has done a controlled trial in primary care on this point.

GPs in most areas can now send patients to clinics, not necessarily in a hospital, for quick and easy diagnosis of angina. The GP must do certain basic blood tests and send the results online to the clinic where an appointment is automatically made for exercise testing on a treadmill within 2 weeks. A cardiologist then looks at the result, and if the test is positive the patient is given an appointment at the hospital. A good system for channelling the right person through as quickly as possible is a marker for good cardiac care, but not all areas have such a system at the moment.

In the UK there is a continuous audit to see how well different hospitals are doing in getting their cardiac patients into hospital early,[66] and treating them with the best up to date methods, and treatment is changed according to how success-ful it is. It is evidence-based medicine at its best, with clear end-points (patient survival) and robust data. There are two ways of treating angina once it has been diagnosed; an operation on the heart itself to improve the blood supply to the heart, and medical treatment with drugs.

So as far as operations are concerned, there are two operations commonly done for coronary artery ischaemia – which is a term used for a lack of oxygen to the heart muscle due to narrowed coronary vessels caused by atheroma (cholesterol and fat building up and blocking the arteries). One is coronary artery angio-plasty, which is done through the skin via an artery in the leg and consists of putting a stent in to improve the circulation to the heart (percutaneous coro-nary interventions, PCI); and the other is coronary artery bypass graft surgery (CABG, known to medics as Cabbage), which of course is open-heart surgery. Both are very safe, and angioplasty, as mentioned above, is used as an emergency treatment for an acute heart attack, improving survival rates.

But in chronic stable angina, an operation does not save lives compared with medical therapy, which consists of one or two anti-anginal medications plus drugs for the secondary prevention of cardiovascular disease. Nevertheless more and more patients are getting an operation done early. Patients getting a PCI often think they are going to live longer by preventing another heart attack. But this is not so – it is done to relieve symptoms. Trials have compared the two operations, per-cutaneous angioplasty and CABG for angina patients, and there were similar rates of MI and death at 12 months in each group, and no difference from medical therapy. Of course the medication-only group do have to keep taking the tablets!

NICE guidelines state that patients with angina should not be offered acupuncture, TENS or EECP (a mechanical procedure which is said to 'milk' blood from the legs to the heart). All these treatments have been in vogue at various times. If angina does not respond to drug treatment and revascularisation, patients need to be reviewed 'with the consideration of other causes for their pain, and an exploration of psychological and social factors, which might contribute to their symptoms'. You wouldn't think chest pain could be a psychological problem but sometimes it can be, although more usually this is another way of saying we don't know what causes it so therefore it could be psychological (which may be rather hard on the patient).

Anginal symptoms can also be caused by coronary artery spasm (smooth muscle constriction of the coronary artery). Coronary angiography may reveal a focal area of spasm but frequently demonstrates apparently normal coronary arteries. However, coronary spasm typically occurs near an atherosclerotic plaque so probably is a symptom of heart disease, and so patients need secondary preventive therapy and coronary risk factor management such as aspirin, beta-blockers and other drugs to lower cholesterol.

We had two patients during my time at the practice who suffered from very severe chest pain at intervals, and always had to be admitted to hospital, but no damage to the heart was ever found. At that time we GPs were supposed to visit them at home each time they called for heart pain, but it always seemed so unnecessary as whatever we found when we got there and however many times they had been admitted before you could never just reassure them, and we had to call an ambulance. This must have been very upsetting for them as doctors often thought they were malingering, but in retrospect they must have been suffering from either cardiac syndrome X or coronary artery spasm. Both patients, who were in their 40s and 50s when they first developed symptoms, lived to good ages, and one died of something else in his early 80s!

Another problem GP see a lot of is cardiac arrhythmias, where the heart becomes irregular. Atrial fibrillation (AF) is the commonest sort of irregular pulse and is due to the electrical signal becoming so disorganised that the atria (the smaller chambers of the heart where the blood enters the heart) no longer beat, but are in a constant state of random contraction, called fibrillation. Only the occasional signal gets through to the bigger chambers, which actually do the pumping (the ventricles) so that the heart beat is completely irregular. The commonest cause of atrial fibrillation used to be damage to the heart following rheumatic fever but as the incidence of that has declined, nowadays no definite cause is found in most cases. It is very common in the elderly. It may be symptomless but it greatly increases the risk of a stroke. This is because the lack of regular emptying of the atria causes stasis in the blood and clots can form. If any of these clots break off the first place they will land is the brain. Not a very nice thought.

Recently a conference of stroke specialists called for a national screening programme for people over 65 to identify those with AF,[67] which they say will prevent up to 2000 premature deaths per year. Apparently about 1 in four people will have it at some time in their lives (but usually as they get older) and AF contributes to 15% of strokes. However are they going to set up a separate system to screen people, such as calling people in to clinics? No, it seems that the most cost effective method of screening would be opportunistic, that is for GPs to check the pulse of everyone who comes to them for whatever reason. Now that isn't what I call screening. GPs will only be able to do that if they have time and that is what most of them don't have (although a GP or nurse is able to pick up AF whenever they check the blood pressure, which of course they do on most people regularly). I think may be that the specialists would like it to be a task rewarded by the Quality and Outcomes Framework. To my mind it would have to be combined with advertisements to the general public to check their own pulses and go to their GP if they think it is irregular. While it seems superficially at least to be a good idea to run a screening campaign you would have to be absolutely sure it did save lives. So often these initiatives when eventually subjected to a proper clinical trial turn out to be ineffective.

However there are other benign causes of irregular pulse, the most common of which is sinus arrhythmia. This is common in younger people where the pulse slows when you breathe in and quickens when you breather out. Try it yourself. If anything it is a sign of a healthy heart! So you can imagine GP surgeries being even more crowded with people coming in for this. That said, a stroke is a terrible thing and if money could be found to set up a proper screening service (the specialists say that screening would satisfy the UK National Screening committee's criteria for a screening programme) it should be done. Atrial fibrillation can be treated of course with anticoagulants – warfarin usually, although this isn't an easy treatment because blood levels have to be measured regularly, a time consuming and tricky process usually carried out by GPs in conjunction with the local hospital. There are newer treatments being developed, which even if expensive may well save money if there was no need for blood monitoring.

Of course GPs need lots of expertise in reading electrocardiographs (ECGs), as this is the test which will prove it is AF. Sometimes if an ECG is particular difficult to read GPs can sent the ECG to the consultants, saving the patient from having to go there. That can be extremely helpful for everyone. GPs in our area also wanted open access to exercise testing, ECHOs, and access to 24 hour monitoring tapes. These are the sorts of thing GPs commissioning groups could set up, if they had the money.

So now we need to discuss statins, those ubiquitous wonder drugs. Despite the wonderful new treatments for heart problems, it has been preventative drugs that have changed the world of heart disease more. Statins are said to have saved millions of lives. These drugs were developed in the late 90's and have been amongst the most successful drugs ever developed. They lower 'bad' cholesterol (low density lipoprotein) by inhibiting a very important enzyme (HMG-CoA reductase) that regulates cholesterol metabolism in the liver. They are absolutely life-saving for people we know already have heart disease (people who already have angina or have suffered a heart attack) and are also used extensively for people who have never had any such problem before but are at risk because they have a high cholesterol, and usually other risk factors such as obesity or a family history of heart disease. So far so good – this certainly gives a huge pool of people to medicate who may so far be symptomless. But we never stop there do we? Remember the premise with HRT – that because it was a good treatment for hot flushes it should be given to every woman past the menopause? Now doctors are advocating that everyone should have statins and even that statins should be put in the water or a poly-pill. Yet we do not know for certain whether drugs such as statins and other drugs which will raise the good cholesterol (high density lipoprotein, HDL) actually do increase life expectancy – the true outcome needed. Large trials are under way but haven't yet been published.

People over 70 regularly used to come in to my surgery wanting statins. So we would test their cholesterol and try to work out their risk of heart disease. We had all sorts of computerised algorithms to help us decide who should be prescribed them. But the trouble was none of the original research work had been done on older people, and of course people's cholesterol levels always rise, as they get older. So the cholesterol tests would say either that yes, these people should have statins, or more honorably that the algorithm didn't apply. That didn't stop us having to prescribe them though. I remember one woman in her early 80's, who was very fit, and both her parents had lived into their nineties and her mother to 100, with no sign of heart disease in either of them (they both died basically of old age). Her cholesterol would have been slightly abnormal had she been in her early sixties, but was probably normal for a woman of her age. But it was no good. She had read the columns in the newspapers about how marvelous statins were and insisted on having them. I felt very uneasy over this. I might have drawn a line and refused but she was actually a friend of mine, and I didn't want her to think I was being mean with the NHS' money. In fact I overheard someone saying later that she had praised me as being an excellent doctor because I prescribed them. Of course she will live a good long time – but I don't think statins will have made a bit of difference to her life chances.

There are of course side effects of statin use. Many people get quite severe muscle pains while on them – at least 10% in most studies, and sometimes this can be serious. Everyone when they start a statin should have a blood test called a CPK (creatinine phospho-kinase) taken to make sure there isn't going to be severe muscle damage. Recently the FDA in the USA has just added warnings to statins regarding their risks of increasing diabetes, memory loss or confusion as well. The risks are low, and undoubtedly if you have already had a heart attack this should not prevent you taking a statin. But if there is nothing wrong with you? Again this could be a case of over medicalising the ordinary population, especially the elderly.

There is also a darker side of the biochemistry of statins, promoted by Stephanie Seneff.[68] Her conclusion, from a closely argued article which does really need a considerable knowledge of biochemistry to understand, (and she is not primarily a biochemist) is that while there are short term benefits from statins on the heart due to lowering LDL (low density lipoprotein) in blood, the long-term effects on the muscles, heart, kidney and brain are likely to be deleterious. Her argument is that cholesterol is extremely important to the body and there are bad effects from preventing us synthesising it. She predicts that in the next couple of decades it is going to be obvious that people taking statins will have a much greater incidence of kidney failure, chronic neurological diseases, and short-term memory loss. Not at all what people were expecting. This is only a theory and there is no evidence that any of it is true, but it is interesting. Only time will tell if she is right. Her suggestions for a healthy life are plenty of sun (she postulates a direct effect of sunlight on cardiac health), plenty of exercise, eggs, and milk, and no fructose. There's a surprise then!

What we need of course is evidence that primary prevention of CHD actually works. Primary prevention means that you give everybody the intervention. So here you need to give statins not to people you know to be at risk but to everyone, in a controlled trial. The authors of a paper recently did a meta-analysis of studies, which have done just that. The age of recruitment was from 51 to 75 years, and the results showed that there was no decrease in all-cause mortality between those taking statins and those not taking them.[69] If statins had an effect on heart attacks in everybody then you would expect there to be a decrease. Included in this study were some patients who did have an increased risk of heart trouble, and even then the results were negative, and there was some evidence of a poor quality of life due to side effects. Unsurprisingly I see no publicity given to this study.

Yet it was headline news when recently a meta-analysis, combining the results of many smaller trials, indicated that statins do 'work' for people with a risk as low as 10%.[70] That would include everyone over 50 with a slightly raised cholesterol ratio, and will include 60% of the elderly (over 70). So should everyone who might benefit take statins?

Firstly, as explained in Chapter 7, the NNT would be very high – 99% or more would not benefit. Some would be harmed – one in a hundred would develop diabetes as a result (the same as those who benefit). Secondly, the load on primary care worldwide would be huge. As people can be harmed by statins, you can't just take them and hope for the best. You would need to be checked for muscle damage and diabetes regularly. Thirdly, there may be more side effects than we know about now. Fourthly, there is the problem of medicalising people and illnesses. The psychological impact of going from some one who considers themselves healthy to someone who is 'on medication' can be large, the daily reminder of your own mortality when you take your morning pill. What of its effect on life insurance, and travel insurance? Also it now strays into philosophical realms. What do you want to die of? You do in fact have to die of something. Although heart disease in a young person is a tragedy, in a person in their nineties it is a 'natural' way to go, like pneumonia. Though not painless, it can be quick. Would you prefer cancer? Or a neurological condition such as Parkinson's? What about dementia? Think carefully before you try to exclude a heart attack from the long list of things you can die of.

I feel there is a wrong presumption here. Statins undoubtedly do something useful in people whose metabolism isn't absolutely finely tuned on the cholesterol front, but that doesn't mean that it will do anything if there was never a problem in the first place. That said though, personally I think that a family history of heart disease (i.e. that a close relative suffered a cardiac event under 65) is very important and is sometimes not considered enough in the commonly used algorithms. I would certainly recommend statins in these people regardless of their cholesterol level.

Manufacturers and some specialists though are going to promote these drugs to everyone if they can get away with it. To me though, if there ain't a problem, don't fix it.

Part 4

Common problems encountered in general practice

Diagnosis, evidence for therapy and vested interests

Chapter 12
The GP encounter: consultation, investigations, reaching a diagnosis and gaining patient trust

How to make a diagnosis – guidelines and algorithms – appropriateness of investigations – the Internet – honesty to patients – patient lists – sick notes and fit notes.

So, back to the GP and the patient in front of her. What actually goes on in a consultation?

You may have a problem. You think it is a medical problem, because it pertains to a part of your body or mind, and is causing distress. So, before you do anything, you try to work out for yourself what it is, whether you need to see a doctor or pharmacist, how to explain the problem to them and what the pharmacist or doctor is likely to do about it.

This may seem simple, and in many cases it is. You have a sore throat. So it must be an infection and if it doesn't get better soon you might need to see a doctor or get some medication from a pharmacist. But even in that scenario there are lots more questions to which you might want the answer. What proportion of sore throats will get better by themselves with no specific treatment in 5 days? Will antibiotics make it better more quickly? Are antibiotics needed to prevent complications? Is it OK just to take paracetamol or would it help to go to a Pharmacist to get something to relieve other symptoms? How long does it have to go on before you can see a specialist?

In fact it is far from simple and people vary as to whether they will try to access knowledge from friends, family, books, magazines or the Internet, or seek help from a professional.

But many consultations with GPs are straightforward and may not even need a diagnosis. The patient wants a prescription, a sick note or a check-up for a known condition and both sides can agree on an outcome quite quickly. When a things are not that clear, there are several ways in which your doctor would arrive at a diagnosis or at least a strategy for dealing with your problem. The process of diagnosis does not often fit the HOUSE method (on TV) of firing possible diagnoses into the air and coming up with more and more bizarre solutions, entertaining as the TV series is. (The series really did have a seductive appeal to medics because it managed to put just enough real diseases with long eponymous titles in to make you think for a moment that it was real – until they overdid it and you laughed at yourself for thinking that. And of course the hapless patient always proved everyone wrong by vomiting large amounts of blood or having a spectacular fit at a dramatic moment). The ways doctors actually make a diagnosis are much more mundane.

The easiest is a 'spot' diagnosis – the patient walks into the room and the doctor immediately knows what the problem might be. These would be conditions where there are obvious clinical signs – jaundice, Parkinson's disease, etc. That only works though if the patient has actually come because of that. Many times they haven't and then the problem will be whether to broach this problem to the patient, who may indeed be happy to discuss it but this may just lengthen the consultation, as they have actually come about a sore throat, say.

One dilemma that sometimes comes up on doctors' chat sites is – what would you do if you saw someone on a bus with something obvious that needed treating – like a malignant melanoma for instance? Would you go up to the person, and draw attention to it? Even if you were 100% sure of the diagnosis it would be slightly risky as the patient might know about it, have treatment, lined up and may not be at all happy for you to remind them of it. But it is equally a risk not to do it as it might save their life, and doctors have blogged about doing just that with happy consequences for everyone!

GPs most commonly use the presenting complaint such as a pain in the shoulder, ('Doc, my shoulder is stiff and sore'), and then collect enough information to make a working diagnosis. Or a doctor may take the diagnosis the patient has come up with, ('I've got arthritis, doc') and work with that if it seems reasonable, and may use pattern recognition as a trigger – the mixture of presenting complaints makes a pattern the doctor is familiar with. Of course common things occur commonly so that the doctor will have seen this pattern many times before. But probability-based reasoning (shoulder pain equals arthritis, because it often is), although essential to some extent, can be misleading in primary care.

Sometimes it leads the doctor astray, like the lady who went to her doctor 39 times with pain in her shoulder and was given physiotherapy for weeks before a chest X-ray was done which showed lung cancer. Shoulder pain can, very rarely, be a presenting symptom in lung cancer, as the pain can be referred from the neck, back or chest. For instance, shoulder pain can be caused by problems in the diaphragm area or from a tumour in the periphery of the lung (so called Pancoast tumour which every medical student learns about but would hardly ever be seen in a GPs lifetime). A chest X-ray is not one of the recommended investigations for shoulder pain in any guideline that I have seen so it was understandable that lung cancer was not considered first time, but after so many visits a doctor would need to consider other possibilities. So often diagnoses have to be made in a stepwise fashion, using test of treatment (physio in this case), test of time (to see whether it gets better quickly or not) or further investigation. But in this case the recommended investigations are unlikely to include a chest X-ray until the condition has failed the test of time.

It is of course part of a doctor's training to think of the most serious diseases to rule out first and then do step wise refinement in his mind, asking questions all the time. Knowledge of guidelines and clinical pathways (algorithms, flow charts and step by step logical procedures) are essential to make sure that doctors are up to date with their knowledge but can't easily be referred to during the consultation because the GP doesn't want to spend valuable patient contact time looking at the screen. So GPs are much more likely to use pattern recognition, but that depends on the doctor having seen the pattern before. In this case of shoulder pain the doctor hadn't, and would have to rely on knowledge learned in medical school.

A doctor will learn the most common causes of the presenting problem and a shortlist of the more serious diseases to rule out, then refine the possible diagnosis step by step based on either the anatomical location after a thorough examination of the area in question, or by doing more tests to work out what pathology (disease process) might be going on. For instance, if both your shoulders are very sore and stiff and you are older than 60 then a test for inflammation in the blood (ESR) might prove beyond doubt that you have polymyalgia rheumatica, a quite serious disease which will need steroids to treat it.

The role of a clinical examination has changed a lot since I qualified. At that time a clinical examination was the gold standard for diagnosis. Heart murmurs, chest signs the doctor could hear while listening through the stethoscope, the exact point at which the patient shouted 'ouch' while a joint was put through its movements, these were the basis of all medical practice. A breast examination, even a routine one when patients had no complaints of a lump, would take at least ten minutes to do properly, and might be very unpleasant for the patient. That was what we were taught and indeed there was no alternative. Tests to demonstrate abnormalities early had not been developed. But almost all these clinical examinations only picked up gross abnormalities when the patient was probably already very ill. Nowadays it is rare for a GP to pick up a 'physical sign' – a positive sign on examination that will tell the doctors at the very least that there is a problem and which system it is in. It is crucial sometimes especially for internal examinations like vaginal and rectal examinations, and the art of general practice is knowing when a full examination is likely to help. But for many common self-limiting illnesses like coughs and sore throats it is often not helpful at all. A person can be complaining of a really dreadful sore throat and you look inside and see very little abnormal. There is no correlation between what the patient feels and what you see. A good history from the patient and a liberal use of simple tests is mostly a much better bet. And if you do find an abnormal sign it is likely that there has already been a considerable delay – from the patient or the doctor.

But many patients still have this rather simplistic notion that a doctor can find everything out by examination, and many was the time when I sat on medical service committees when a patient had made an official complaint where the main problem seemed to be that the doctor had not examined the patient. Never mind that it was extremely unlikely that the doctor could possibly have picked up any thing abnormal at the stage that mattered. But it was important to patients and because of this I was always punctilious in examining the chests of patients with colds, the abdomen with people with indigestion and joints which moved fully without pain. Towards the end of my career I felt there was a very strong element of 'laying on of hands' in a spiritual sense, that it strengthened the bond between doctor and patient, and will be sorely missed when doctors finally give up the pretence that in some cases it is doing much good. The art of knowing when you really do have to examine the patient thoroughly and when you don't is one that takes a long time to learn. Sometimes it is essential – a rectal examination for prostate cancer, for instance.

In hospital practice the problem will have already been narrowed down by the GP to a particular speciality, and in over 95% of cases (certainly in our studies) the GP will done that correctly. This makes it relatively easy to start on the next stage of further investigation, which is usually done nowadays to a menu of things that clinical guidelines recommend, and almost all patients going to a clinic will get certain tests regardless of the actual problem.

But in general practice the range of possibilities is so wide, and the time so limited that it can be much more tricky. The patient coming in with a painful shoulder might have strained their shoulder doing some DIY the day before, may know perfectly well what the problem is and may only want some anti-inflammatory tablets on prescription (especially if otherwise they would have to buy them), and investigation would be a waste of time.

Knowledge of guidelines and clinical pathways are essential to make sure that doctors are up to date with their knowledge, but are difficult to use consistently during the consultation because of time constraints. There are many computerised and on-line aids to help a GP during the consultation, but this risks the doctor spending more time looking at the computer than at the patient, and the quality of the consultation takes a nose-dive. A GP will be bombarded with complicated guidelines from specialist doctors each thinking theirs is the only important one for the GP to know about.

If the doctor is not sure of the diagnosis she will arrange further tests, and here there may be a problem if the test recommended is not one available to the GP. Many people have to be referred to hospital, not for the test, but to see a specialist to arrange the test, and this causes a bottleneck. There has been no way of deciding which tests should be available to GPs until recently because often the ability to do the tests was jealously guarded by specialists. This is fully discussed in Chapter 20.

Sometimes the GP is really not sure what is going on and will use other strategies, such as recall for further review, or use a 'holding' prescription such as a painkiller or anti-inflammatory medication. The doctor thinks that it might do some good but in any case will enable the consultation to be continued in a few days with the benefit of using time to see how the condition develops, or reassurance with the invitation to make another appointment. The doctor may or not share the clinical uncertainty with the patient and whether to so or not depends on the relationship between doctor and patient.

Once a working diagnosis is reached, then the doctor will start treatment if available, or explain the problem so that the patient can then manage the problem (often this is another way of saying 'live with it'). Everybody needs an explanation.

It is always a problem keeping to time in surgery. Some consultations really need far more than the allotted ten minutes to make a diagnosis, but there is never going to be enough time, in any healthcare system to do everything. In some other European countries consultations are often longer but the GP will not have an army of helpers – nurses, phlebotomists, receptionists, as in the UK, so the GP has to do these things herself, thus reducing the real time with the patient to the 10 minutes or so available in the UK.

When the condition is vague, undefined, or complicated, too often a consultation is a game. The patient has a rough idea of what is bothering him, and also usually an idea of what he might want to happen. But he knows that there is only going to be a short time in which he has to explain the problem and he does not know what the alternatives are. The doctor maybe running late by this time and want to get things over quickly. So it might become a 'game' in an effort to best fit the immediate objectives of the patient and doctor as quickly as possible, but the real understanding can get lost.

If anything, when the doctor is under time pressure or uncertain how to proceed, it is more likely that a patient gets more investigations or treatments rather than fewer, and some of these may not necessarily be needed according to up to date guidelines. In these times of straitened finances for all health service in the world this may be of concern.

In a recent study,[71] a significant minority of clinical examinations (15%), prescriptions (19%), and referrals (22%), and almost half of investigations (46%), were thought by the doctor who arranged them to be only slightly needed or not needed at all. If 22% of referrals were indeed not necessary this would indeed be a huge waste of resources. In my work I found the proportion of referrals which the doctor thought to be probably not necessary was much less than that, between 4% and 12% depending on speciality. Perhaps this discrepancy is due to the definition of need. In a study done in our area,[72] these referrals were classed as 'Patient Demand' when the doctor could not quickly convince the patient that they were not needed or the patient would not be satisfied otherwise, which is a rather tighter definition than 'maybe not needed'. Whatever the figures, the doctor perceives that the pressure is coming from patients for 'something to done', and does 'something' other than give time and expertise, even though the presenting complaint may not be one that would require these actions according to guidelines. This amounts to a failure of communication and doctors really should directly ask patients about their expectations, in order to limit unnecessary resource use and to prevent things going wrong as a result of the unnecessary referral (iatrogenic problems).

However most cases are much more straightforward than this and the doctor usually does what he thinks the patient needs, solely as a result of a thorough analysis of the problem in the consultation. Anything that can speed the information gathering can help, and fortunately nowadays there is the Internet. Both sides use it – the patient to get an idea of what may be the solution (diagnosis by Google), and the doctor to check up on points she might have misremembered. I feel that the Internet, for all its faults and inaccuracies, is a much better source of medical information than the popular press. If you google a common condition such as shoulder pain, the first few pages you reach are those which are quite reliable, at least in the UK, such as NHS Choices, Arthritis Research, Wikipedia, and GP Notebook (although you may also get advertisements for injury compensation lawyers at the top of the list). Further down you will get more sponsored sites encouraging you to have various sorts of treatment, which may or may not be relevant.

The authentic sites will give you an indication of what you might need, and your GP, after confirming by clinical examination what the problem might be, is in the best position to help you decide how to proceed. The popular press such as newspapers and magazines, on the other hand, are interested only in headline-grabbing information and can completely distort things. In a newspaper you may see that there is just around the corner a new breakthrough in treatment for arthritis (or prostate cancer, or diabetes), which immediately takes you several steps away from any problem you might have in this area. The new treatment is likely to have been taken from a recent paper published by a scientist working with mice or a drug company with a product which has not even been tested on humans yet, and any development is years away, if ever. The reasons for publication are obvious – the scientist wants recognition of the work he is doing, knowing that this would make it more likely that he will get funds from research bodies to continue his work, and the papers want to sell copies, and anything that will attract readers will do. The press story may not even be a good account of what the scientist is trying to do, or may be a direct plug by a company with a vested interest. In no way are these stories designed to give the public an unbiased account or information about this new development, and all should be taken with a pinch of salt. They are interesting dreams but are not relevant to current medical treatment. Unfortunately, many is the patient I have seen clutching a cutting from a newspaper with such a story and it takes valuable time out of a consultation in explaining the reality that this is not going to change anything any time soon, and probably never will.

Of course one of the main ways in which people appreciate a GP consultation is in the nature of the doctor himself. Doctors vary of course in how they interact with patients. There is the 'matey' doctor, the more formal doctor, the paternalistic doctor and the empathetic doctor, to name but a few, and of course many doctors are all of these things at different times and with different patients. While most patients nowadays prefer a patient-centred approach, where doctors constantly ask what the patient understands about the problem and discuss what choices the patient has in detail, some patients, up to a third in some studies, actually prefer a doctor-centred approach where the doctor makes the decisions and the patient accepts what the doctor says ('doctor knows best'). The style of doctoring comes from an interaction between the doctor's personality and their training.

I surprised myself recently when I found myself on a tropical island on a package tour. A Russian lady was lying on the beach near where we were sitting and her boyfriend was getting very agitated because she seemed to be ill. He called the tour leader (a Thai) who called for some coffee to revive her, and when that didn't work he began to cast around to see if there was any other help around. So I thought I should go over to see what I could do. It appeared that she had had an injury to her leg few days ago and now was feeling unwell and had a pounding in her head. Her boyfriend told me in very limited English that he thought her pulse was racing. Immediately I found myself clicking into consultation mode. In real life I am quite an impetuous sort of person who comes to conclusions very quickly and does things directly without too much agonising about it, but here I sat back carefully considering the options in my mind. She did not look shocked, wasn't sweating, her colour was good, and I thought she was probably OK. But I was worried about the relationship between the two of them. He had the most awful sunburn on his shoulders and right arm and had obviously taken no notice of the fact that we were very near the equator. I didn't know who was looking after whom and why! Anyway I carefully enquired whether it was OK to examine her, and when she nodded, I felt her pulse and checked her breathing. Her pulse wasn't racing and was absolutely normal and her breathing was slow and deep. I was sure she was hyperventilating, but I know from experience that people can feel very ill indeed when they are doing that.

Over-breathing is a natural response when adrenaline is produced because adrenaline is the flight and fright response – you see danger and immediately your body responds by increasing your pulse rate and respiratory rate. What happens is that when people over breathe is that the acidity in the blood alters and this does make you feel ill – dizzy nauseated and generally unwell. Often people cannot believe that this is due to over breathing and they can get quite angry when you say that it is due to stress on the body. So I went quite carefully talking it through with the boyfriend who immediately seemed delighted that the situation was now under control. I expect he was thinking of all the consequences of her being ill (helicopters to take her to hospital, medical expenses, loss of rest of the holiday) as well as being concerned for her. But she was not yet satisfied and said she still felt ill and had the pounding behind her ears. However after I explained that it could be due to excitement as well as actual stress she appeared to accept it and soon after she said her headache had gone and sat up. So I left them. Soon afterwards I saw her carefully applying sunscreen to his badly burnt neck and shoulders, and all was suddenly well. I was surprised at the training I had over all these years about being careful, taking things step by step, not rushing to conclusions and explaining carefully what was happening, kicked in even after several years of not seeing patients at all. But of course it was what I had done for 34 years so perhaps not so surprising.

There are few other walks of life when a person will convey his greatest worries or fears to another person, and there has to be complete trust on both sides. Are doctors always honest with their patients? When I first qualified the answer was an unequivocal 'no'. Paternalism was very strong, and there was a belief that patients did not want to hear bad news, and indeed to be told that you had an incurable illness or were dying was actually going to harm your spirit, and perhaps make you 'give up' so that you died earlier. I was taught that you never told the patient he was going to die, but always put as positive a gloss on it as you could. Thus, bladder cancer was 'warts on the bladder', stomach cancer was a 'bad ulcer', and lung cancer was a 'shadow on the lung' – as of course was TB. Even when it was clear that the diagnosis was cancer, for instance breast or skin cancer, the patient was told 'it has all been taken away' and shouldn't come back.

We always told a relative the true picture of course, heaping on that person all the strain of dishonesty. I don't remember patients ever asking me questions in those early years; if they did we would always put as positive a gloss as we could. I think it must have been a reflection of the fact that so little could be done, and a doctor's success lay in her being able to inspire devotion and belief from the patients in a time when a doctor had to compete for patients far harder than they have to now.

This changed of course only three or four years after I qualified, and before I started work as a GP. Gradually it became absolutely essential to tell the truth, but for many a year we (and I was certainly guilty) did not necessarily tell the whole truth. It took a while for medical schools to realise that telling patients bad news was something that doctors needed training in, and for courses to be put on for GPs. In a way it was possibly easier for GPs, as we dealt with uncertainty all the time and were rarely absolutely sure of our diagnoses as specialists were; in many cases to frighten a patient with bad news when it wasn't true was always a risk. Later generations of doctors though seemed to positively relish telling the patient of all the awful things they might have even if rather unlikely, on the assumption that a patient would forgive them if everything turned out OK but wouldn't be pleased if they didn't warn them and it did turn out to be something nasty; also of course to protect them against legal action. I think it is a fine line that has to be trod here, but the doctor should always be as honest as possible.

Even nowadays doctors sometimes admit to being economical with the truth. In a recent survey in the USA[73] about a third of doctors admitted to not always informing patients of serious medical errors or disclosing financial relationships with drug and device companies, and 10% admitted to sometimes telling a patient something that was not true. Surgeons and Paediatricians were most likely to report being completely honest with prognosis while internist doctors in family practice and psychiatrists were the least likely. But an Ipsos MORI survey of 1,026 people in the UK in 2011 found that 88% trusted doctors to tell the truth, with the profession beating 20 other professions on honesty, including judges, clergyman and priests, and the police. Just 8% of respondents felt doctors did not tell the truth. So we must be doing something right.

In the past, GPs had an individual relationship with patients registered with them, which dated from pre NHS days, and this was certainly the case when I went into practice. One of my partners had an extremely loyal list of patients who would see only him, to such a point that it was very difficult for any to the other doctors to look after his patients when he was away. At that time a doctor's individual list of patients was his power – he could take his patients off with him in the event of disputes with other doctors, although many practices tried to stop this happening by putting legal covenants into the practice agreement. They turned out not always to be legally enforceable and one of our local doctors did take his list of patients and set up his own practice, very successfully. Now the individual list system has all but disappeared as the payment for patients is made through the practice and a patient does not have to be individually registered with one GP. The personal link is weakening with practices being more impersonal and with the growth of so many other clinicians such as nurses, seeing more patients.

The system in the NHS of each person having to register with one practice has great strengths but also some weaknesses. The biggest advantage compared to the system in the USA, for example, is that a GP record is a lifetime record which will follow a patient wherever he goes, so that doctors can look up what has happened in the past, what treatment has been tried and so on, very easily. This saves a great deal of time, compared with the USA where there is no such record and a new doctor has to take everything from the patient himself with no corroboration from notes (a patient's memory may not be that good, and sometimes a patient want to conceal or deny information). It leads to good continuity of care, even when a patient does not see the same doctor each time. When asked in surveys patients say they want to have a primary care doctor they know and trust wherever possible, and this is because both patient and doctor can relax having a shared history of how things have panned out on the past.

Certainly for me as for most doctors, a good proportion of people I saw were people I knew well in that context and I could tailor my recommendations to what I knew the patient needed. It is really nice to be told, 'you are the only person who really understands me, doctor' even though you know that – oops – you had better be careful here. This may be the honest truth, and a wonderful compliment, or it may be a prelude to 'you are the only doctor who will prescribe this for me/ give me this sick note/visit me at home' which ought to ring alarm bells. Why would this be so – why would other doctors not do this? Is it perhaps because it goes against all guidelines? It may be of course that it is because you know what has happened in the past (a patient suffered because another doctor would not visit, refer, prescribe steroids or antibiotics when in retrospect this would have been obviously the right treatment) but it may be that you are straying into dangerous waters. However in most cases there are lots of advantages, if you are a patient with specific or multiple problems, to seeing the same doctor when possible. Unfortunately the structure of general practice is changing rapidly and this relationship is not so easy to achieve.

What do you do if you cannot find such a doctor, if no doctor will take you seriously, or if you have had a bad experience in the past and really cannot trust your family doctor any more? The system at present makes it easy to shop around, so long as you aren't in a rural area or have to go to a particular practice for other specific reasons. However it is time-consuming and unpleasant to have to change practices, having to get used to new systems and faces. This problem should not be the patient's problem; it should be the doctor's. For the vast majority of patients, the problem lies in the personal relationship with the previous doctor, and a careful teasing out of what went wrong can mend things and allow a new relationship to develop. This may take time, but is essential. The most important part is an acknowledgement of the problem, an explanation if possible – which may include a reassurance that such a thing should not have happened and won't happen again. If the problem boils down to unrealistic expectations by the patient, then it may be possible to correct these. Sometimes not though, and unfortunately the doctor has then to go on defensive mode, which means making sure that every action is explained and documented very clearly in the notes. Good communication is vital at every step.

The worst outcome here is usually that the patient sees a different doctor every time, often the most junior registrar, and may get inappropriate investigations or referrals, and not the ones that are really needed. If the patient is right and the problem really is one which should be taken seriously and isn't, and the doctors really are being unhelpful, then sometimes a well respected and well qualified nurse can help. Such a nurse often knows the patient and the doctors very well and may be able to see a path through.

It is all the more important to clarify the understanding of patient and doctor when the consultation might result in a referral to another service, either within the practice, or to a consultant led service or to a service led by other health workers such as Physiotherapists or Optometrists. However most every day problems are dealt with entirely satisfactorily within the practice.

All in all the system of 'one patient one practice' for most situations works well in the UK. It should allow any patient who wants a personal relationship with a GP to get one. General practice surgeries are in general well equipped and well run, with a team of nurses, healthcare assistants, and sometimes midwives, health visitors, physiotherapists, counsellors, and psychiatric nurses attached. So many problems that used to be managed in hospitals can now be easily managed in the surgery.

Another change in doctor behaviour over the years was our attitude to 'sick notes'. When I first went into practice my senior partner took me aside and told me that 'only the patient knows when he or she is fit for work. You can't know how he was feeling. So in general unless you are sure the patient is faking it, you give the sick note'. So that was what I did, through almost my entire career. Many jobs at that time were hard, accident-prone, and often very boring, and we used to see lots of men in their fifties with back pain and arthritis. So we thought that giving the sick note was only fair. It was only later that we began to understand that actually work is nearly always good for you. People who are out of work or on incapacity benefit report worsening health even when they are entirely healthy when they first go on sick benefit. Putting the unemployed on to long-term sick benefit did their health no favours whatsoever. But that was what we were all exhorted to do early in Mrs Thatcher's Government. Its policies led to large increases in unemployment and we were suddenly faced with (usually) young people who had been 'sent' from the benefits office to get a sick note, often when there was no reason whatsoever for them to have one. This was a method of keeping the unemployment statistics down. Once or twice I rang up the benefits office, but they denied that was why they were doing it. Anyway it was very difficult to refuse if one 'arm' of the State had said they needed a sick note. The result of that was a whole cohort of young people remained on benefit for a very long time. As is likely to happen again now. The fact is that with Health and Safety legislation these days, jobs are almost always safe and often conditions of work are good, so we can reasonably say that to have a job is extremely therapeutic.

So eventually I did try occasionally to tease out what was actually happening in a young person's life. Now the emphasis is on 'fit notes' to emphasise what a person can do rather than what they can't do, and a lot of long-term certification is taken out of GPs hands altogether, which is right and proper. GPs don't have the training in Occupational Health to make these decisions.

That doesn't entirely let the GP off the hook though. I do remember one man in his thirties who had worked for about five years after leaving school, then lost his job and had been on benefits ever since. After ten years he was certified as fit to work, and he came back time after a time asking me to write letters for him in support of his appeals. He seemed very anxious and I tried to find out what he saw the problem as. He said 'I'm too slow. Whenever I do anything at work they harass me. It's horrible'. I wondered if he really did have a problem with anxiety, but then I was told that in fact he was a pigeon fancier and had a very nice lifestyle with his hobby, and had no intention of doing any work. In his previous jobs he found the answer was always to do everything extremely slowly, and this ensured his eventual dismissal. So he didn't get a letter from me that time.

The thrust of reforms to all UK health systems at the moment is to make sure that as many problems as possible are dealt with either within the practice, or in community-based services near to the patients' home. It is the referral to hospital step that overloads the system, and it is in both the patients' interest and the Exchequer's to ensure that only conditions that have to be referred to hospital are treated there. Most areas are setting up a raft of services in local communities that can be accessed through GPs, and often directly without seeing a GP first, and those services that have always been available locally such as pharmacists and optometrists are now getting powers to extend their range of skills.

Practice-based commissioning groups should be those driving the changes, and while hospital specialists are needed to advise on these where is no need for them to run the services as part of the hospital remit. This frees up the system to be more flexible, so long as there is good evidence behind the news developments, and fail safe governance to protect patients.

Chapter 13
Is the patient really ill?

Fibromyalgia/myeloencephalitis (ME) – convincing the GP; tiredness and chronic pain; alternative therapies – where's the evidence?

Most diseases now have clear, evidence-based pathways for treatment. However there are a group of common conditions where the definition is blurred, there aren't easy pathways to follow, and patients complain that they are not taken seriously. These include irritable bowel syndrome, fibromyalgia and of course ME (myeloencephalitis, or chronic fatigue syndrome), but there are lots of others. Some patients with these and similar conditions find themselves in great difficulty with the medical profession in getting a diagnosis, understanding it, and even more in management and treatment. The reason is that they are sort of sink diseases – patients fill up out-patients clinics, never get better and may remain unsatisfied for years. Not much is written in the serious medical literature, and no solutions are ever found. These people have my greatest sympathy. There is nothing quite so demoralizing than having a condition that may be painful and distressing and may completely mess up your lifestyle, yet isn't taken seriously. People can be left feeling a nuisance, unsupported, and feeling that they have to turn to one more health professional after another in search of answers, and sometimes even just for sympathy and understanding.

From a doctor's perspective, these are not easy patients to deal with precisely because the conditions are not, and will not become, life-threatening, and there are so many methods of management, only a few of which have a robust evidence base behind them. Some are not even diseases – the menopause was in this group for years, until a 'cure' was found and then people didn't stop researching it, or at least the precise form treatment should take.

So it is important to look a bit deeper into the relationship between people with such conditions and the medical profession as a whole Fibromyalgia is an example and is seen very often in Orthopaedic and Rheumatology clinics. It is a chronic painful muscular problem, which affects mostly women and again can be very debilitating. Wikipedia says 'it is a medical disorder characterized by chronic widespread pain and allodynia, a heightened and painful response to pressure. It is an example of a diagnosis of exclusion. Other symptoms include debilitating fatigue, sleep disturbance, and joint stiffness. Some patients may also report difficulty with swallowing, bowel and bladder problems, numbness and tingling and cognitive dysfunction'.

There is no specific test or treatment that will cure it, so it is important to give a very detailed explanation for the symptoms. While it is associated strongly with anxiety and depression it is important not to think that it is caused by these psychiatric conditions. It is completely unhelpful to dwell on this when a patient is suffering real pain and distress. I think the explanation again lies in the concept of inappropriate contraction of muscles causing mild but long lasting spasms, similar to the sorts of muscle ache you get when you have done unaccustomed exercise. There may also be a metabolic cause from anaerobic metabolism – I am no expert. But I like to give an explanation for these sorts of symptoms and this one is borrowed from a wonderful local consultant.

The story goes like this (and it is just a story but it is a good one). In Paleolithic times, stress was a constant companion for early hominids. Lives were short, illness often fatal and there were big predators and other hostile tribes around. There was a survival advantage to hyper-alert people who would be aware early of such dangers, not only to the individual but also to the group, which might be saved by such an individual. The genes for this hyper alertness were therefore selected for in a population. Not surprisingly the hyper-alert people in such a society were often the females with dependent young, with a heightened protective instinct. You can imagine at night in a cave the young mother, not sleeping well because of the demands of her young, lying awake and hearing the sounds of approaching predators or dangers from other tribes. She would then alert the others, but her own adrenaline would then be running very high. Because the initial recognition comes from her but the decision for action would came from the men she might be in a state of heightened tension for some time. Men also could be in this position if they preferred to slowly take stock of the situation rather than act immediately.

In modern times the prevalence of anxiety and tension is high. Anxiety leads to the production of adrenaline. But adrenaline is a flight-and-fright hormone and causes physical changes – rapid breathing, and re-distribution of blood supply to muscles from stomach and intestines, and is designed to help you to run away. In modern life stress isn't solved by actively getting on your running shoes and running several miles as if from a tiger (although in fact that would help a lot), but you stay still and worry in your head, and the bodily symptoms are misinterpreted.

So today, the fright and flight response is maladaptive to some extent. All these symptoms are produced by disturbances of the sympathetic and parasympathetic systems and over-production of adrenaline, and they are common in everyday life. Hyperventilation, from the adrenaline causing increased breathing rate, makes you feel as if you can't get enough air in, and also causes a reduction in acidity in the blood causing paraesthesia (pins and needles), weakness and nausea, and increased muscle pain from increased blood supply. The trigger points for muscle pain are always the back of the neck, shoulders, and small of the back and these points can be very tender when touched.

So my point is that there is never going to be a 'cure' for these problems, which are due directly to the way we are programmed to deal with stress. Some people, perhaps with a double dose of these alertness genes, which were so useful to our early survival, are now suffering from them, but it can get into a vicious circle with the stress of the fear of serious illness making the symptoms worse.

People who have received a diagnosis of fibromyalgia will have accessed websites and learnt a lot about possible causes, treatments and general management. But making the diagnosis, or not making it, is important and is initially in the hands of GPs, or occasionally physiotherapists. There are several points that I used to take into account. Firstly, though it may provide a label and an explanation of sorts for the problem, it is no panacea. It is a rotten condition to have, and people's quality of life is lower than if they had something like rheumatoid arthritis. Yet theoretically as there is no obvious damage to joints or muscles that can be seen, it would never do any harm to encourage exercise and positive thinking when people are having symptoms like neck pain and generalized muscle pain. I would never rush in to diagnose it or refer to a rheumatologist unless it was unavoidable. The label can be non-productive and lead to people thinking of giving up work and getting disability benefit. There is so much evidence now that work is good for you, and that people on benefit for whatever reason develop further health problems. If people are so desperate that they feel a diagnosis of fibromyalgia will help, they may be destined for a life of invalidity anyway. So I always used to prefer to encourage people to soldier on with support, sympathy, encouragement and medication where necessary rather than refer to hospital. Then of course patients might complain that they were diagnosed 'too late', but I always countered with: too late for what?

ME, myalgic encephalitis, post-flu debility – it has lots of names – is a very important related condition. It is a real problem for the medical profession because some patients have got so angry with the lack of research into infective, biochemical or metabolic causes that they have targeted doctors doing research into the psychiatric side of ME, or researching into the effect of graded exercise, by sending hate mail and even tried to hurt them physically. This of course is indefensible. Such people think that ME is an infection, perhaps like brucellosis or TB (or even HIV), which has no primary psychiatric aspect, and that exercise is always bad for patients and should never be encouraged. To be advised to have cognitive therapy (CBT) or graded exercise therefore seems like a slap in the face. I can understand why people who feel so tired and in pain might feel that exercise is too hard, but to blame the people trying to help seems perverse. Suffice to say that the most recent study[74] showed that graded exercise (with physiotherapy input) and CBT both help reduce fatigue and increase physical function much more than either management by a hospital specialist, or 'adaptive pacing therapy APT' (pacing yourself – matching your activity level very carefully to the amount of energy you have, sometimes under the guidance of an occupational therapist). The percentage of people who appeared to get worse was the same in each group and was very low.

So as with fibromyalgia, support, encouragement, advice on keeping active, and referral to these services where available is what primary care can provide when making such a diagnosis.

Tiredness is known in medical circles by its acronym – TATT (tired all the time). It is a very subjective symptom. You can't measure tiredness very well, it overlaps with fatigability, which can be measured, but it also overlaps with low motivation that is more difficult to measure. Sleepiness and the need for sleep are also interrelated. We don't understand what sleep is nor what tiredness represents. But undoubtedly there are many pathological conditions which cause them.

Cancer, and its treatment, chemotherapy and radiotherapy, almost invariably cause tiredness. This can easily be understood in terms of the work the body has to do in order to for its natural defences to overcome the insult it has suffered. Infections again need to be overcome by the immune system and if that is working overtime you can see there must be less energy for the rest of the things the body needs to do. Metabolic or endocrine diseases also commonly cause tiredness – lack of thyroid of course as the body's metabolic rate is dependent on thyroid hormone to keep going at its usual rate, and also Addison's disease, a lack of cortisol and other related hormones secreted by the adrenal cortex. Cortisol is crucial to the sensation of tiredness. Addison's disease is quite rare but is a killer so must be picked up early, yet the tests are very specific. If you don't ask for a serum cortisol to be done at a certain time of the day (as there is a big diurnal variation) you won't pick it up. There are other symptoms, such as low blood pressure and pigmentation, but they are non-specific too. Without cortisol, your blood pressure will drop and eventually you will die.

The value of steroids (cortisol and other steroids produced by the adrenal glands) can't really be over-estimated. When there was no other treatment for cancer after it had spread we used to give quite large doses of steroids, and the patients, from being feeling awful, ill and tired and reluctant to eat anything, used to improve dramatically after a few days. They would have an inordinate appetite, put on weight and feel full of energy, and would give them a window of life again. It did not last of course and soon the cancer would take over, but the end would be quite swift. I never regretted giving them those few weeks of life, although it was sad when the patient did not realise it could only be temporary.

Degeneration such as in extreme old age, is also associated with tiredness and lack of energy, but this is usually very benign and most people accept it as due to 'old age'. Depression and chronic anxiety, though, are probably the commonest causes of the tiredness we see in general practice. The cause is unclear, but there seems to be a cycle of guilt, despair and low motivation leading to the subjective symptom of tiredness.

So what is the cause of tiredness in fibromyalgia, chronic pain, IBS and ME? I don't know, but I would have thought it would contain elements of all of these. The overpowering tiredness of severe ME when people can't get up, wash, and feed themselves is a particular challenge to understand. It is much worse than seen in even severe depression. There must be an underlying cause for this, but nothing has ever been found. If you have a young person, perhaps in their late teens who stays in bed, can't get up or do anything yet continues to eat so doesn't waste away, and gets some enjoyment out of being attended to, then it is easy to think this can't be due to any of the pathologies that we come across. It is such a subjective symptom we then think it has to be a problem with the 'wiring' – how the synapses are connected – in the brain. Or so we would think, but of course some ME sufferers disagree with this profoundly.

So what should people do who have lost faith in their doctors to help them? It is easy to complain and doctor-bash, and all doctors have had their share, but that is part of the job. From the patient's point of view the most important part is to find out for himself or herself how best to manage their condition. Keep things simple; once it has been made clear that there is no easy solution but that the condition is not going to get worse or kill you, get as much information as you can and try to find one health professional that you trust and will give support. This could be a trusted GP or other health professional. I would advise you to approach people with a positive attitude, and things may improve. But it can be hard. GPs should be the ones to help, as specialists have to confine themselves to patients whom they think fall into their sphere of expertise, and if your problem doesn't do that then you will need to think again.

Many people of course turn to complementary medicine in these circumstances. This may bring you support and sympathy, and this can be worth having, but you should be aware that apart from a very few conditions – hypnotherapy for smoking cessation, acupuncture for knee pain, some herbs – there is little evidence that it works. I have gone into some forms of complementary medicine in detail later on in this book. If you do improve with any other treatments then this may be a real effect or due to chance, a change in your circumstances or the placebo effect. Should those therapies with an evidence base be available on the NHS? Yes, if the evidence is sufficient to fit local criteria. Otherwise I would say no. Anyway people who can afford it often really don't mind spending money on their health, and sometimes they may get better quicker when they do! But the Health Service really has to stick to funding treatments that are proven to be useful, so that everybody has access to those that are really needed.

However primary care can do more to help such patients. There are two distressing components of these diseases, pain and tiredness.

> Pain is a complex sensory and emotional experience. The way in which we perceive pain is a complicated and dynamic interplay of inhibitory and excitatory neural events involving many parts of the peripheral and central nervous system. The relationship between pain and tissue injury is not straightforward.[75]

This introduction to a guide which aims to help GPs deal with patients' chronic pain is important because it emphasises that pain is not only due to 'tissue injury' – where there is a damaging process going on in your body and pain is an indication to you that you should do something about it – move your hand away from the fire, or see your doctor in case you have cancer. Chronic pain can be due to other things that are extensions of what normally goes on in your body – spasm of muscle, dilation of blood vessels, or over-stretching of your air cells in your lungs, which will stop happening in the normal course of events, or may feed back on itself so that your mental reaction to it may make it worse. It is a perception that only you are experiencing and there is no easy way of measuring it. And if you can't measure it you can't easily treat it effectively.

Pain clinics, and the appreciation of some of the causes of chronic pain, are quite recent developments. For most of my time in general practice, all we usually did was to dish out painkillers, usually depending on the latest drug rep to satisfy those patients who kept coming back. In my early days Solpadeine was a winner, but then this got taken off the list as it contained caffeine and codeine – stimulants and really strong analgesics. Later we used various combinations of paracetamol and codeine and also non-steroidal anti-inflammatory drugs such as ibuprofen. We spent millions on the latest Big Pharma products which were all much more expensive than the ingredients would ever be. For a long time we were strongly discouraged from using opiate analgesics – morphine and its analogues – for anything but cancer pain, but even this taboo was broken when it became acceptable to use opiate drugs for severe arthritis, severe headaches and so on.

This was about the time when more understanding of the nature of pain was developing, and things like pain analogue scales were introduced to try to capture pain severity. You had to ask each patient where on a scale from one to ten, he or she would describe their pain at the moment, with 10 being the worst they have ever experienced. This may have worked in specialist departments when the specialist knew what sort of pain the patient was experiencing, but it didn't in general practice when, though we probably knew what was causing the pain and had tried to cure it many times before, we had no idea what it meant to different patients. We knew that Mrs Bloggs always wanted the latest opiate type medication because nothing else worked, but we also knew that Mrs Smith never took anything other than paracetamol despite her illness generally being considered much more painful than Mrs Bloggs' illness. We really didn't know whether Mrs Bloggs' very real pain was being helped by analgesics or whether we should be doing something else for her. It was all very frustrating.

So the idea of pain management clinics in primary care is an attractive one. The main benefit to the patient is in a better understanding of the mechanisms of pain by the primary care team, involving professionals such as doctors, physiotherapists, specialist nurses, occupational therapists, or psychologists, who can give many different sorts of treatment. Physiotherapists and occupational therapists can help with relaxation, exercises, hot and cold packs and transcutaneous electrical nerve stimulation (TENS), which works by electrical stimulation of the skin to 're-align' the pain messages (it must be used continually for 90 minutes or more to work.) Rarely, counsellors, psychologists or community health nurses are needed to help with CBT or a psychologically based rehabilitation programme, especially if anxiety or depression is a problem. Specialist nurse often coordinate the treatment plan and are invaluable and very knowledgeable about pain. It was necessary for all of us to re-learn our medicine and debunk many myths.

For instance, the amount of pain is NOT proportional to the injury or pathology, even for acute pain in Accident & Emergency departments, or in the simplest of experimental pains, and certainly not in chronic pain where the pain experience becomes altered by many complex modulating processes in the brain and nervous system. Also that Mrs Bloggs is not (usually) exaggerating the pain she feels, and Mrs Smith may be trying hard not to show her pain and is worried that others might disbelieve her. When patients say that strong painkillers, even opiates, do not work they may well be right. There are different sorts of pain which need different sorts of pain relief, for instance neuropathic pain (neuralgia), which is pain due to stimulation of the nerve itself rather than pain just being transmitted through the nerve, does not respond to any opiate and need medications that work on the nerve itself to dampen down the heightened activity in the nerve. Dental pain is one of the worst pains we experience because it may be caused by inflammatory pain due to infection, and no painkiller will ever touch that, as well as neuropathic pain if it affects the nerve.

Getting together many professionals in a team is very helpful as it is then possible to give a 'holistic' (to use a well-worn phrase) approach, which will help to tease out the many different aspects of a patient's chronic pain. Improving their social situation with financial help, or with family worries can help concomitant depression and anxiety and this will help the patient herself to reduce the pain. Advice on developing activities that the patient can do will help to distract her from the pain. We all know that a headache can suddenly disappear when an interesting event or problem enthuses us – for a while at least.

It is clear that the earlier patients at risk are helped the better the outcome is. Once pain has become really chronic it is very difficult to treat. The most important thing is to talk to the patient and help him towards a better understanding of what is making the pain more severe in his particular case, then going through the various strategies to help. Keeping active and maintaining social, work and family activities is important. The focus is on symptom management rather than diagnosis of the cause of pain as in many instances no cause is found or the cause is untreatable.

These clinics can help to bridge the gap between a patient's expectation that all pain can be cured by referral to a specialist – an 'ologist' who will investigate, diagnose and cure with little or no input from the patient, and the reality, which is that in many cases the pain is unlikely to be cured and must be managed, and that the patient has to do a lot of work to ensure a good outcome. The patient will be well on the road to a better life once this is understood. GPs though have to be supported in doing this with both education and financial help, as all this costs money. But it may be money that will be saved by not referring the patient for endless investigations that may keep everyone busy but is unlikely to help the pain.

Sometimes it is necessary to refer to a hospital pain clinic for further investigation and management. Unfortunately, chronic pain is complex and we do not understand the mechanisms for all pains, but we can do our best to try to help the patient live with it.

The onus on GPs is to diagnose any condition that can be treated effectively and quickly. The patient must be convinced that the doctor has done everything possible to exclude some of these treatable diseases, and to continue to trust the doctor if nothing is found. That is a very tricky art, and many of us have failed to do that as the patient gets angry, hostile and disillusioned. The well-known progression from denial, anger, depression, and finally acceptance is as applicable here as it is with a diagnosis of cancer or bereavement. After that all we GPs can do is give general advice and support people as best we can. For families affected by this though it must be a dreadful condition.

Chapter 14
Bowel problems: causes, investigations and treatments: what works?

Irritable bowel syndrome – investigation and referral – probiotics – food allergy – coeliac disease – food intolerance

Irritable bowel syndrome (IBS) is another difficult condition to manage, in a similar way to fibromyalgia and ME. The Wikipedia dictionary definition is 'It is a functional bowel disorder characterized by chronic abdominal pain, discomfort, bloating, and alteration of bowel habits in the absence of any detectable organic cause.'

'Functional' in medical terms means that it is assumed to be due to a malfunction of a part of the body, as distinct from when there is a progressive disease process, which causes anatomical abnormalities such a cancer or obstruction. The difference that the label 'functional' puts on an illness is that it is not likely to have any serious consequences, and therefore some people – including, sadly, some doctors – sometimes use the label to mean 'all in the mind' – quite wrongly of course. It is certainly not 'all in the mind' in the sense that people aren't really suffering but just think they are (!), but such conditions are not as exciting to treat as when there is a serious pathological process going on. IBS is a common condition and affects all ages from 15 upwards, usually starting in young people and continuing with ups and downs until old age. Its importance lies in the fact that it is easy to diagnose but almost impossible to confirm with any objective test, and so people may be left wondering if there isn't something more serious going on. It can also be a great mimicker of other conditions, as symptoms are very general, such as stomach ache, wind, bloating or altered bowel patterns. A cardinal symptom is abdominal pain or discomfort that is either relieved by defaecation or associated with altered bowel frequency or stool form. Some but not all people experience passage of small amounts of mucus.

There are some tests that are usually done to exclude more serious diseases such as coeliac disease, diverticulosis, pelvic infections and sometimes ovarian cancer.

So patients are right to wonder whether there may be something else going on, but with a careful history and a few simple tests it should be diagnosed accurately by a GP and managed within primary care. According to the latest guidelines the blood tests that must be done after a careful history to find out the background are a full blood count (FBC), tests for inflammation in the blood and antibody testing for coeliac disease. Other tests, such as endoscopy and scans and tests for lactose intolerance are **not** necessary to confirm diagnosis in people who meet the IBS diagnostic criteria.

However there are certain 'red flag' i.e. danger indicators which should be investigated straight away. These are

- Rectal bleeding (this would need immediate referral to a gastroenterologist under the 2 week rule – in case it is cancer)
- A change in bowel habit to looser and/or more frequent stools persisting for more than 6 weeks in a person aged over 60 years – this would usually mean referral for further investigation
- Anaemia, which would be diagnosed with a blood test and if positive would require immediate urgent referral
- Abdominal or rectal masses on examination at the first consultation, or
- unintentional and unexplained weight loss over several weeks, which would need emergency referral.

If there is a family history of bowel or ovarian cancer then further investigations should be done with these in mind, and certain other conditions such as coeliac disease or inflammatory bowel disease, should be excluded by testing the blood for various inflammatory markers.

In a person with typical IBS symptoms and negative tests, treatment and self-management can then be started. Lots of medications such as laxatives, anti-spasmodics (medications which relax the gut), and small doses of amitriptyline (see under depression) can be used. People with IBS should be discouraged from eating too much insoluble fibre, for example bran, though for a long time we doctors advised people to do just that, as it was thought it gave the bowel muscle something to 'grip' on. Later trials proved that bran actually can make IBS worse, and soluble fibre such as ispaghula powder or foods high in soluble fibre such as for oats are better. Most people nowadays get expert at managing their condition and are happy with the diagnosis. All the usual treatments – antispasmodics, peppermint-based substances, and amitriptyline – are out of patent and very cheap.

This is an extremely unsatisfactory situation for the Pharmaceutical industry and considerable effort has been made to develop new drugs. Fairly recently, we GPs were suddenly seeing advertisements for IBS saying that there was to be a new treatment very soon. Obviously the drug company was paving the way for a blitz with this new wonder drug as soon as it was licensed. I was interested enough to read the latest research on it and it seemed that the new drug did indeed show promise, but of course was going to be extremely expensive (to reflect the work that had been put in to develop it). Then a bit later I found that it had been refused a licence. The problem wasn't that it didn't work, but it had some rare side effects. Of course the problem with treating IBS is that because it does not have serious consequences, no side effects of any importance can be tolerated, unlike for life-threatening or progressive illnesses.

However, it can still be extremely painful and doesn't go away, so some patients, often those under stress, which is known to exacerbate the symptoms, may ask for a specialist, usually a gastrointestinal, opinion. This may be perfectly justifiable but we have to be very careful about what happens next. Specialists are specialists, and they have their own pathways of investigations for all patients coming to their clinic, so for completeness many tests may be done. If the diagnosis is indeed IBS these tests will be normal, but it is possible to pick up other unrelated conditions, which are unimportant – incidentalomas we call them. An '-oma' is a tumour of some sort (such as a dermatoma on the skin) so this would be an incidental tumour, almost certainly harmless but must be investigated for completeness. This is especially likely to happen if a relatively junior doctor in specialist training sees the patient in clinic. The patient then may make a round of visits to hospital to see other specialists such as Gynaecologists or rectal surgeons. Whatever the outcome it does not help the IBS and can be frustrating for everybody. Doctors in many specialities are used to seeing such patients turn up again and again in their departments, often convinced that doctors are misdiagnosing them. Well, of course in a few cases this may actually be so, and eventually the truth is discovered and there is another medical negligence case, and every one wants to make sure it never happens again. Medical science is not perfect and even if doctors follow all guidelines occasionally things do go wrong. But most patients who remain unconvinced by repeated investigations in secondary care are in fact suffering from incomplete explanation of the symptoms and anxiety, and this needs to be tackled in primary care, not in the hospital setting.

IBS can and should be diagnosed in primary care. The history of colicky abdominal pain, with loose or rabbitty stools, and distension, with no other red flags, should suggest the diagnosis. Sometimes in a thin person you can actually feel the spastic bit of bowel under your fingers and I always tell the patient if I can. After the necessary tests have come back negative, I try to spend some time explaining the cause of the problem. I usually put it like this. People are normally unaware of things going on in their digestive tract as there is no mechanism for this – you don't want to be aware of every detail of the passage of your food down the intestine. The workings are regulated by two opposing systems of nerves (sympathetic and parasympathetic), one of which causes contraction of the smooth muscle of the bowel and the other facilitates relaxation so that normally food is passed smoothly along. But if something disturbs that balance then you can get spasm of the muscle, which does not then relax, and that spasm causes the pain. It can be a short spasm or it can go on for hours but always gets better on its own. The things that cause that are many but the common ones are intolerance of food, infections and stress.

When I was in practice I used to play down the stress bit and concentrate on diet and simple lifestyle changes, but now I think stress is actually is an important precipitant. Anyway, once diagnosed and the patients told the fact that it is a problem about how the digestive tract works rather than anything actually wrong with it, most patients can learn to manage it themselves with lifestyle changes, diet, tablets and better management of stress. A trick some patients find helpful is to consciously trying to relax the lower abdomen muscles and even massaging the tummy can help a lot. But if this is not explained in detail and patients can't believe that this amount of pain can be caused by something so simple then the merry go round can start, increasing stress.

Stress can cause the same flu-like symptoms in IBS as in fibromyalgia and ME, such as headaches, muscle and joint pains and chronic fatigue. These are sometimes put down to an alteration in the immune response, (see below) presumably heightening it because of a hypersensitivity syndrome. But to me these latter symptoms are pathognomonic of extra adrenaline and an overactive stress response as in fibromyalgia. Others disagree and a paper has been published[76] giving data which seems to demonstrate that altered gastrointestinal (GI) microflora can influence immune upregulation (i.e. enabling the immune system to fight infections better) in patients with IBS, suggests that this could potentially play a role in the aetiology of IBS. This paper has not got widespread support, and seems to me to complicate things unnecessarily. IBS is not an infection and the immune system, which is there to fight off severe infections and some cancers, does not seem to be involved. Incidentally 'upregulation' of the immune system in otherwise healthy people seems to me to be a bad idea. Apart from serious diseases which directly cause the immune system to malfunction such as leukaemia and other blood diseases, HIV, and rare genetic diseases where the immune system never develops, the most usual problem with the immune system is when it doesn't recognise what to attack and attacks the body's own cells. These are known as autoimmune diseases and are very unpleasant diseases to have – rheumatoid arthritis, asthma and MS are the most well known. Upregulation of the immune system would seem not to be without risks. People with IBS don't have anything wrong with their immune systems on testing.

Some patients report that their symptoms started following an episode of acute gastritis. A longitudinal study[77] of a town in Canada that experienced a widespread outbreak of *Escherichia coli* gastroenteritis following contamination of the water supply found that, two years later, rates of IBS were three times higher in the affected population than in the unaffected population of the same town. There was also a theory that ordinary bacteria normally confined to the large intestine may expand into the small intestine, prompting uncomfortable bloating and gas after meals, and a change in bowel movements. I would dispute the causation here; as if you alter the motility of the gut (because of the imbalance described above) you would undoubtedly alter the bacterial flora, which is very specific to the conditions in its environment. Anyway, enter stage left, probiotics, whose sales have rocketed over the last few years with massive promotion of their benefits.

The use of 'natural' remedies has an intrinsic appeal to many people. Probiotics have been heavily promoted as 'good bacteria' which are essential for the healthy bowel. Any imbalance must be 'corrected' by taking probiotics in yoghurts and other foods and there are claims that these will help IBS and many other conditions such as infective diarrhoea, antibiotic-associated diarrhoea, and *Clostridium difficile*. However these claims miss a very important point. As with herbal medicines, the studies on probiotics have all been done on specific strains or species of probiotic bacteria and these may have profoundly different immunological and antimicrobial effects, such as altering GI transit, reduce hypersensitivity in the bowel and/or reduce colonic inflammation.

These properties are often (although not always) unique to a specific strain. So certain strains have indeed been shown to ameliorate IBS symptoms in some patients, but not others, so taking a mixture of different strains will may very well cancel each other out and have no effect. On a doctors' website recently, I came across an article which gave the evidence for many different strains of probiotic in various different diseases, but many of these strains are only available in the USA and others are difficult to get hold of. While health food shops will sell lots of perfectly good probiotics they will be a mixture and so there will be no scientific evidence for them working as general 'good bacteria' for IBS or any other condition. You can certainly experiment with different types of product to see if any does help, but it would seem to be a long-drawn-out process. I would have thought that if a certain probiotic strain had been definitely proved to help IBS then it would be heavily marketed and easily available.

Food allergy is a complicated subject, because there are so many different sorts of 'allergy'. An immune reaction happens when a protein in the surrounding environment gets into the body and provokes a defensive reaction by the body. This is what should happen, as some of these substances would be damaging, especially viral proteins, bacteria and poisons. The first time your body comes into contact with any foreign protein there may be no discernable reaction because the cells, which mediate the reaction, have to learn to recognise the protein, and then learn how to react by producing antibodies. Antibodies are a special sort of protein, called globulins, and each is specially designed to fit with an allergen like a lock and key forming an allergen–antibody complex that then causes cell death, so neutralizing the foreign protein. This means that there will be a delay before the body can fight this particular protein. Once the biochemical pattern is recognised by the body, it will make the antibody extremely quickly so that after this delay the body gets very good at overcoming the challenge. The next time a person comes into contact with this substance the response can be immediate, and the types of immune reaction or 'hypersensitivity' are classified according to which cells the body uses to develop these antibodies and how quick they are at doing it.

So an allergy is a by-product of the body's ability to fight off substances that might cause damage, such as infections and poisons. But this process itself can cause harm to the body, and this will include allergies when the foreign protein is not necessarily usually harmful. Most allergies are mediated by mast cells, which are one type of white cell in the blood, and they produce antibodies called immunoglobulin E or IgE for short. These reactions can be very rapid and can be fatal, as the chain of antibody reaction can cause anaphylaxis, a condition where there may be swelling of the lips, (angio-oedema), difficulty in breathing and airway obstruction. Nausea, abdominal pain, vomiting and diarrhoea are also IgE-related symptoms. Peanut allergy is the best known of these, and once the allergy has developed people need to carry an adrenaline injection to use if the allergy starts. Adrenaline and steroid injections are lifesaving.

This is all well known, and many people, especially parents of children who have come out in rashes or severe hay fever, can get very worried about it. Every time a child has a severe reaction there is usually a great deal of publicity, so despite the fact that such severe allergies are extremely rare, parents tend to think the worst will happen to their child.

I was often contacted when on call by panicking parents who thought that their child was going to die, and of course it is often very difficult to sort out on the phone whether it is likely that something serious is going on. The crux of the matter is – has your child any swelling of the lips or mouth? Or do they have any breathing difficulty? Any other symptom is not an emergency. In fact the only advice that is sensible is to take the child to the nearest primary care centre or emergency department as soon as possible, yet in every case that I dealt with by the time the family arrived there it was obvious that the child was fine.

The treatment for anaphylaxis due to a food allergy is intramuscular adrenaline, and this is what GPs and emergency doctors give if they see a case. However since 1991 devices have been developed which allow for self-injection, or injection of adrenaline by any bystander or carer – epi-pens. (In the US adrenaline is called epinephrine, hence the name). These can be prescribed by GPs for children or adults with a proven serious allergy, and over 100,000 people have been receiving them over that time. In the UK they are supposed to be prescribed initially by an NHS paediatrician or allergy specialist who has confirmed that the person does have a serious food allergy. But in my experience many children and young adults are being prescribed them regularly without such assessment. This seems to be as a result of patient or parent pressure; because of course it is a very emotive subject. How can you refuse to prescribe if it might save a life? Yet they are expensive (£60 each) and have a short shelf life so a new one needs to be prescribed when the old one is time expired even though it has not been used. I remember trying to persuade a mother who arrived on my list with a repeat prescription for an epi-pen without any NHS authorisation (she had taken her child to a private non-medical allergist) to see a paediatrician locally for assessment, but she flatly refused and implied that I would risk her child dying to save money. I did refer her, but of course she did not turn up for the appointment, and I knew that if I did not put it on a repeat prescription some one else would. A bit later I saw the child for an unrelated matter, and casually asked whether she had her epi-pen with her. No, she said. She thought it was in school. The prescription seemed to be a comfort blanket for the mother, but not one that was needed often!

So how well do they work? Do they in fact save lives? A paper published in 2011 casts doubt upon this.[78] If they worked then theoretically the death rate from acute anaphylactic reactions should have reduced but in fact it has remained the same. There have apparently been 110 deaths worldwide attributed to acute anaphylaxis due to food allergy (about 5 per year) since the introduction of epi-pens. 67% of those dying had not been given epi-pens because their previous reactions had been so mild, and of those who had been given pens, around half used the pen late or not at all because they were not carrying them at the time of the attack, and the other half had used the pens correctly but still died. This last group is the most worrying. Why should this be? No-one is sure but possibly there may be a problem with the delivery system in that many of the injections will not hit the muscle, but go into the subcutaneous tissue, especially in fat people. This is being investigated further, but it is obvious that just having a prescription for an epi-pen is not on its own going to be enough It may even give a false sense of reassurance. Patients who are prescribed them must be educated to carry them at all times, and this may be difficult as the peak age for deaths from food allergy is not childhood, but in young people between the ages from 18 to 24.

However, most allergies aren't nearly as dramatic as this. IgE-mediated allergies are those such as hay fever, urticaria, itching, vomiting, or wheeze, and these are a nuisance rather than dangerous. Food allergies are usually mediated by IgE, and can cause abdominal pain, vomiting, respiratory symptoms, and rashes. Up to 10% of children can have no reaction to the usual tests for IgE yet have un-doubted problems when they are challenged with the food in question. These non-IgE-mediated symptoms are slower in onset, and can be reflux, loose stools, colic, food refusal or aversion, constipation and faltering growth, so can have a big impact on health generally. Eczema is also non-IgE mediated.

The diagnosis of food allergies can be done in three ways: a skin prick test, or atopy patch tests, or you can have a RAST (radioallergosorbent test) blood test to test for the presence of specific IgE (actually RAST tests have now been super-seded by more accurate fluorescence enzyme-labelled assays). These are now very accurate, giving a scale of the likelihood of an allergy. With any test it is essential only to test for substances which you know you get symptoms from. The com-mon method of sending a blood test off for every substance you can think of re-gardless of symptoms is futile. If the test shows a reaction to strawberries but you can eat strawberries normally without problems then you do not have an allergy.

If however these tests are all negative, indicating that the allergy is not IgE-mediated, and you still suspect a food allergy, then you need to do a food chal-lenge. In its purest form this would be done by the person taking a pill containing the food substance to be tested, and they would have to be watched carefully for any reaction, as theoretically it could cause an immediate and very serious aller-gic reaction such as anaphylaxis. For this reason it should take place in a setting with resuscitation facilities available.

In the eighties, our nurses often used to give a series of a proprietary injection called Migen to desensitise people from the house dust mite, which causes so much hay fever and breathing problems, until a 14 year old girl died in a nearby surgery because of anaphylaxis. Although it was being done in a GPs surgery the adrenaline was not immediately available. Now the rules are very clear – any such challenge or desensitisation has to be done with everything to treat anaphylaxis near to hand. Skin prick tests and patch testing for allergies are often only available in dermatology outpatients and there are sometimes long waiting lists. So blood tests are most commonly used nowadays.

Trials of subjects taking part in allergy tests to determine whether they really have a food allergy or not are usually done using double-blind, placebo-controlled food challenge (DBPCFC), and then there is no doubt what is going on. Usually, the only realistic treatment of an established food allergy is avoidance of the culprit food, and I often used to advise people on exclusion diets (for between 2 to 6 weeks) and then adding in the suspect food to see what happened. For children, as severe food allergies can cause poor growth and development, NICE has issued guidance on what parents and GPs should do, starting with a full examination and history, and this guidance is available to parents so that they can check on what should be asked. In most cases it is then fairly easy to work out what to do, and most can be managed in primary care. In many areas the NHS is not good at helping people with allergies. It is time-consuming and complicated to take a full history and examine the patient, then do the various tests, so unless a GP has an interest, time constraints make it difficult to give a full service.

I remember one man who came in saying that he had an allergy to sugar. So which sugar, I asked, thinking he would say lactose. Lactose intolerance is common as it contains glucose and fructose joined together in one compound, and you need an enzyme called lactose dehydrogenase to split them. Glucose and fructose are the main source of energy for cells (they release energy through a complex pathway called the Krebs cycle, which absolutely fascinated me when I first learned about it at school), and failure to split these two causes lots of problems, mostly due to the accumulation of un-split lactose in the bowel. It is therefore intolerance not an allergy). 'No' he said, 'I am allergic to glucose'. 'That can't be', I said, 'you can't be allergic to glucose. You would be dead if you were – it is such a fundamental source of energy.' 'Yes I am' he said 'I have tried eliminating it many times and I always come back to that – it is definitely sugar. I feel weak and ill and get itching of my mouth.' I am afraid the argument got quite heated, as I really could not believe him. I could not test him for glucose – there is no such test – so I agreed reluctantly to do some other tests – a simple full blood count I think. He left feeling very dissatisfied. Fortunately he did come back the following week after I had had time to look it up – glucose allergy is actually a corn allergy due to impurities in the sugar, and then of course we found that he did indeed have a corn allergy. It just shows how a GP needs to take every problem seriously however daft it appears.

There are certain tests NICE definitely disapproves of.

- Vega test – this combines traditional acupuncture theory and classical homeopathy theory.
- Applied kinesiology – kinesiology practitioners place samples of the potentially allergic foods in the patient's mouth whilst tests for muscle weakness are performed.
- Hair analysis.

All these and many more are covered in detail in Ben Goldacre's book 'Bad Science'. There are indeed many people wanting to make money out of private allergy testing, so be very careful to go only to a reputable set up. The main problem with all food exclusion regimes is that you can be left with a diet which excludes essential nutrients. Certainly with children and anyone with lots of problems, a registered dietician will be a very good person to consult.

Coeliac disease is another condition which causes all the usual non-specific and annoying symptoms we associate with gastro-intestinal upset, diarrhoea, bloating, loss of weight, and also anaemia. The symptoms of the fully blown form include too much fat in the stools which has not been absorbed and this is often very smelly and greasy. It can also cause no symptoms at all. It is not an allergy to wheat, even though wheat causes the disease, as it is a reaction to a product of the enzyme transglutaminase on the gluten protein. This reaction damages the lining of the bowel and causes atrophy of the villi, the small polyp-like formations on the lining that actually absorb the food. Without these, food which has been digested cannot be absorbed. Coeliac disease is therefore classified as an autoimmune disorder, and it is an important and serious condition, which can have links with other autoimmune diseases.

The diagnosis has been revolutionised by the development of an accurate blood tests, the first of which was for anti-tTG antibodies. Before that the problem could only be diagnosed by asking the patient to swallow a very large capsule, which would take a sample from the lining of the bowel, and then pass out in the stool. The capsule then had to be found in the stool and analysed by the laboratory. Many of my patients were very unwilling to do this test, so not many people were properly diagnosed and there must have been a lot of undiagnosed chronic ill health in sufferers. So it is very important to exclude coeliac disease before one even thinks of food allergy or intolerance.

Food intolerance is not an allergy, is not hypersensitivity, not a food poisoning and not coeliac disease. It is an adverse reaction to a food because the body cannot deal with the substances in that food, usually due to lack of specific enzymes. The commonest is lactose intolerance, as described above, due to a shortage of lactase, the enzyme that breaks down lactose into glucose and fructose, and there is a strong hereditary element. Babies can often be affected. Lactose is present in cow's milk; so affected children are prescribed soya milk instead. Gastrointestinal infections can also damage the lining of the bowel in infants and they then can get a temporary lactase deficiency, which is treated by removing dairy products from the diet for a while. Lactase deficiency can be diagnosed using a lactose tolerance test, a hydrogen breath test and a stool acidity test, and all these can be done in general practice if there is doubt. Often though it is easy to diagnose just by excluding dairy products from the diet.

The severity of symptoms varies depending on the amount of enzyme the person makes and how much of the food has been consumed. Some people have adverse reactions to chemical preservatives and additives in food and drinks, such as sulphites, benzoates, salicylates, monosodium glutamate, caffeine, aspartame and tartrazine.

So GPs can find it very difficult sometimes to sort out people with vague abdominal symptoms and general ill health. Add in people who think that children's behaviour problems are due to additives in the diet, and an industry that thrives on unproven remedies, and it is not surprising that some people are dissatisfied with NHS services. What we eat is very important but we have to remember that it all gets broken down to very small molecules and in wealthy societies like ours a varied diet will give you everything you need for good health. If you do have symptoms then your GP is the best one to try to help.

Chapter 15
Psychiatry: when to refer and to whom, whether and what to prescribe, and how to follow up

Depression and antidepressants – CBT – anxiety – somatization – sleeping tablets and drugs for anxiety – OCD,

All GPs have to be expert in psychiatry. Psychiatric conditions probably represent more than 30% of a GPs workload and psychiatric consultations are different from others. They are longer, often more intense, yet often very frustrating. It was rarely possible to feel that anything much had been achieved, because so often the doctor is not sure of what the patient will do as a result of the consultation. Does he believe you? Is there anything you can really offer?

Psychiatrists have always had to be very discriminating in what cases they will see. The burden of mental illness is huge, so they have to make sure they only see those in which they think they can make a difference. If they offer an appointment it may be five or six weeks ahead, yet the patient may be in a desperate state. So the GP, being always available, has to take up the slack. Community psychiatric nurses were an enormous help, but they too had the luxury of being able to say, 'no, my appointments are full. I can't see you till a week next Thursday'. The GP can never do that; at least, we always had a rule that if a patient wanted a same-day appointment they would have one.

I saw a lot of sad people in my time at the surgery. The fact is that some people have awful lives, and one has to have sympathy, and help and support as far as possible. Some people have bad luck thrust upon them, while others make terrible choices. How many of these suffered from clinical depression was another question, and if their life circumstances had been different they may not have suffered from 'depression'. There is a limit however to what healthcare can do to improve a life situation, but medical treatment may be helpful. Depression then becomes a medical condition. There is no doubt that clinical depression runs in families, and will influence how successful people are in their lives.

I had also trained as an anaesthetist and in my early days in practice I was an anaesthetist for Electro-Convulsive Therapy (ECT), of 'One Flew over the Cuckoo's Nest' fame. In the film, ECT, which puts a large shock through the brain using electrodes, was done without anaesthetic, a terrifying and rather barbaric procedure. But in reality it was almost always done under a full general anesthetic. We used to give a short acting drug to put the patient to sleep, and then a muscle relaxant to protect the muscles from the severe contractions that would then occur from the stimulation of the brain. Unfortunately that meant the patient also stopped breathing, and so the technique was to pre-oxygenate the tissues beforehand by pumping the lungs full of oxygen with a hand mask connected to an oxygen supply before the shock was given by the psychiatrist, then once the muscle relaxant had worn off (about 3 minutes) giving them oxygen to breathe as well. That way the patient was completely unaware of the shock.

Although ECT had a very bad reputation even then and was considered almost a punishment, there was absolutely no doubt that it could be life-saving. Some patients suffered terribly from very severe depression in those days before effective anti-depressants and I remember patients coming in almost mute, withdrawn and completely disabled by their illness, yet after three or four treatments of ECT, improved dramatically. The side effects, especially memory loss, were quite severe, but even recently there were some people who would respond to nothing else and would willingly agree to have the treatment rather than suffer such severe depression. People who had both depression and quite severe physical or painful diseases such as Rheumatoid Arthritis would tell me that the physical illness was always much easier to bear then depression. Fortunately medication such as anti-depressants and other therapies such as Cognitive Behaviour Therapy (CBT) have now made ECT unnecessary in the vast majority of cases.

Severe depression, to the extent that patients will commit suicide, is really a dreadful disorder. The worst case I came across was a teacher who had the most awful bouts of depression in which she several times tried to commit suicide. At first she tried to take overdoses, but each time her husband, who was very caring, found her and she was treated as well as possible with just about everything available at that time (this was in the mid eighties). Then in a particularly bad bout of depression and having no other method, she just walked out of the house into the mountains (they lived way out in the country with no neighbours) in her nightclothes in atrocious weather. It was snowing with temperatures way below freezing and her husband was unaware she had gone. When he realised and raised the alarm it took many hours to find her in the mountains, and by that time she was suffering from extreme hypothermia and frostbite. She eventually lost a leg and part of her hands. What awful distress she must have been in to do that. After that her life was even more unbearable and eventually she did manage to kill herself with an overdose. We were sometimes desperate for any treatment that might help.

From my earliest days in practice I prescribed antidepressants. I always held to the notion that established clinical depression is a biochemical disorder of the brain, which can just appear without obvious cause (idiopathic), or can be provoked by stress. My mental picture, admittedly a very simplified view, was of stress, or lack of proper sleep, or worry, burning up your biochemical transmitters. If you worry about something which you can't do anything about, your neural networks will go on firing in the same old grooves, and your thoughts never get anywhere. Therefore eventually you run down your stores of transmitter substances, which enable messages to go through your synapses, and this depletion leads to depression. This was why I believed that antidepressants, which cause the stores of transmitter substances to build up again, would work, and also when cognitive behavioural therapy came in, I was a great supporter, as this is based on stopping you thinking these same old thoughts which never got anywhere. This is in fact current thinking, that depression is rooted in the patient's own thoughts, and it replaced the previous ideas that psychodynamic forces (inner conflict) were the main problem (ideas first put forward by Sigmund Freud).

Whatever the rationale, antidepressants were promoted from very early on in my career. The tricyclic antidepressants, such as amitryptiline, were discovered in the 50s, and were found to work in severe depression. However they were very 'dirty' drugs and had dreadful side effects. This was because of the multiplicity of biochemical actions, such as being anticholinergic, which means that they work against certain transmitter substances in the synapses of nerves controlling the automatic systems of the body such as heart rate, bowel movements and so on. They caused dry mouth, enlarged pupils, and bladder effects, and also severe sedation. You needed to know the drugs very well and tailor them very carefully to each person. I soon stopped using the full recommended dosage of amitryptiline, as it was totally incompatible with leading anything like a normal life outside hospital. Also some people seemed to be extremely sensitive to it – I reckon at least 20% of the population. So I never started with more than 10 mg and though the recommended dose was 70 to 150 mg I don't think I ever prescribed more than 50 mg despite guidelines saying this was not an effective dose.

In hospital it was different of course and severely depressed people did need 150 mg or more, and they did slowly get used to it. But in general practice I found people would stop taking the drugs quite quickly as the cure was worse than the disease. But 10 mg tablet of amitryptiline was good for helping people sleep, was not at all addicting (people stopped it if they thought they could) and was something that people thought might help, while we talked about their problems. This was what really helped of course, even though counselling people was in its infancy then. It was something GPs learnt along the way – to use the doctor as the drug and be interested in the patient and their problems. This was the most interesting part of psychiatric treatment for me, and if nothing else people did get the sense that they were listened to, and we could discuss what other courses of action they could take to lessen the problems they faced. I suppose though the fact that we GPs could prescribe something that might help gave the consultation an added meaning, and in a way could justify the discussion of intimate details of the patient's life.

The original anti-depressants had lots of other uses – Nortriptylline was also very good at treating bladder dysfunction such as bedwetting, though how much of its effect was actually due to helping children sleep better was a moot point. Nowadays, small doses of tricyclics are often used as an adjunct to painkillers in certain types of severe neuralgia and some other sorts of pain, and they work very well. However, very soon more powerful antidepressants, called second-generation antidepressants, became available. There were two main types, SSRIs (serotonin re-uptake inhibitors) and SNRIs (noradrenaline re-uptake inhibitors), which differed according to which neural transmitter substance they affected. Of course we all began to prescribe them, though I was never sure whether they were in fact any better than the tricyclics. It is now thought that they may not work very much better, but they do usually have fewer side effects at equivalent doses and are less dangerous in overdosage. A problem with these new drugs is that patients get all the side effects, which though much milder than with tricyclics in full dosage are nevertheless a nuisance, and the beneficial effects of the new drugs don't kick in for 10 days. This is a long time if you are desperate for relief from dreadful feelings of despair. So I always arranged to see the patient again after 7 days to make sure they were still taking the tablets and to adjust the dose if necessary.

Each new expensive antidepressant would be strongly advertised and promoted by the manufacturer, and the idea was that we should stop prescribing the older drugs, which were out of patent and very cheap, but the claims were often way over the actual research evidence. However it was finally concluded that the newer drugs should be used in preference to the older ones, not because they worked any better, they didn't, but because it became clear that that some effects on the heart which had been known about for years, could be really severe and people could die if they took them in an overdose (which of course depressed people sometimes do). The use of tricyclics in full doses was then stopped.

However there are similar problems when people overdose with some of the newer drugs too, but they occur far less often. As usual as you use new drugs more and more other side effects come to light. It is now known that these drugs that affect serotonin are associated with an increased risk of suicidal thinking and self-harm in people under 30. So you have to be very careful about using them in young people; you need to warn them that these drugs are associated with an increased risk of suicidal thinking and self-harm in a minority of people, and see them within 1 week of first prescribing. NICE guidance is that doctors should monitor the risk of suicidal thinking and self-harm weekly for the first month.

Although I always sympathized with the patients' lobby that tried to stop patients taking psychoactive drugs with such severe effects, mental illness and especially depression are so unpleasant that it is often very necessary to treat with drugs. But it is important to identify those people who really need them. Recently there has been a big emphasis on effective diagnosis of clinical depression to make sure that only patient who would really benefit from medication are prescribed them. GPs should use a validated questionnaire to do this asking such questions as 'During the last month, have you often been bothered by feeling down, depressed or hopeless? and ' During the last month, have you often been bothered by having little interest or pleasure in doing things?' A positive answer to both questions makes clinical depression very likely, a negative one unlikely. The severity of the depression should then be gauged using scoring systems such as Becks Depression Inventory. This contains 21 questions, on symptoms of depressions such as hopelessness and irritability, guilt or feelings of being punished, as well as physical symptoms such as fatigue. PHQ-9 is a similar one.

Nowadays the rule is that antidepressant medication should only be used for severe depression. In this way it should be possible to restrict its use to those who really will benefit. The sort of person who doesn't usually benefit is someone who has what is called a 'reactive' depression (we used to call them 'nervous breakdowns') to stresses such as marriage break up, job problems or a death in the family, and are prescribed antidepressants, but they only take them for a week, and then stop them as soon as they experience side effects. Hopefully with help from their friends, family and talking to health professionals they improve. However for those who really do need antidepressants it often necessary to take them for a long time. Antidepressants don't necessarily treat the cause of the depression or take it away completely. Without any treatment, most depressions will get better after about 8 months so it is recommended that they should be taken for six to twelve months after the patient starts to feel better. However depression can recur so sometimes it is necessary to take them for years, and people shouldn't feel guilty about doing this. There can be a problem here, as one of the symptoms of depression is feeling excessively guilty about things and sometimes taking tablets is one of them. Then it can be difficult to stop patients having recurrent depressions.

Although there have been reviews which question the efficacy of second generation antidepressants, the latest evidence does seem to support it, which is good news. However there is no evidence that one tablet is any better than any other (there are over 20), so the choice of drug now should be based on side-effect profile and cost.

We have often advised patients that exercise helps depression. It is always very difficult to persuade patients who are depressed to exercise – that is the last thing they usually want to do. Nevertheless it was recommended by NICE for people with persistent sub threshold depressive symptoms or mild-moderate depression, but unfortunately a recent study which assigned groups of depressed people to either exercise or normal care, found that there was no effect.[79] It may be that the people in this trial were more severely depressed than the people we see frequently in general practice, and of course exercise is always good for you, but for now we cannot say for sure that exercise actually helps depression. (Though this trial didn't actually prove that exercise didn't help, only that advising them to exercise did not help.) That is a shame though no doubt a bit of a relief to our depressed patients!

Anxiety and depression often go together, and people with depression can be very anxious and vice versa. NICE now recommends psychological therapies such as CBT as first line for both anxiety and depression. All such therapies focus on the patient learning to control his own unhelpful thoughts. The patient needs to works with the therapist to identify the types and effects of his thoughts on symptoms, and feelings, and develops skills to identify, monitor and then counteract problematic thoughts, beliefs and interpretations related to the target symptoms. The aim is to learn a repertoire of coping skills appropriate to the thoughts, beliefs, and behaviours that appear to be contributing to the problems the patient has.

In its simplest form, the patient uses written or electronic self-help materials, for example a book or workbook, provided by the practice (individual non-facilitated self-help). Sometimes a therapist can be asked to contact the patient by a short telephone call of no more than 5 minutes, to support and help. These low-intensity psychological interventions appear not to do any harm and may work for some people (it certainly worked for people in prisons in one study).[80] The next stage up for people with more severe symptoms is guided self-help, which also involves a trained practitioner whom they see or speak to on the telephone for 20–30 minutes every week or fortnight for five to seven sessions. There are also supportive written electronic self-help materials. Group therapy can also help usually with trained practitioners (ratio of one therapist to 12 participants). Despite these recommendations from NICE, the availability of CBT in any form is very patchy, and there may be long waiting times. There is a big push to increase the funding for all sorts of psychological therapies.

Excessive anxiety is more common than depression and is a big problem in general practice. We all think we know what anxiety is. For instance, suddenly you realise something is not right with your health (or any other worry come to that). You may develop a short-term common condition you have had before – a sprain, a headache, a cough – and you know what you need to do about it. You know that most things get better by themselves and you don't worry about it. But if it gets worse or lasts a long time, the effect of the daily reminder – pain, discomfort, or whatever – can be distressing in itself and makes you think that you need to do something more active to stop it. Pain or discomfort will inevitably increase anxiety in most people – you don't have to be an anxious person for this to happen. The problem just needs to be persistent and continually interrupting your thoughts, even if it doesn't affect your lifestyle. Usually anxiety subsides on its own but in some people it gets out of control and messes up their lives. Of course anxiety is sometimes very justified but when the situation is resolved for good or ill, the anxiety then subsides.

People who have a problem with anxiety often show what are called 'somatic' symptoms – that is, their anxiety shows itself not only in feeling anxious but in pain and discomfort in many parts of the body – head, back stomach and so on. These symptoms can be very distressing and of course from the doctor's point of view it is not necessarily at all clear that anxiety is at the root of the problem. It is very rare for people to tell a friend or doctor that they 'have anxiety'. In almost all cases they will say what they are anxious about, and then it is the friend or doctor's job to work out whether anxiety plays a role in the patient's problem. It is often very difficult for the advisor to do that. You may have to ask yourself: would I worry about this particular problem or not? It is difficult to be objective without knowing the patient's background, life style, and attitudes.

All sorts of people can 'somatise' in this way. People whose lives are miserable and especially people without any power over their own lives – women with a dominating husband for instance – are especially prone to this. Then, the GP's job is firstly to realise that this is happening, so that she can see the context and not assume every symptom is life threatening, and then to listen and sympathise, suggesting simple practical ways that might help. It sounds easy, but this is probably the most difficult thing a doctor has to do. She has to recognise the serious symptoms that really need immediate further action and differentiate them from those symptoms that are likely to be somatic manifestations of anxiety. There is a huge overlap of course, and if a GP errs on the side of caution (as is often necessary) and takes action, such as invasive further investigation or referral, and the result is negative, the patient is not any better off and may be made even more anxious after a round of hospital attendances and negative investigations. And when she misses a 'red flag' symptom or the patient turns out to have a serious disease then that is a disaster. This situation, faced daily by all GPs, causes anxiety in the most phlegmatic of GPs and I often used to wake up in the night in a panic, thinking 'Have I missed a possibility there really is a serious disease here?' and torment myself till morning. Then in the cold light of day I would reappraise the situation and work out whether I really ought to contact the patient for further tests. The panic never survived the resulting review and if I missed anything it was usually something I had not been concerned about at the time. That is the only reassuring thing about intense anxiety – what you worry about hardly ever happens and what nasty thing happens is usually something completely unexpected. My patients never appreciated this of course.

People don't have to be downtrodden and powerless though to be anxious. People with high-powered jobs, people with plenty of money, almost everyone at times can suffer from excessive anxiety and it can sometimes be very difficult to manage.

A farm worker came to me once complaining about a pain and pins and needles in his arm, so I examined him to see whether there was an obvious cause. I couldn't find anything so reassured him. In this case he came back repeatedly for pain and numbness in his arm up to the elbow, and I eventually realised that he was very worried because he had been putting his arm into sheep dip while on the farm, and he thought that sheep dip may have damaged his arm in some way. Sometimes the patient may worry about things such as the effect the problem might have or might come to have on one's job, (back pain in someone who works as a labourer is a common problem). I repeated the tests which were negative again, but actually I couldn't reassure him completely as sheep dip contains extremely toxic substance. However the distribution of numbness did not correlate with any dermatome so it was unlikely to be caused by anything affecting the nerves to the arm. (Because of the way nerves develop in the body, the areas they serve – dermatomes – are not necessarily near to each other in the skin and it's easy to find out whether a peripheral nerve is damaged by working out whether the symptoms the patient is complaining about do fit the developmental pattern.) I referred him to a neurologist even though there were no actual neurological signs at all, but there was a very long waiting list at the time and before he was seen the symptoms disappeared. He later developed other symptoms that were much more anxiety related, and I discovered that he was also having problems with his long-term girlfriend. I do wonder though what caused his symptoms in his arm. He certainly wasn't making it up. Did the sheep dip cause an irritation in the skin (rather than in the nerve) and his brain misinterpreted the sensation as pain? We will never know but it is likely that his anxiety was fed also by his problems with his love life.

I was of the generation of doctors that went through the Valium debacle. When I first qualified the only medication that worked for anxiety was phenobarbitone, a long acting barbiturate that caused extreme sedation and was also addictive. (It was also used as an anaesthetic for a while). It was originally combined with Dexedrine, an amphetamine, in a tablet called purple hearts, and several of my elderly patients were on these. They were called uppers and downers, and they were originally prescribed but then got on to the black market. The dangers of these tablets were obvious and people died after taking accidental overdoses. We were all told how dangerous barbiturates were and exhorted to get patients off them as soon as possible. This proved very difficult though as people had become addicted to them.

When Valium was first put on the market it was hailed as the perfect solution for anxiety and was said to be totally safe. As is well known, Valium was prescribed with gay abandon, not only in general practice but also by consultants who weren't psychiatrists at all. It took years before the real effects of Valium showed up. It was dangerous, caused respiratory depression and so could kill quickly on overdosage, and was a highly addictive drug. It helped anxiety all right, by blocking the receptors in the brain that fed the anxiety but it also created many, more receptors so that more and more Valium was needed to get the same effect. Valium was one of a class of drugs called benzodiazepines and many drug companies rushed to get on the bandwagon with similar drugs – Librium, Xanax and so on – each with their own little niche (for duration of action, side-effect profiles etc.) which were jealously guarded and marketed by their manufacturers. So we were in the same position again of having made people into addicts by prescribing innovative new drugs and again had to try to get patients off these drugs. They found it just as difficult as the previous generation of patients who took barbiturates. One patient told me that stopping Valium was by far the most difficult thing she had ever done in her life, and there were quite a few patients who were still taking it when I retired 30 years later.

Temazepam was another benzodiazepine, which was promoted for insomnia rather than to treat anxiety during the day, until it was found that not only was it equally addictive but also caused lots of problems of cognition the following day, so that driving and other mental tasks were affected. It also caused falls, due to balance problems and lack of concentration, which was desperately bad for the elderly people who were the main consumers. A fall easily led to fractures and hospitalisations which would not otherwise have happened, and was an immediate cause of deterioration and death. You would think by this time drug companies would be a bit more circumspect about developing new drugs for anxiety and sleeplessness. But people never learn.

The next generation of anxiolytics (as they were called) were the z drugs, Zopiclone etc., used as sleeping tablets and these went through exactly the same trajectory, promoted as wonder drugs: short acting, did not give you a hangover, were perfectly safe in overdosage, until when their usage grew it was found that none of these claims were true. Now GPs are given targets to get people off the z drugs. It is very difficult though. Most people hate not sleeping. They get panicky because they can't sleep and this alerts them even more. Elderly people are very much at risk, especially when they aren't very active during the day. I have had many, many consultations when people have begged me to prescribe them, and I always felt a bit of a heel in denying them a good night's sleep. Short-term gains stoking up long-term problems is what hypnotics actually do, and now the emphasis is on finding other ways of helping people who have trouble sleeping.

Actually a friend who was also a patient told me about an excellent way to help when you wake in the middle of the night and fail to get back to sleep. You get a radio, fit an earphone (well you have to if you are married!) and listen to Radio 4, a podcast, or anything. It seems to be the monotony of the human voice that does the trick but you will have to experiment to find out exactly whose voice is best! Remember reading stories for children at bed-time? I have absolutely no evidence that it works in many people, but at the very least it enables your mind to get off those useless tracks, usually downbeat ones, that we all excel at in the middle of the night. For those with MP3 players there is also a nice little app which will turn itself off after a pre-determined limit, usually 15 mins!

A relatively new term for anxiety that is all-encompassing is generalized anxiety disorder (GAD). About 5% of a GP's populations will have it so GPs will see a lot of it. It usually starts in early adulthood – mean age about 21, but some had it since childhood. It tends to fluctuate and in many cases does improve on its own with time. However it represents a big workload for GPs as many patients are frequent attenders and many also get referred to hospital (most often to gastroenterologists) much more often than people who do not suffer from anxiety. So it has a large economic cost. A few patients with severe symptoms come back time and time again, and are never reassured and it is important to make the diagnosis of anxiety as early as possible. Often in truth patients are likely to have had this condition for some time prior to diagnosis, often years.

The important thing is for the patient to recognise that this is the problem. GPs have always spent time exploring the diagnosis with the patient, the effect it has on their life and the different treatment options available. This simple intervention in itself can be helpful, and also such things like reducing caffeine intake, and offering basic relaxation techniques. If the symptoms continue, as in depression, psychological therapies are recommended as first line treatments as it is recognised that drugs have a very limited role in anxiety.

Just for completeness, I should include psychoanalysis, the original 'talking therapy'. It never caught on in the UK though it is still popular with some groups of people. Freud originated his theories of the id, ego and suppressed memories, and called them Psychodynamics, the dynamic relations between conscious and unconscious motivation. This was said to be important in understanding sexual abuse and other symptoms that have their origin in early childhood, but Freud himself may have misunderstood what his patients were telling him (some think that many of his patients were ladies who actually had been abused by their fathers or other members of the family). It is still popular in the USA as a treatment, but is anything but a quick fix. Some people in the USA are 'in therapy' for years with little to show for it at the end. It certainly assured people of plenty of attention.

Obsessive–compulsive disorder was probably the most difficult to deal with. Patients with this were young, as it often starts in childhood, and a GP may follow a patient for years through the ups and downs of a chronic distressing illness. I am aware that some patients with this condition never come to see a doctor, as they may not trust a doctor to understand, and think that they can deal with the problem themselves. But GPs are often the only professionals that patients will turn to, precisely because there is no stigma in going to a GP, unlike psychiatric clinics.

I looked after many people with OCD, often for years. One person was particularly memorable. I first met her when she was home from college many years ago. She was panicking because in her gap year, she had had unprotected sex in Thailand and was certain she had HIV. It took a while to calm her down and to arrange the necessary testing, but it wasn't an unusual sort of problem as at that time, HIV was untreatable and lots of young people did things they regretted while on their gap years, away from parents for the first time. So when the test came back negative (and she had been back a while) I thought the problem would be solved. However she wouldn't be reassured and came back time after time with symptoms that she thought might be due to AIDS. An additional factor was that she was studying Pharmacy and was interested in medicine, and had obviously read up a lot about HIV and AIDS.

I tried to take her symptoms seriously but then realised that her anxiety levels were way out of control. So I set aside a double appointment for her and went into her background. It appeared she was always an anxious child, and also a high achiever who set her very high standards. She had also had a problem with obsessive thoughts and compulsive actions, which started when she was 13, and had a particular problem with cracks on pavements so that she often had to re-trace her steps ten or more times when walking outside. Her mother knew about all this and had arranged appointments with child psychiatrists many times, but she had always refused to go. As was always the case the symptoms waxed and waned depending on her stress levels and sometimes the time of the month. I felt she needed expert psychiatric treatment and of course I wanted to refer her myself, but again she refused. She said it would cause problems with her course and she was adamant that I could not tell anyone, but promised to go to the college counselor when she was back, to get some support (although she said she wouldn't tell her very much).

So that started many years of her coming home in the holidays and getting me to do more and more tests to 'prove' she did not have AIDS. Eventually I told her that I would continue to see her but I could not organise any more tests, and she did accept that. However I found myself colluding in her fears to some extent because I was always having to examine her – usually she insisted on an abdominal examination to prove that her liver and spleen weren't enlarged, and to examine her skin in minute detail for putative rashes. I gave her medication, anafranil, an antidepressant that was a standard treatment at the time and this took the edge of some of her symptoms. But then in her last year of college she took an overdose and ended up in hospital where she had to see a psychiatrist, but again refused to cooperate, so I had to liaise with him and his secretary to tell him of the treatment I had given. She then got some help at a clinic near the college, but her fears were substantiated when the placement in a pharmacy that had been lined up immediately after graduation was withdrawn. She then blamed me and I didn't see her for a while.

I heard that she did graduate and after a while got a job in a pharmacy elsewhere in the country, but it didn't last long and she came home to be near her parents. That was a terrible time for her as she was really quite ill, but fortunately did go to see a psychiatrist now and then. Her old habits of coming to see me regularly were resumed and she consulted about twice a week at some times. During that time we talked through her problems at length, sometimes rationally but sometimes not, and sometimes she got very angry with me. The psychiatrist she was under gave advice on medication but she never took it for long, although I knew at times she was drinking alcohol to reduce her symptoms. She then met a young man, a very nice lad who was extremely understanding, and for a while things improved a lot and she got a part-time job. I saw her from time to time and felt that she was making good progress. Then I saw her because she was pregnant, and she had an uneventful pregnancy and had a lovely little boy. Sadly some months later her OCD, probably triggered postnatally, got really bad and she was admitted to a psychiatric hospital. Her mum took on the baby and it was months before she was well enough to go back to family life. After discharge from hospital an excellent community psychiatric nurse in whom she had complete trust treated her with cognitive behaviour therapy, and I only saw her for the usual GP consultations, which was much better for everyone.

OCD is a terrible affliction. Though I often tried to help her control the thoughts, which would pop into her head with no reason, and to help her to overcome the anxiety without repetitive counting or behaviours, I could see that she really couldn't control them. They came from nowhere and would completely incapacitate her. It seemed to me that it had to be a biochemical problem triggering it – I couldn't see how anything she had done in the past could have caused this. In retrospect while I felt it was absolutely necessary for me to see her so often, I really should have insisted on proper psychiatric help as a condition of her seeing me. But general practice is like that – there are very few boundaries, very few patients you really should not see because you could do more harm than good, and young doctors can be drawn into this sort of situation very easily. There is always a shortage of good trained psychiatric staff and it is such a shame. I would like to think that some method of preventing it in young people could be found. It does seem clear that once patterns of anxiety have become entrenched it is very difficult to see how they can be altered permanently. However the disease does seem to abate somewhat as people gets older.

This is an example of a serious psychiatric disorder, which is quite clear-cut in most cases. But some psychiatrists have become more and more dissatisfied with the diagnostic labelling that goes on at International Conferences, which seem to expand definitions of psychiatric illness and bring more and more people into the net, with all the difficulties and stigma that can go with it.

One British psychiatrist, child psychiatrist Sami Timimi, has founded a network for psychiatrists called the Critical Psychiatry Network,[81] which is calling for the abolition of formal psychiatric diagnostic systems because he says they have failed to advance our understanding or treatment of mental disorder. He says that unlike in the rest of medicine, psychiatric diagnoses have failed to connect their diagnoses with any causes. There are no physical tests that can provide evidence for a diagnosis. Diagnoses in psychiatry are descriptions of sets of behaviours that often go together. By itself a psychiatric diagnosis cannot tell you about the cause, meaning or best treatment. He says that improvements in a patient's condition is more often due to a change in the patient's social circumstances, and in treatment the best outcome comes from developing a good relationship with the clinician. Matching the classification of disease to a specific drug has minimal effect. So this petition is trying to act against the authors of psychiatric classifications of diseases such as the ICD-9 codes (the International Classification of Diseases, 9th Revision, an American classification also used in hospitals in the UK), with a call for 'No more Diagnostic Labels', especially for young people, whose lives can be altered forever by such a label, with lowering of their expectations and increasing their dependence.

When you look at the history of drug usage in psychiatry you can see that there are definite limits to what pharmaceutical treatment has managed to achieve in psychiatry and it is right that people should focus on other ways of managing the symptoms. So this petition is a welcome wake-up call for all clinicians to focus on supporting people in their lives and improving their social circumstances rather than medicating them. That is what GPs have always wanted to do, I suppose.

A seemingly more 'natural' way of treating depression is with so-called herbal medicine, and I have given details on some of the most commonly used in the Appendix.

Part 5

Medicines

Chapter 16
The pharmaceutical industry: effective research and patient care versus profit

Regulation of breakthrough treatments – GPs as targets – tricks and subterfuges used by Big Pharma – drug patents – conflicts of interest

It is very easy to knock Big Pharma, and I certainly do my share. But first I would like to pay tribute to some of the achievements of researchers and scientists in both academic institutions and pharmaceutical companies, which have transformed the lives of so many during my working life.

There were at least three big killers at the time that I qualified in the early seventies. Treatment of infections was being improved, so it was rare for people in their 40s and 50s to die from pneumonia as they had done previously. But heart attacks very commonly killed men in their prime, and breast cancer was a death sentence for women in nearly every case within two years. There was also something that sometimes killed and always produced a lot of misery and hospital admissions in the early 70s – peptic ulcer disease. When I qualified I first worked in the surgical department of a big teaching hospital in London, and there, after every 'take' – when all the emergency admissions were allocated to our firm – the wards would have a few people having been admitted with gastro-intestinal bleeding, nearly always from peptic ulcer disease. These patients – usually men – would be admitted almost exsanguinated when an ulcer in their stomach or duodenum suddenly bled. They would need to have massive blood transfusions to stabilize them and then they would have an endoscopy to define the source of the problem – where the ulcer was and how big it was. They were then sent home and treated with antacids such as Magnesium trisilicate and Rennies, and advised on a diet which excluded lots of nice things to eat – fatty foods, spiced foods, alcohol and so on. Patients were usually pretty frightened by this time – losing so much blood is a nasty experience, so they adhered to the dietary restrictions. But ulcers still recurred and so eventually many of these patients were allocated to have a vagotomy and pyloroplasty, (an operation to cut the nerves to the stomach to prevent the production of the acid) or sometimes even a partial gastrectomy (removal of a large part of the stomach) – both operations with nasty side effects.

The problem was that the acid in the stomach (the normal acid level, pH, is 2.1, which is really quite strong acidity: it is necessary to have it like this in order to digest food) in these people was eating in to the lining of the stomach, and it was a long-term condition. I felt sorry for some of these people with very restricted diets and yet still having regular and rather nasty hospital admissions. There was one man in particular who had recently married again, his first wife having died of cancer, and he came in with a particularly nasty bleed and died post operatively. He left four children aged between 4 and 12 (families were bigger in those days) and two children belonging to his second wife. It was really dreadful having to break the news to the family, and I felt very inadequate, having only been qualified six months. However those that survived the bleeds and the subsequent operations had a miserable time sometimes. The vagotomy and pyloroplasty caused something called a dumping syndrome, where after eating the food just eaten passed into the duodenum too quickly and stimulated the production of insulin (the hormone lacking in diabetics) which is normally timed to coincide with the moment the food arrives, but because the food had moved through too quickly there was now no food to process and people got symptoms of low blood sugar from insulin overdose – feeling faint, sweaty and very ill, about an hour after eating. Also later on it was found that there was a much higher incidence of cancer of the stomach in people who had had this operation. So altogether it was a very unpleasant condition. The causes were thought to be firstly stress (the ambitious stressed business man working all hours was supposed to be the prime candidate), but it was also known that smoking and drinking too much alcohol were factors in its causation.

Then sometime in the early seventies, when researchers were beginning to understand exactly how acid synthesis in the stomach was regulated in the body, a new class of compounds was discovered – H2 antagonists (H2 receptors in the stomach were the mechanism by which acid secretion was produced). The first of these, cimetidine, was developed by Smith Klein and French team using a rational drug-design structure starting from the structure of histamine – the only design lead, since nothing was known of the then hypothetical H2-receptor. Sir James Black got the Nobel Prize for this and it revolutionized the treatment of peptic ulcer disease. I was sceptical at first, but soon I was prescribing tons of the stuff. It really worked and soon many people with this problem were able to live a more normal life. Then a bit later, came an even bigger breakthrough. In 1982–83 an Australian researcher, Prof. Barry J. Marshall, came up with the idea that the cause of the problem was neither stress nor alcohol, but a bacterial infection with a hitherto unknown bacterium called *Helicobacter pylori*. However despite publishing many papers he was getting nowhere – most people thought it was a stupid idea and no one believed him. It was thought that no bacterium could survive in the very acid environment of the stomach. So he decided to test the theory once and for all – on himself, by drinking a concoction full of helicobacter bugs. He proved his point and suffered symptoms exactly like peptic ulcer disease, while his co-worker, Dr J. Robin Warren who also did this was very ill indeed.

Helicobacter pylori is a corkscrew-shaped Gram-negative bacterium which is found to be present in the stomach lining of around 3 billion people around the world (i.e. nearly half the world's population) and is the most common bacterial infection in humans. Many of those carrying the bacterium have few or no symptoms and are apparently well, but all without exception have inflammation of the stomach lining, a condition that is called 'gastritis'. Gastritis is the underlying condition that eventually causes ulcers and other digestive complaints. If a person has had a Pylori infection constantly for 20-30 years, it can lead to cancer of the stomach. This is the reason that the World Health Organisations (WHO) International Agency for Research into Cancer (IARC) has classified Pylori as a 'Class I Carcinogen' i.e. in the same category as cigarette smoking is to cancer of the lung and respiratory tract.

This was therefore a momentous discovery and led to them (Prof. Barry J. Marshall and Dr J. Robin Warren) being awarded the 2005 Nobel Prize for Medicine & Physiology. So nowadays people with gastritis or ulcers are tested for *Helicobacter* and if positive are treated with antibiotics and H2 antagonists (or the newer proton pump inhibitors such as omeprazole) together, thus eliminating the bacteria and curing the patient. So no longer do patients have to suffer and have unpleasant surgical operations, and medical treatments are extremely effective.

Breast cancer was another killer. Women in their 40s and 50s would come in immediately (or sometimes not so early as they were all terrified) with their breast lumps and get often mutilating surgical operations to remove their breasts but would still die of metastases within two years. Now with drugs like Tamoxifen, developed in Britain, women can live for years even after their cancer has spread to other parts of the body. My cousin's wife in South Africa survived over 12 years after the cancer had already spread – long enough to see her girls grow up and go to college.

Herceptin was one of the drugs that caused great controversy when it was first licensed, as NICE would not recommend its use, and campaigns in the popular press, highlighting the cases of women who had been refused the medication, led NICE to reassess its use much earlier. Since then successive government have had to bow to the campaigns run by the popular press on several more treatments for end-stage cancer, some of them with not a lot of merit at all. NICE had been charged with calculating the value of new drugs as to the number of 'quality-adjusted life years' (QALYs), that would be added. This is an indication of the number of years longer that you would live as a result of the intervention, reducing it if the added years were not of good quality (for example if you lived longer but were in more pain), and 30 years was decided upon initially.

However, as so many of these very expensive drugs were coming through over this limit the government raised it to 40, so that it would now include drugs which gave people a maximum of an extra two or three months to live. This was a purely political decision and many medics and others cannot see the benefit to the NHS as a whole for so much to be spent on drugs that add such a short time to life, often not with a high quality of life either. Which brings us to some of the problems with having a very powerful and profitable drug industry, which knows how to get the media on its side.

Despite the undoubted benefit we have all gained from the pharmaceutical industry, there have been many problems of regulation over the years and it is well known that the industry has sometimes been very unethical in its relentless drive to maximize profits for its shareholders.

GPs are at the sharp edge, the main target of a great deal of advertising by the drug firms, because in the UK firms are not allowed to advertise directly to the public. This contrasts with America where most health advertising is direct to patients and I am sure everyone who visits the USA is amazed at the volume and persistence of advertising of medicines. It changes the dynamic completely, and doctors there daily have to deal with patients wanting the latest very expensive treatments. The only way this can be managed in the USA is with regulation from the Health Maintenance organisations and insurance companies, so the more you agree to pay for your insurance, the more drugs you can get. Even then though there is a co-payment – the patients have to pay for part of the cost themselves. I don't think people in the UK realise how incredible it is that for most people most of the time prescriptions are free, and how important it is that medicines should be cost-effective. I personally think that advertising medicines to the general public is totally wrong in any society that aspires to equality and effectiveness in health care. Only if the target audience – the patients – is fully informed of unbiased evidence would they be able to make an informed choice and this is rarely the case. The more people know about the evidence base behind their medications the better but until that happy day comes advertising direct to the patient causes endless problems in ensuring equal access to everyone on basis of need not wealth.

In the sixties and seventies we GPs were shamelessly courted, wined and dined by the drug reps, and 'drug dinners' in expensive restaurants were almost a standard way of getting a nice night out – even with your non-medical spouse. There was very little attempt to be 'scientific' about it; the main qualification for a 'rep' seemed to be (in our area) that you were an ex-rugby player! It was all very matey and it was accepted that this was how you got to know of new drugs. Gradually these perks were phased out and a strict code of practice such as no non-medical spouses, and a limit on hospitality and gifts, was introduced, together with a ban on promoting brands within scientific lectures. The 'reps' all became graduates in biomedical specialties and very knowledgeable about the science behind it all. But even so the advertising was relentless. The costs of doctors' prescription writing spiralled very quickly after the inception of the health service and so government inspectors from the late 80s on monitored prescriptions by GPs. Doctors were employed by the Department of Health to visit GPs who had high prescribing rates, though they had very few powers to make GPs change.

Then came the 'black list' in 1978 where whole categories of drugs were removed from the prescribable list (such as cold and cough remedies of dubious effectiveness). There was a huge fuss from patients' groups at the time as it removed many very popular drugs such as caffeine-containing drugs, and for us GPs it was a very difficult time with many patients coming back again and again to try to get 'free' equivalents, which weren't available. After that, again primarily to save money, came targets such as for the proportion of generic drugs prescribed. Generics are drugs that are now off-patent and therefore can be made much more cheaply than the brand named drugs from the big companies, so make for more effective prescribing. This is an area that all countries are now looking at very carefully. In the USA drug costs are way out of control because of the strength of the pharmaceutical lobbying, and the cost is getting unaffordable. Most European countries are also now looking at increasing the amount of generic prescribing. Most health authorities in the UK now employ many highly qualified pharmacy graduates as prescribing advisors to monitor prescribing by GPs, but it is a constant battle to keep the costs down. Drug companies are past masters at getting round regulations to make sure that their more expensive product continues to be prescribed.

One of the tricks to ensure profits are maximised is to develop a drug with a very minor modification to a drug that is about to go off patent, and get it licensed. The company then vigorously promotes this new drug, which may have very few, if any, better properties than the one about to go off patent, to GPs and in the popular press (using articles about it rather than direct advertising as that is not allowed) and try to get GPs to switch patients over to it. Then shortly before the patent is about to expire they will stop manufacturing the original drug, so that for a while (before generic manufacturers can get in on the act), GPs have no choice but to prescribe the expensive new drug. Once the patent expires obviously GPs can switch patients to the new, cheaper generic but by this time patients may be established on the new drug and may be reluctant to change. Indeed the drug companies rely on this. Hard-pressed GPs may also be reluctant to bring the patient in specifically to make the change-over and so the new drug will be prescribed for some time despite being much more expensive and no better than easily obtained generics.

Of course if a new drug is a great advance it may save hospital readmissions and there may be other savings, but in many cases this is not so. Of course nothing should stop patients being prescribed drugs that have the potential to revolutionise people's lives and save lives, and of course pharmaceutical companies need to make a profit. But only a small proportion of the new drugs licenced each year are in this category, and a great problem is the proliferation of 'me too' drugs. Once a new drug is licensed and is prescribed extensively because of its good effects, all other firms will try to develop similar drugs by altering a molecule there or a difference in formulation there. Some of these turn out to be improvements, but many aren't; yet they would be extensively advertised to us GPs as being much better. The evidence is often sadly lacking, misrepresented or even falsified, and important side effects may be minimized or denied, but it is very difficult for a GP make an informed judgment. Many people think this is a problem of licensing and regulation and that new drugs should only be allowed on a formulary when they have definite proven benefits over existing drugs, but at the moment this is not the case. There is little time for GPs to look up the small print even if the information is available.

Painkillers and anti-inflammatory drugs have been the favourites for 'me too' drugs. These represent huge profits because so many people take them. Yet at bottom very few of the new drugs were much better than the originals. When I first started in practice I remember being astounded that a man who came in with such severe neck pain so that he could hardly turn his neck at all, reported being better in six hours after taking phenylbutazone, the only anti inflammatory drug available at that time. I had thought he would need physiotherapy at least. Phenylbutazone was indeed extremely effective but unfortunately a small minority of patients developed severe blood problems with it, sometimes life threatening, so it was withdrawn. Ibuprofen, which was the next drug on the market, did not have this drawback and has become the standard anti-inflammatory, and despite many claims by manufacturers of very expensive newer drugs such as COX2 inhibitors (which inhibit an enzyme called COX2 thus reducing inflammation), is still one of the best. However for a long time I, in company with so many other GPs, would prescribe the latest non steroidal anti inflammatory drug thinking that it would definitely be an improvement. It rarely was. Ibuprofen is now cheap and can be bought over the counter.

There has been a lot of publicity about the new drug Lucentis for age-related macular degeneration (AMD – for details on this see the section on Eyes), and that there is a much cheaper alternative (Avastin), which nevertheless is not used. The story behind that is very interesting. Avastin was developed by

Genentech, an American company that specialises in molecular research, in 2004. It is an anticancer drug licensed to treat bowel cancer and has been very successful drug for the company. It is a monoclonal antibody which works against vascular endothelial growth factor (VEGF) and some ophthalmologists reasoned that scientifically, as increased blood vessel growth was responsible for the damage done in macular degeneration, it might offer hope to those going blind because of AMD. As I understand it, some of them tried it experimentally, off-licence, injecting it into the eyes of patients suffering from early AMD. It was remarkably successful, and one would have thought that the company would have been delighted. However, the company saw dollar signs in this development and decided that they would not apply for a licence to use Avastin to treat AMD because the price of Avastin was by now not all that high, and profits could be made much bigger by developing a new drug. So they developed another very similar drug, which they said would be more suitable because the molecule was smaller, and therefore could enter the eye tissues more easily. That drug is Lucentis. So far so good. However the price tag on Lucentis was at that time (2006) put at $2227 per injection, while Avastin cost $50 per injection. This is an incredibly high difference in price, especially as the amount of work the company had to do to develop the drug was not very much. The company then had to prove that Lucentis was better than Avastin at treating AMD in controlled trials, which they did with a randomised controlled trial. Drug regulators in the US and in the UK therefore felt they had to approve Lucentis despite its additional costs.

It was soon clear however that the costs were threatening to siphon off public funds, and some ophthalmologists were very unhappy. As patients in the USA often have to pay at least part of the costs themselves, some ophthalmologists were recommending to patients that they use Avastin instead. There were many arguments in the scientific world about which was the better drug and many clinicians decided that Avastin was actually better because it was longer-acting and therefore fewer injections were needed. This was, paradoxically, because it was a bigger molecule. So Avastin was continuing to be used, off-licence, but of course the company that now markets the drug (Novartis in the UK) was not willing to licence Avastin for this purpose because that would be the end of all those marvelous profits from Lucentis. The company claimed to be concerned about the safety of Avastin, but ophthalmologists reasoned that as the dose of Avastin used in the eye is 1/300th of the dose used in cancer (where it had been safely used for years) safety concerns were not likely to be large.

If Avastin could be used instead of Lucentis this would save billions off the health care budgets of countries all over the world. In the US in 2006, it was said that the total cost of Lucentis was $9 billion, whereas the *total* Medicare Allowed Charges for *all* of ophthalmology was $4.77 billion.[82] This meant that savings undoubtedly needed to be made elsewhere, and other treatments might not be available. In the UK, NICE has approved Lucentis and so here too there is a lot of money having to be spent when there is a good alternative drug. One problem is that Novartis cannot be forced to apply for a licence for Avastin, and so Avastin cannot be considered in the same way as a licenced drug.

In May 2010 a randomised controlled trial was started, comparing the two drugs directly against each other. The two-year results therefore came through in May 2012, and they proved conclusively that both drugs were highly effective in treating AMD.[83] 'The dramatic and lasting improvement in vision with these two drugs is extraordinary. At two years, two-thirds of patients had driving vision (20/40 vision or better). With previous treatments, only 15 percent of patients retained similar visual acuity,' said the researchers.[84] The risk of serious adverse events was slightly higher with Avastin than Lucentis, but as the range of conditions was large this was thought to be due to chance. So that should be the end of the problem. Shouldn't it?

Well, not quite. Novartis, which markets Lucentis in the UK, asked a UK court in April 2012 to stop NHS organisations in Southern England using Avastin. The reason they can do that is because Avastin still only has a licence to treat cancer. It can't have a licence to treat AMD because the company hasn't applied for a licence. And doesn't intend to.

Currently in the U.K., Avastin for eye disease costs about £60 per dose, versus £740 for Lucentis, according to NHS sources. You can see that Big Pharma will fight for its profits right to the end.

There is a view that the current method of keeping the costs of drugs down in Europe—price controls—adversely affects both the public health and the health of European research. Drug companies need to sell their products to higher-paying American consumers to recoup their costs, they say. Well, indeed, American consumers do indeed pay a very high price. A recent study of the 50 top-selling prescription drugs found that US pharmaceutical prices were at least 60% higher than those in five large European countries in 2007. Because of the lower price some new drugs never reach European patients, and Europe is losing many jobs in research and development. However the fact is that the USA cannot afford these prices either, and the situation is only likely to get worse. As stated previously we already have very good drugs for most conditions and to produce even better ones may never be cost effective, because the costs are going up and up.

There may be another way of funding new developments in treatments. In Sweden there is a new political party, the Pirate Party, which gained two of Sweden's 18 seats in the European Parliament in the 2009 elections, winning 7.1% of the vote, and there are similar parties being established in other countries. Although the party was initially concerned with file sharing, it has expanded its focus to include three areas that are especially relevant to doctors: reform of copyright law, respect for patients' right to privacy, and the abolition of drug patents. The movement, which has spread to the UK, wants to alter the copyright laws as they relate to scientific research, as it sees knowledge as having intrinsic value that should not be owned. It thinks that reform could dramatically speed up the rate of discovery in many disciplines and change the scientific process radically. Similarly, they say, researchers will need to rise above their petty rivalries and be prepared to share their data with others. The Internet provides tools to facilitate this.

They argue that, thanks to universal health insurance, government subsidies account for most of the income of drug companies in Europe. Only 15% of this income actually goes into research, with most of the remainder being spent on marketing. Instead, they say, governments should allocate 20% of today's drugs bill directly to the universities for research. More funds should produce more research results. Without the need for drug companies to undertake the research themselves, there would be no need for medical patents to protect their investment. The price of drugs would drop if they were manufactured in a competitive market, rather than by patent protected monopolies. People in developing countries would also benefit because their governments wouldn't be forced to buy expensive patent drugs.

Theoretically it would also be possible to abolish drug patents altogether, they say. The reason this could work is that governments actually subsidize the income of pharmaceutical companies in Europe, because of universal health insurance. In the UK the government is almost the only buyer of drugs because of the NHS.

It seems a big step to consider removing patents altogether but in fact they are only a tool of the financial system and not necessarily useful for systems like the NHS. Many people agree change would be a good thing but there will have to be a lot more public awareness of the issues before it is likely to happen. I doubt it will catch on. There are far too many vested interests that will protect such a powerful revenue earner as the pharmaceutical industry, especially in the UK. But the scientific research community does need to clean up its act by making more research easily available and making sure that the data on all research studies is published accurately. This alone would make the claims of Big Pharma more easily scrutinised. At present many companies seem to get away with not publishing evidence: a recent example is the refusal to publish details of the studies on the anti-flu drug Tamiflu which has made billions for the companies without being used very much (the UK government bought large stocks of it in the face of a possible epidemic which did not materialise), and also without enough evidence for its effectiveness ever having been published.

More and more organisations that fund research are now insisting that the results of this research be made 'open access', and many journals have adopted revenue models where the authors (or their employers) pay to enable this to happen. This movement also would like to empower patients more by transferring the control of medical records to the patients themselves, and would ensure better security and privacy (they say). For instance, they are against giving insurance companies access to medical data, as it is difficult to keep the data entirely secure.

Restless legs syndrome and L dopa drugs

I referred to restless legs in the introduction, as an example of where a drug that I thought was a good treatment for a condition turned out to be completely useless. Restless legs syndrome (which is also sometimes referred to as Jimmy Legs, spare legs or 'the kicks') may be described as uncontrollable urges to move the limbs in order to stop uncomfortable, painful or odd sensations in the body, most commonly in the legs. Moving the affected body part eliminates the sensation, providing temporary relief. The main problem patients had was poor quality of sleep. I saw a few patients, usually elderly, complaining of these symptoms, but not many. When I discovered that my preferred treatment was useless, I changed to advising patients to take more exercise during the day and not to get too warm at night, to avoid alcohol and caffeine. I have no idea whether that advice was helpful, but again I can't remember patients coming back to see me about it. It seemed to be one of these conditions where patients want an explanation or at least a reassurance that it was not a serious condition that would get worse and cause problems. Once that was clarified they were happy to put up with it or found remedies for themselves that appeared to work.

But around 2003–2004 there was suddenly a lot of media attention about restless legs. Articles were appearing about it in magazines for the general public, and we doctors began to get a lot of information about it in our mailboxes. It was obvious that an 'awareness campaign' was in progress. There was no talk of treatment for it at first – the campaign must have gone on for several months before finally a treatment was identified. It turned out to be a drug related to the L-dopa agonist, called Ropinirole, which is usually prescribed for Parkinson's disease, which as most people know is a severe mobility disorder not uncommon in elderly people. This drug, however, has some quite severe side effects when used for Parkinson's, including appearing to make the symptoms worse, (augmentation), and in some cases it can cause pathological gambling and eating, so it seemed to me that to try to market it for something like restless legs was going over the top. Yet the campaign went on for months and I knew several GPs who tried it on patients. What tended to happen was that a patient who may or may not have restless legs came to her doctor and if her description was good enough the doctor thought, 'Oh yes, there is a treatment for this now – let's try it.' For young doctors who had not seen the natural history of patients with this problem – that in general all they need is reassurance – it must have been a temptation.

I personally doubt many patients were taken in by this and most would have stopped the treatment pretty quickly once they realised what it entailed, but even so some patients may have an unpleasant time, far worse than the actual symptoms they were complaining of. There are I am sure some people who experience major disruption of sleep and significant impairments in quality of life from restless legs (although I never met any). But they are not drugs that should be prescribed with gay abandon. When the available evidence was reviewed, it was noted that substantial numbers of patients were improving with placebo, possibly reflecting a natural tendency for the disease state to wax and wane, (which was exactly what I had noticed all those years ago). Another medical review suggested that only a few people (less than 20% of sufferers) actually wanted medical treatment, and some of these stopped it quite quickly. Some may indeed benefit but an awareness campaign to the general public and a relentless campaign to GPs is pure market economics.

Most of the health-related articles that you read in the press are actually 'awareness campaigns' so that people who have conditions that so far have not been medicalised can go to their doctors to get treatment. They are usually fronted by 'experts' who are paid directly or indirectly to do this. First a disease that has a treatment that would create a profit for the company needs to be highlighted. If it is a well-known disease, such as diabetes or heart problems, that isn't a difficult job, and a few national advertisements and mail shots to doctors are enough. If it is less well known then many companies will work through patients' organisations. They set up and fund such organisations, which consist of sufferers and their families who want as much money spent on 'their' condition as possible (very understandably), but often don't make their sponsorship clear when they advertise. Then doctors are targeted, GPs by mail shots and the funding of relevant meetings, and soon the new product becomes well known and prescribed.

Another fact that is now better known is the role of 'ghost-writing' mentioned in Chapter 6. It is now unusual for drug firms to take out direct advertisements for their drugs. Instead they rely on articles written ostensibly by medical experts, which depend on seemingly respectable academic review articles, original research articles, and even reports of clinical trials, which one might think ought to depend on unbiased science. However the 'authors' of these papers may not have written the papers at all. Under these circumstances one cannot be sure that the evidence is unbiased, and they can mislead so that patients are harmed. To get rid of these practices altogether, in the future it would mean that editors should enforce policies stating that 'involvement with ghostwriting is a serious and punishable breach of publication ethics'[85] and authors who do it would be banned from any subsequent publication in the journal and their misconduct reported to their institutions.

You might think that there is always good evidence behind the product at this point, but it isn't necessarily so. It is difficult to get good data that a new drug is better than an established treatment, which is bound to be much cheaper and has a lot of evidence behind it. So the trick is to develop guidelines, written by experts, which will be accepted by doctors as valid. However it is clear that often these 'experts' are not impartial.

In a recent study,

> Six of 12 named chairpersons of the experts making the guidelines had a conflict of interest, as did 138 of the 211 panelists who provided a disclosure statement; 12 more failed to disclose an interest, and 10 others received research funding from industry. Only 61 (29%) had no potential financial ties.[86]

In other words the guidelines are being written by people with a financial interest in the treatment in question – either they have had their research funded by the company, have been given 'honorariums', or even paid directly with the money transferred in a way that cannot be traced.

The author of this paper concludes that only when the medical profession itself cleans up its act and no doctor agrees to sit on a committee deciding on guidelines when they have an interest, will things change. 'Conflicts of interest, including fee-for-service arrangements, are at the heart of the astronomical increases in healthcare costs in the United States, and transparency is no substitute for more substantive reform.'[87] And just as the US health system thinks of ways to get out of this hole, our British political masters are determined to push us into it.

After decades of uninterrupted progress and massive profits however, the big pharmaceutical companies are now facing a problem. Their very success has meant that there are now very few avenues where new drugs can be developed. The expected bonanza from the solving of the human genome and individualised medicine has not so far materialized, and as the important blockbuster drugs such as statins and ACE inhibitors come off patent, some drug companies are facing a leaner future. Costs to health systems round the world should drop.

Chapter 17
Prescribing: working out who will benefit from drug treatment

Generics – world wide market – waste – prescription charges

In the UK, GPs do most of the prescribing of medications outside hospital. They initiate many prescriptions themselves in the surgery, and also, as soon as a patient is discharged, they take over medications prescribed by the hospital. This is actually a very time-consuming process and leads to difficulties in the Health Service because historically the two sectors – primary and secondary care – have been funded separately, so the cost of new and expensive medications is quickly borne by the primary care budget. Medical representatives of the pharmaceutical companies ('drug reps') target hospital specialists with their new fantastic drug and the specialist can happily prescribe it without any objection from their managers because the cost is borne by the hospital for only a week or two; after that it becomes the problem for the primary care trust which then has less money to pay for new developments in out-of-hospital care. Even in Scotland and Wales, where the two sectors have been combined administratively, the methods of finance mean that primary care loses out.

In the UK the bill for prescription drugs is not nearly so high as in France (where every consultation leads to a prescription by custom and practice) for example, and nothing like the bill in the US. Fortunately, here, most GPs have a quite small list of medicines they use regularly, and most do not change medications for patients unless there is good reason. That is the advantage of a system where there is a knowledgeable person with the patient's interest at heart coming between the pharmaceutical industry and the patient. Pharmacists are incredibly knowledgeable about over-the-counter medications and it is always worth asking for advice there. There are now many schemes where pharmacists can play a much larger part in helping the public to understand why they are taking the drugs they are.

Prescribing costs are held quite low in the UK. This is because for many years there has been a concerted effort from the government to encourage the use of generic drugs (which are cheap because they are out of patent), by encouraging doctors to prescribe and pharmacists to dispense the generic version of a product. This is necessary because drug reps who want to see GPs about their new drug will always be selling branded drugs and these will be much more expensive. GPs say that though they see reps it doesn't influence them to prescribe the new branded drugs. But this is wishful thinking – of course we are influenced if we see something that our patients might benefit from. So there are incentive schemes whereby GPs are rewarded if they reach a target for the percentage of generic drugs in a particular class. This often means changing the tablets patients receive and as generics are usually made abroad patients worry that the quality is not the same. But apart from a very few cases of a bad batch this does not happen.

There are games that are played around prescription medicines though. For some time now it has been the case that medicines are cheaper in the UK than elsewhere, usually because the NHS is getting better at driving down the prices. But this means that doctors and pharmacist can make a profit by re-selling the drugs abroad, especially when the exchange rate is favourable. This then can mean severe shortages at home and patients can't get their medicines – often critical ones such as drugs for cancer. Unscrupulous firms sometimes cash in on this and buy up drugs in short supply and then re-sell them at a profit, and this has been a real problem in the UK. The government has told firms that UK patients should be supplied first, but it is difficult to see how this can be enforced. There isn't anything to prevent drug companies stopping production of a product (such as insulin) because they will make more profits out of an alternative despite the fact that patients are stabilised on and happy with the original, causing inconvenience to patients and a lot of work for everyone involved with the prescription.

The amount of prescription medication now consumed by the public is enormous and growing every year. Of course the age distribution of those taking medication is greatly skewed, with the elderly taking the lion's share. Most people in the younger age groups consume much less. People with chronic diseases can take 50 or more tablets a day and anyone now being diagnosed with diabetes for instance is immediately likely to be taking at least 4 separate medications, and that is likely to be before they actually start treatment for diabetes itself. They will be advised to take aspirin, a cholesterol-lowering drug, and a drug to protect the kidneys and possibly a weight-reducing drug even before they are given treatment for high blood pressure or diabetes. These drugs should benefit the patient, by allowing them to live longer or have fewer complications.

However usually if 100 patients take these preventative tablets then it is likely that only, say, 10% of them will definitely benefit, and the remaining 90% will not. It is of course impossible to tell exactly which patients will benefit, so everyone has to take them. In this way there have been reductions in overall mortality in the population from conditions like heart attacks and diabetes. For patients to take such drugs day in day out with the possibility that they might not be doing them personally any good, it is essential that the drugs are free of any side effects. This is often not the case of course and it is not surprising then that compliance with the drugs can be a problem for some patients, who do not notice any direct benefit from taking the tablets. Patients may not be fully aware of these facts. There is a simple calculation which was popular amongst doctors at one time – the Numbers Needed to Treat, NNT, which was a calculation of how many patients you needed to treat before one patient benefited, and I am quite sure that of patients were to be given these numbers many would not take the drugs. I am not saying that they shouldn't, of course but I do sympathize with so many patients who have to take so many drugs each with different side effects.

And of course often they don't take them. But patients still sometimes pick up prescriptions, and the amount of waste in the NHS is enormous. I used to regularly look in patients' cupboards to see what medications they were taking, and I was sometimes amazed at what I found – month after month's supply of boxes, untouched. Sometimes it wasn't deliberate; one person in her eighties with failing memory had an arrangement with the local pharmacists, who got the prescription from the doctor every month and delivered it, and the home carer used to put the drugs in the cupboard. Someone was supposed to come in and put the ones she was taking into a drug dispenser, but the list she had did not include two of the drugs, and those were the ones that were building up in the cupboard. We at the practice were partly to blame as it should have been clear that she was not taking those drugs, but the nurse who managed the dispenser could perhaps have noticed them in the cupboard. The cost ran into thousands of pounds before we cottoned on. In many cases the patient is aware they should be taking the drugs but for many reasons don't do so, but they don't tell us. I wouldn't mind so much except that we are not allowed to re-cycle these drugs. If you take them back to the pharmacy as advised, the pharmacists are supposed to destroy them. You can't re-use them even if untouched; neither can you donate them to charity for developing countries. The rule seems to be if they aren't fit for us, no one else can have them on safety grounds. It always seems very righteous to me and I am sure any efforts to change the law would be vigorously fought by pharmacists and pharmaceutical companies who make billions by selling drugs that no one will ever take.

Prescription Charges

I referred earlier to prescription charges, which although expensive in England, are paid by only a minority of patients. In Wales all prescriptions have been free to everyone for about 8 years (you have to be registered with a doctor on the Welsh Performance List so if you live in a border area you may be able to get this even if you actually live in England). They are now free in Scotland as well. People often ask – what is the sense in that? Isn't it just a ploy to get people to support devolution? Surely patients who can afford to pay should – after all if you were on regular medication you could get a season ticket – it works out to be worth doing this if you take more than two items a month regularly. People in England are often rather annoyed that they have to pay when those in other UK countries don't, or might say that they prefer to get shorter waiting times for hospital with the money saved. It is indeed a choice that the individual parliaments will make for themselves. It is, however, often not realised how unfair the current system in England is to some patients and the fact is that the BMA and other medical organisations have consistently supported abolition of prescription charges.

There is a cost of course in giving free prescriptions, with many people asking for prescriptions for things for minor ailments, like cotton wool, that they previously paid for themselves. GPs do not have much choice in prescribing such things, as there is a health justification for most of them even if it was a small cut or a cold, and these items are prescribable. As a GP, you might raise your eyebrows when someone asks for such things but you wouldn't argue or refuse. While people will say, 'why can't the GP just be firm and say no?', it is time-consuming in a busy surgery to argue the point, and the fact is that under the present NHS act you are required to write a prescription if there is a need. This has been a problem for years with so many having free prescriptions under the present system so what is different here? I think it will be much easier in England with the new reforms coming in to issue edicts that patients should not get such things free and some GPs will probably obey and others won't, making the system so much less consistent in different areas.

When the NHS came in, there were no prescription charges in the post-war austerity, but it was soon realised that the NHS budget, far from reducing as people became healthier as was thought might happen, was increasing exponentially. Prescription charges were then introduced but politicians were understandably worried about the reaction, and it was decided that all children and pensioners should receive them free. It was also thought to be sensible to exclude anyone on regular life long essential medications, but the only ones at that time that came into that category were drugs where patients were deficient in essential hormones. Replacement treatment for thyroid deficiency, insulin for diabetes and certain other hormone treatments were to be free. However there weren't any systems at that time to ensure that only those treatments were free, so patients with these conditions were allowed to get all their medications – for whatever condition – free.

In some ways this has proved to be a good thing – people with diabetes now have to take six drugs as a minimum – but people with thyroid problems are still allowed to have free prescriptions for arthritis and painkillers and so on. People with asthma who may also been on essential regular medications have to pay and these are often people in work with families to support. Many were the times patients used to ask me 'I can't afford these drugs doctor – which ones can I leave off?' Also, patients with cancer are not exempt, nor people who have had a heart attack, who are also on lots of drugs. Doctors have therefore for years called for an update of the system, but almost anything you do would be even more complicated and cost more. In Wales and Scotland where the proportion of free prescriptions is higher (due to poorer, less healthy populations), it makes a lot of sense to abolish them altogether. If you are talking about the greatest good for the largest number of people, what is best, to ask a relatively small number of people with arthritis to wait a few more months for their operation, or ensure that a much larger group of people don't have to worry about funding the medications which are helping them live more productive and healthier lives? As I said, it is a choice each government can make.

Chapter 18
Over-the-counter medications

Evidence for effectiveness and the role of advertising – micronutrients – iron, zinc –
other over-the-counter medications – herbal medicine

Of course prescription medicine is only part of the story. The market for over-the-counter medication is huge, consisting of complementary health medications, such as vitamin pills, herbal medicines and other 'extra' nutrients, and drugs which can be bought over the counter for less than the prescription cost (in England) and so on.

There are many micronutrients that may be valuable in keeping people healthy, but I will confine myself to those that I have myself prescribed or that I know many of my patients have bought and say they find useful. Most are dietary supplements rather than essential micronutrients. It is illegal in the US to market any dietary supplement as a treatment for any disease or condition, but not so in the UK and these drugs are extensively marketed.

Iron is the first that springs to mind because it is the vital constituent of haemoglobin, the molecule that transports oxygen from the lungs around the body in our blood. Lack of iron means that we cannot make enough haemoglobin, and so less oxygen can be carried. This puts a strain on the heart, which tries to pump blood harder to ensure that enough vital oxygen gets to the tissues. It is therefore essential to have enough iron in the diet, and this is easy to get because nearly all plants and animals also need iron; there is plenty of it in a normal diet, although is most readily absorbed from red meat so vegetarians can go a bit short. It can be absorbed from vegetables, but ironically not from spinach, despite its reputation, because the iron there is bound to oxalates, which cannot be absorbed.

Iron deficiency nevertheless is common, mostly in women of childbearing years. The menstrual cycle results in a regular loss of blood and therefore iron every month, and unless this is replaced through a good diet, women are likely to become anaemic even without childbearing, which additionally depletes their stores of iron often very severely, after a post partum haemorrhage for example.

Quite apart from in general practice, when of course I saw plenty of anaemia from this cause, it was brought home to me how crucial iron was when we went on holiday one year to Acadia. Acadia is a part of the province of New Brunswick in Canada, and was populated by French-speaking people who migrated from France in the 16th century. They had earlier origins and a different history from the French speakers of Quebec, and suffered a lot when the British gained control of Canada, and because of this they proudly retain a distinct identity. Every house would have an Acadian flag, the French red, white and blue tricolour with a gold star, flying in the front garden to remind you that they are French speaking. We wandered round their cemeteries and communities and heard about the times from long ago when women in their thirties and forties died so young. In those times with no birth control these ladies would have already given birth to 10 or more children by their early thirties and the loss of iron from menstrual loss, post partum bleeding and the normal demands of bringing up a family had shortened their life expectancy considerably. We came across graves of men with two or even three wives buried alongside them. These were fishing communities, and fish is not a good source of iron, so even without constant childbearing these women might have been in trouble, but childbearing was always very hard in areas without much iron. It reminds us that the current trend for women to outlive men is a comparatively recent one.

Still in North America, I did an elective period in the 60s in Labrador, where there were three distinct populations – the original Inuit, the European settlers and a group of Amerindians of the Naskapi tribe. The Inuit had been settled into the community for several generations, but the Naskapi tribe of Indians had only recently been 'given' houses by the Canadian Government (all in good faith). The people told us that the Naskapi were very unwilling to settle permanently in these houses, (single rooms with a stove in the middle, but quite large and with electricity and running water), and only stayed in them in the depths of winter, otherwise resuming their nomadic lifestyle for the rest of the year. As a student I was there to learn, but even so took a lot of responsibility. One woman I remember vividly came in obviously very anaemic, as white as a ghost. Not only did I have to take her blood but I also had to do the lab test to measure her haemoglobin and was shocked to see that it was 5 – the normal would be from 11 to 13 on the scale we were using at the time. So she had less than half of the oxygen carrying capacity that she should have had, and she was very sick.

The next thing after diagnosing anaemia is to decide if it is iron-deficiency anaemia, or another sort as there are two other common causes of anaemia, one of them being folic acid deficiency and the other vitamin B12 deficiency. The two sorts can be distinguished because in iron deficiency the blood cells are smaller than usual (microcytic), while in B12 and folate deficiency the cells are larger (macrocytic). There is a simple test that can be done to determine the size of the blood cells and when I did this, it was clear that this lady had a B12 or folate deficiency. In fact the doctor in charge told me that pernicious anaemia was a common problem (it can run in families) in that group of people, and the woman had to be transferred to St John's, the regional hospital, for further treatment because she was so ill. In fact I learnt later that she had a very stormy ride in St John's and nearly died, but she did eventually come home to her three children, Antuan, Margarite and Marie (the group had been converted to Christianity by French-speaking missionaries some years before). They were such gorgeous kids and everyone in the tiny hospital of 16 beds was over the moon.

Zinc is another essential nutrient and is a co-factor in DNA and protein synthesis and cell division. It is believed to be important in wound healing. We don't store available zinc in our bodies but it is laid down in bones and teeth. There is plenty of it in the average British diet (meat, liver, cereal products, peas, beans, eggs, and seafood, especially oysters, are good sources of zinc) and deficiency is rare, but again people with a poor diet, have malabsorption, or who are generally ill may well suffer from relative insufficiency.

Wikipedia says one-third of the world population is at risk of zinc deficiency, ranging from 4 to 73% depending on the country, and zinc deficiency is the fifth leading risk factor for disease in the developing world. Providing micronutrients, including zinc, to humans is one of the four quick-win solutions to major global problems identified in the Copenhagen Consensus[88] from an international panel of distinguished economists, as deficiency in childhood can cause mental retardation, cognitive difficulties and failure to thrive. Its main importance lies in the fact that diarrhoea from any cause seems to be worsened by zinc deficiency, and in the developing world millions of children suffer from severe diarrhoea every year due to infection and malnutrition, and many die from dehydration due to the diarrhoea. We know that giving fluids by mouth (using an oral rehydration solution) can save children's lives, but it seems to have no effect on the length of time the children suffer with diarrhoea. Zinc supplementation is a possible treatment for diarrhoea,[89] though it can have adverse effects if given in high doses.[90] However it seems a good idea to try to persuade people in the developing world, where zinc deficiency is common, to treat diarrhoea with zinc and oral rehydration solutions rather than antibiotics.

When I was first in practice, we all prescribed antibiotics for gastrointestinal infections and diarrhoea (usually sulphonamide-containing drugs, sulfatriad was one I remember) and it took a lot of campaigning, by paediatricians especially, to stop us prescribing them. It took the general public in the UK a bit longer to stop thinking antibiotics were the answer, but rehydration made so much sense that it was accepted much more readily than the later campaign to stop using antibiotics for sore throats. Unfortunately in many countries in the developing world this process has yet to happen, and people often think antibiotics are the best treatment, even though they are expensive and useless, and can be harmful. They are generally peddled by middlemen wanting to make a quick profit.

Zinc is often thought to help in anorexia and other situations where people have poor appetites, but the evidence isn't conclusive. I was also told it could help when people lost their sense of smell or taste (anosmia), a horrible condition I thought. One patient said that everything tasted like cardboard and she lost pounds in weight. Sadly nothing helped, and the condition was probably due to damage to the tiny nerves at the top of the nose. People also use it for general tiredness and to 'boost the immune system' but there is no evidence that it works consistently. In general people in the UK don't need zinc supplementation, and the doctor treating you will prescribe it where necessary.

Copper – I have to say that copper, either in deficiency or in excess, did not cross my radar much during the time I was a GP. There are several inborn errors of metabolism, notably Wilson's disease, that we checked patients for regularly, and there was indeed one in our practice population. For the rest of the population it wasn't an issue. In the literature there are concerns both of deficiency (but in the USA the recommended amounts are below what most people consume) and the dangers of toxicity due to excess. It seems that it is pregnant mothers, neonates (babies in the first two weeks of life) and young children for whom the balance is most crucial as this is the time that copper stores are used, however it is a rare problem.

Magnesium is again a most important element in the human body. It is the essential ingredient in plant chlorophyll (compare it to the status of iron in blood) and therefore there is loads of it in any green plant food. In animals it is an essential ingredient in ATP, which is the biological substance that stores energy and releases in the muscles. So it is marketed as something that will improve your muscular activity, but I have seen no evidence for this. Magnesium has been considered to help in treatment-resistant depression but I don't know of anybody who has tried it and our psychiatrists certainly don't. I would think we generally have enough of it in our diets.

Of the other micronutrients, **Cobalt** is a constituent of vitamin B12, and has been used, as a treatment for anaemia, but very little is needed. Excess cobalt is toxic to humans – in the 1960s, some breweries added cobalt salts to beer to stabilize the foam. It caused heart problems in some people who drank a lot of beer (8–25 pints/day) and some died (of the cobalt, not the beer, it is presumed). Just recently it has been reported that people who have had metal-on-metal hip joints implanted, made of a cobalt–chromium alloy, have been found to suffer from cobalt poisoning. After many months of no problems with their new joints, patients began to complain of pain in the hip, anxiety and depression, tinnitus and hearing loss, and cognitive decline, and the levels of cobalt in the blood were grossly raised. It is now known that trivalent cobalt ions are released into the bloodstream and there are have been cases of genotoxicity and concerns about cancer. So far they are still being used. One hopes that better joints will be developed.

Radioactive cobalt of course is extremely dangerous.

Boron, occurring in borate salts, is similar to common salt, and is not toxic, but also no deficiency has ever been noted. **Chromium** has no verified biological role and has been classified as not essential for mammals.

Fluoride of course is best known for its effects on teeth. Dental caries is still a problem in most countries, affecting 60–90% of schoolchildren and most adults. Fluoride in water prevents cavities in both children and adults by improving the mineralisation of tooth enamel in the early stages of cavities. Certainly when I was at school some of my schoolmates had lost many of their second teeth, including front teeth, from caries, which was awful for them. Nowadays all toothpastes are fortified with fluoride, and some areas put low levels of fluoride in the water supply. The latter will reduce tooth decay by about 40%, over and above those using toothpaste only.

Fluoridation is still controversial of course, partly on health grounds, as fluorides can causal dental fluorosis and can be dangerous to health in high dosage, but also on the principle that people cannot consent to taking fluoride when it is in the water supply. This argument will never be settled and each area makes its own decisions, but where the incidence of tooth decay is very high it does seem a sensible way forward. There are no schemes at present in Wales, although there is a water fluoridation scheme in the West Midlands and their rate of dental decay in children is much lower. Fluoride is not considered to be an essential nutrient, as it is not used in the body.

It may be noted that we don't usually know how much fluoride there is in bottled water, so people who mostly drink bottled water rather than tap water don't know what they are getting.

Manganese is an essential nutrient as it is a component of many co-factors and enzymes in many cellular functions. It is widely available in our diet, and no deficiency in humans has been described, though some animal studies have indicated it might cause skeletal problems. It is toxic in high dosage.

Selenium is another essential nutrient, and acts as an anti-oxidant. There have been claims that taken regularly it can help prevent cancer, but a Cochrane review of studies concluded that there is no convincing evidence that individuals, particularly those who are adequately nourished, will benefit from selenium supplementation with regard to their cancer risk. However, there is evidence that selenium can help chemotherapy treatment by enhancing the efficacy of the treatment, reducing the toxicity of chemotherapeutic drugs, and preventing the body's resistance to the drugs. Actual deficiency does not appear to cause disease but in AIDS patients it has been found that depleted selenium levels and selenium deficiency does strongly correlate with the progression of the disease and the risk of death. On its effect on type 2 diabetes, one study correlated higher levels of selenium with the high prevalence of type 2 diabetes and so in the USA supplementation in well nourished people was not recommended. Nevertheless another study has indicated that selenium may inhibit the development of this disease in men only. More research is obviously needed on selenium's role in the human body, however there is no doubt it is toxic in high amounts.

Molybdenum is another substance which is classified as an essential nutrient, and dietary molybdenum deficiency from low soil concentration has been associated with increased rates of cancer of the oesophagus in a geographical band from Northern China to Iran. However a controlled trial giving people their extra molybdenum did not reduce the cancer rate. There is plenty of molybdenum in soils in the UK.

Most of the other micronutrients mentioned by Wikipedia have no proven uses, though those with money to burn can try them for their supposed benefits. There are many other drugs available from pharmacies OTC.

Caffeine is a well-known stimulant, used in tea and coffee, and is also a constituent of many OTC medications. In my early years in practice half my practice population seemed to be taking caffeine derivatives such as Solpadeine on prescription, usually in a proprietary preparation together with codeine for its pain relieving properties. It was difficult to resist the request for such prescriptions as patients were extremely persuasive and of course they were useful as painkillers. But most patients took them for their stimulating effect. It got to be such a problem that these combinations were excluded from the list of medications doctors could prescribe in 1985, along with so many untested and over-promoted medications. Now caffeine is never prescribed as a medication and people have to make do with coffee to get their kicks. In fact it is a stimulant which improves concentration and idea production, but it hinders memory encoding and also produces jitters. Caffeine used to have a very important role in special care baby units, as it was thought that caffeine given to very premature infants with breathing problems could reduce the rates of cerebral palsy and cognitive delay at 18 months. Sadly follow-up at 5 years showed that any benefit disappears with time.[91] So, the authors said, there is little point giving it to the babies, only to the NHS staff!

1/5-hydroxytryptophan is a precursor to serotonin in the brain, and was in vogue in the late nineties when prescribed antidepressants got a bad name because of adverse publicity about side effects. It was quite heavily promoted then and I certainly prescribed it for patients with mild depression, but I have to admit

I thought of it as a safe placebo. Sometimes a tablet can work as an adjunct while you talk through people's problems and show interest. Tryptophan can still be prescribed but my British National Formulary (BNF – the doctors' bible of drugs available to patients in the NHS) tells me that it is licensed as an adjunct for people resistant to standard antidepressants but has been associated with eosinophilic myalgia syndrome, (don't ask!) and therefore should be initiated under specialist supervision! So not really something people should just pick up at a supermarket.

Theophylline is a drug I remember well, and was marketed OTC for asthma. It can be extracted from tea leaves and early on was found useful as a bronchodilator, that is it will relax the smooth muscles in the walls of the small tubes within the lungs called bronchioles, which are the ones that get constricted in such diseases as asthma and chronic bronchitis (chronic obstructive airways disease). Asthma was a dreadful problem in my early days in practice: there were many patients with really severe asthma, which is basically an allergic or autoimmune phenomenon, not associated with smoking though would be made worse by smoking. There wasn't much effective treatment around in those days – we hadn't started using steroids or inhalers then – and theophylline was one if the best drugs we could use. It had to be given by injection, and the dose had to be just right, as overdosage was easy and could cause heart irregularities and even death.

Well do I remember one particular woman with severe asthma who called me out one summer afternoon. We all knew that she would not call us unless it was an emergency and I was on call, so I headed out there. However she lived on a farm way out in the country and I got lost getting there (no mobile phones or sat navs in those days). So when I arrived her breathing was very bad, and she wanted me to treat her there rather than go into hospital (she had been sent in many times before and hated it). Anyway the ambulance would have taken an age to reach us, so I gave her an intravenous injection of theophylline. You had to give a large amount (about 20 ml) very slowly indeed, feeling her pulse all the time. There were several times when her heart rate jumped up and I was terrified her heart was suddenly going to stop. But once started I had to continue, and soon her breathing eased and she was so grateful. I felt so happy, but I got lost again on the way back and arrived nearly an hour late for evening surgery. All the staff did, instead of congratulating me, was to tell me off for being late! Nowadays with inhalers, oral steroids, and other effective drugs, theophylline is never used, but it saved many a life back then.

Chondroitin sulphate is important in maintaining the structural integrity of bodily tissues, especially cartilage. Wikipedia says, 'The tightly packed and highly charged sulphate groups of chondroitin sulphate generate electrostatic repulsion that provides much of the resistance of cartilage to compression. Loss of chondroitin sulphate from the cartilage is a major cause of osteoarthritis'. However this does not mean that giving chondroitin orally is going to do anything to the joints and recent evidence indicates that it is useless.[92]**Glucosamine** is a precursor to a substance that is a component of cartilage and therefore has been promoted for years as a treatment of osteoarthritis, often with chondroitin. At one time lots of my patients used to buy both these preparations as they are intensively marketed in the UK and indeed I used to – rather reluctantly – recommend them myself. When NHS budgets are squeezed it can be tempting to recommend that patients buy such preparations to reduce the drug bill for non-steroidal anti-inflammatory drugs, which can be very expensive, but I am not sure of the ethics of doing this! There was evidence at that time that they worked, as studies done by the drug manufacturer showed that they helped not only pain and stiffness but also improved the X-ray appearance of affected joints. Later many independent studies were done and you won't be surprised to learn that the results weren't as good. Overall, large meta-analyses of large numbers of trials have not shown conclusive benefit[93] and therefore they are not recommended by NICE and not available on the NHS. If you want to buy something extra for arthritis (and it is such a painful condition that lots do) I would have thought some of the herbs would be a better bet.

Herbal Medicine

So what is the evidence that herbal medicines work?

Herbal medicine may be broadly defined as the use of plants and plant extracts to benefit human health. Most GPs that I know, including myself, are vaguely sympathetic to the use of herbal medicines (in a survey 75% believed that herbal medicines are 'helpful in some circumstances'[94]) – if only because if people treat themselves for minor ailments they won't come consulting us! However only a few GPs (less than 20%) described their own knowledge of herbal medicines as 'quite good' or better, and less than 40% routinely asked patients about herbal medicine use. This is unsatisfactory, as many people use herbal medicine in combination with orthodox medicine, and some herbal medicines interact with mainstream medicines,[95] so theoretically there could be some dangerous interactions which GPs need to know something about. For instance, surveys in patients taking warfarin[96] (to prevent excessive clotting) found that 15-43% took complementary medicines which might interact, such as garlic and ginger, and there have been some instances of patients reporting excessive bleeding, though no reports of real harm.

Using plant extracts to treat illnesses has a very long history. There is documentary evidence from The Medical Book of the Physicians of Myddfai in the 13th century about using herbs such as the following:

§34. For headache or pain in the joints. Take cakes of pounded wheat, and grind into fine meal. Then take wood sorrel, dandelion, betony, and red wine, bruising them together in a mortar well, then mixing them thoroughly together on the fire, adding ox tallow and salt thereto freely. Let this plaster, spread on thick cloth, be then applied to the shaven scalp. This will induce the breaking forth of boils, thereby extracting the venom, and relieving the patient.

This was of course treatment by counter-irritation, and in those days patients must have accepted that they were going to feel a lot worse before they might feel better! Actually something of this goes on today, as many treatments, for instance antidepressants, do this and it is true for many operations as well. Legend has it that the physicians of Myddfai got their magical skills from 'the lady of the lake' – their mother, who was a fairy; at any rate the three brothers used their skills to treat the royal household. You can see some of the plants they used in the botanical gardens of Carmarthenshire. Even nowadays people use dock leaves to treat nettle stings or suck peppermint to relieve indigestion.

There is a biological reason why plants can have useful properties to treat illnesses. Some have evolved to synthesize chemical compounds such as phytochemicals; tannins and alkaloids, which may have antimicrobial activity that helps them defend against attack from a wide variety of predators such as insects, fungi and herbivorous mammals. Sick animals will forage such plants, and some birds will select nesting material rich in antimicrobial agents that protect their young from harmful bacteria. And of course penicillin itself is a naturally occurring substance manufactured by certain fungi, which presumably had a need to discourage too many bacteria around them.

Many drugs developed by pharmaceutical companies have their origins in plant species. In 2001, researchers identified 122 compounds used in mainstream medicine, which were derived from 'ethnomedical' plant sources. Many new drugs even now are found by researching the traditional use of medicines.

As prescribed drugs of all sorts get negative publicity, it is understandable that some people would prefer to use more 'natural' therapies, and the industry at present is booming. A recent survey estimated the UK retail value of complementary medicine at £213 million, with an 18% growth rate between 2007 and 2009.[97] Examples of the most popular herbal medicines include garlic, echinacea, St John's Wort, ginkgo biloba, ginger, ginseng, peppermint, chamomile, valerian, milk thistle, black cohosh and saw palmetto. Patients use these for specific conditions, from acute self-limiting illnesses such as colds or stomach upsets, to chronic, severe conditions such as asthma, diabetes and cancer. They are also used for broader health-related goals such as enhancement of relaxation, sleep, memory, concentration, energy and immune function.

Estimates of herbal medicine use vary depending on the survey population and the definition used. A UK random telephone survey found that 20% of the adult population had used a complementary therapy in the previous year.[98] A national survey in the United States found that 18% of adults used 'non-vitamin, non-mineral, natural products' (mostly herbal medicines), with a corresponding figure of 4% in children.[99] Factors associated with herbal use in surveys have included female sex, higher educational background, age (45-64), ethnic and immigrant background, herbal use among family members, and use of prescription medications or OTC medications.[100]

However we know that people will also often treat themselves with complementary therapy not for general health improvement or minor illnesses but for specific medical problems, sometimes quite serious ones. For instance, a survey of asthma in UK primary care[101] found that 14.5% of patients used complementary medicine (mostly homeopathy, herbal medicine and relaxation techniques), with half the patients not having disclosed this to their GP. For hospital outpatients with inflammatory bowel disease the corresponding figure was 26%, nearly half of whom were using herbal remedies. It is certainly big business that the medical profession might usefully know more about.

In the UK, people obtain herbal medicines mostly by buying them from pharmacies, health food stores or online. You can also visit private herbal practitioners including Western medical herbalists and practitioners of traditional systems such as traditional Chinese medicine and Ayurvedic (indigenous Indian) medicine, several thousand of whom practice in the UK, although almost none within the NHS. As well as giving lifestyle and nutritional advice, often after a prolonged consultation, herbal practitioners, whether practising according to European, Indian or Chinese tradition, typically prescribe an individualised combination of several herbs with the aim not only of inhibiting the disease process but also of making bodily systems work better. For example, for a patient with osteoarthritis, a Western herbal practitioner might give analgesic and anti-inflammatory herbs, herbs to 'get rid of toxins' using mild laxatives and diuretics, and herbs to enhance bile production and flow, herbs to optimise immune function, and adaptogens (herbs to optimise the stress response). The herbs used within these traditions have a history of empirical use over hundreds or even thousands of years. There have been studies of individualised herbal medicine, but none have shown any definite benefit over placebo. This is not surprising given that studies of the actions of individual herbs have shown a variety of results with some herbs working well and others to be completely useless.

Herbal medicines are usually prepared from one part of a plant, for example leaf (ginkgo), root (ginger), flower (hawthorn) or fruit (agnus castus) or from the 'aerial parts' – everything above the ground (passion flower). These may be presented in dried form without further processing to be boiled as a tea (traditional Chinese medicine), turned into powder, capsules or tablets, or extracted in alcohol to make a 'tincture' (often prescribed in Western herbal medicine). In a few cases the active ingredients of herbal medicines are known and also how they actually produce their effects. In principle herbal medicines can just as effective as conventional medicines but also can have the same potential to cause harmful side effects.

So do we know what works?

Everyone who uses herbal remedies obviously thinks or hopes that they will work. We all have heard stories of a cold or a temperature which disappeared a few hours after taking a remedy, of bruising that cleared up much more quickly than expected after taking a homeopathic preparation, of tiredness that magically disappeared after a session of reflexology and so on. I have no problem with any of this – if it appears to work and people can afford the treatment then there has been some benefit. But for serious diseases, infections, cancers – is there really any role for treatments that have no evidence at all behind them? To use such treatments instead of scientifically proven treatments seems perverse, until we realise that a lot of people have no real understanding of science and don't care either. It is entirely a matter of faith for these people and they won't thank me for telling them what to believe. But for those who would like to see what is scientifically proved to work here is the evidence – and there is a lot of it.

There are approximately 5,000 randomised controlled trials (RCTs) of herbal medicines available on PubMed, with 550 registered on the Cochrane database (search carried out July 2011). They aren't all useful; often there are insufficient numbers and size of studies, and differences in outcome measures, doses and types of herbal extracts used for the same indication. But some conclusions can be drawn.

Many herbal remedies are discussed in the Appendix (with references). In summary:

- Herbs to treat anxiety and depression: **St John's Wort** probably works in mild depression and there is the biggest body of evidence behind it. There is weak evidence for **camomile**, but there is no evidence that **ginseng** works and it can interact with warfarin to cause bleeding.

- Herbs to help Premenstrual syndrome: **Agnus Castus** may help.

- Cognitive function in the elderly: **Gingko Biloba** can help (discussed in section on care of the Elderly).

- Benign prostate hypertrophy: **Saw Palmetto** was thought to work but latest evidence says not.

- Pain killers: **Cat's Claw Vine**, **Devil's Claw Root**, **Boswellia Resin** and **Turmeric** may well be helpful, and **Comfrey** (seven seas) cream might work as a pain killer for arthritis.

- For Cholesterol lowering: **Garlic** and **omega-3 fatty acids** do work up to a point.

- Colds: **Echinacea** – Guaranteed Immune System Supplement! At one time most of my patients used to buy Echinacea to ward off colds, but there is no evidence that taking it regularly over the winter will prevent colds. Of course there is no treatment known to do this anywhere – **vitamin C** has been shown to have only very small effects even at high doses. There is poor-quality evidence that it might reduce symptom severity with a cold with some studies showing it works, but others not. Whereas the OTC preparations for colds and flu do work very well indeed to relieve symptoms.

- **Kava, Black Cohosh** and **Aristolochia** have all been shown to cause medical problems directly, and there are many interactions between herbs and conventional medications that could cause harm.

Of course one big problem with recommending herbal medicines is that none are available on the NHS and so they all come at a cost. Until very recently, herbal products available over the counter were classified as dietary supplements and subject to food regulation, requiring very little quality assurance. Recently there have been concerns about contamination of imported Chinese and Indian products with orthodox drugs, and it seems that traders have been enhancing their products to make them work better. For example, fenfluramine (a standard western slimming medicine which has now been withdrawn because it can cause serious heart disease) in herbal slimming pills; sildenafil (the active ingredient in viagra) in herbal aphrodisiacs; topical steroids in skin creams and, more seriously, contaminants such as heavy metals and herbs containing aristolochic acid which are very damaging to people's kidneys and has resulted in death. So the Traditional Herbal Medicinal Products Directive (THMPD), under EU law that came into force in the UK on 30 April 2011, regulates marketed products on the basis of traditional use, safety studies and quality of manufacture. But unlike orthodox drugs, clinical studies demonstrating efficacy are not required.

The new regulations are designed only to make sure that herbal remedies are safe, but are not concerned at all with whether they are effective. But not many people are aware of this. In the UK, the Directive is administered by the MHRA. So there will be fewer products available to the public, since such licensing is expensive, but these should be of better quality. Customers however who have been happy with existing formulations over the years are less than happy about big increases in price, and sometimes withdrawal of some products such as those for vegetarians. However, some herbs with a tradition of culinary as well as medicinal use (such as garlic, ginger and turmeric) may still be available as food supplements. The new regulations are onerous and companies have to decide whether to tool up to provide the new formulations and to pass on the cost to the consumer, or to bow out of the market. As companies sell out of their old stocks customers may notice a very large increase in the costs of their favourite herbal remedies.

At the moment anyone may practise herbal medicine, as there is no regulation of non-medically qualified herbal practitioners. However there is voluntary participation in registers maintained by professional associations. For Western herbal practitioners, the longest-established registering bodies are the National Institute of Medical Herbalists (with 500 members) and the College of Practitioners of Phytotherapy (150 members). Their registers give some assurance of adequate training, fitness to practice and participation in continuing professional development. For traditional Chinese herbalists (the largest group, with several thousand herbal shops in UK high streets), the longest-established organisation is the Register of Chinese Herbal Medicine (450 members). But most people use local knowledge and word-of-mouth recommendation to identifying practitioners with a good reputation. The government has now said it recommends statutory regulation of herbal practitioners under the Health Professions Council, the body which already regulates physiotherapists, occupational therapists and dieticians. This is expected to take 2 or 3 years, but should reassure the public about the standards and accountability of practitioners.

So would I use herbal medicines? Firstly I would not go to a herbalist, because there is no scientific evidence behind their methods. If people want to do so however, it would seem to be harmless, although I would recommend you tell your GP. If you go to a reputable herbalist you may get some herbs that work, and you may well get a lengthy consultation about your concerns and life problems from someone who would listen well – often just as you would from a GP. You may well also benefit from the placebo response, which in most studies is at least a 30% chance. As a GP I often wished I could prescribe a placebo. The recommendation for GPs is that you could but you would have to tell a patient it was a placebo, which would take away much of the point! (Although it is said that it may work even when you know it is a placebo!) It would be an individual decision whether it would be worth the money or not. Be aware though. Some herbs can harm you.

However, given the evidence I have read, if I suffered from mild to moderate depression I might well take some St John's Wort, probably while also going to a trained counsellor or someone with expertise in CBT. For someone needing relief from hot flushes some of the herbs mentioned above might be a good bet, although if the hot flushes were completely messing up my life, I probably would take HRT for as short a time as I could get away with, as this would work a lot better. Otherwise, I like garlic and have every intention of carrying on eating it, and hope it will have some effects on my cholesterol and risk of cancer!

Chapter 19
Vitamin supplements: wonder drugs or profit generators?

What are vitamins? Effects, deficiency and claims of benefit

I really don't know why there is such an industry regarding vitamins. People seem to think that they are special, wonder drugs and that there is something almost magical about them. Actually there is nothing more wonderful about them than there is about a hundred thousand other compounds that whizz around the cells of our bodies, each fitting in exactly to the jigsaw that makes up the cell's metabolism. The only thing special about vitamins is that our bodies can't make them, whereas for the other thousands the body can synthesize them without difficulty. Why this is so is perhaps just chance.

Some vitamins that we have to get from our diet are made perfectly easily by other animals, for example vitamin A, retinol, which is so important to our eyesight, and also vitamin C (ascorbic acid). But it really doesn't matter much because vitamins are widespread in our diets, mostly from plants and some from other animals. Only if our diets are particularly off beam or we are ill, or if we have changed our lifestyle considerably from our ancestors, as in the case of living in these cloudy islands so that we don't get enough sunlight (vitamin D), do we experience any deficiency. A commonly held belief is that we somehow have to have an excess of them, whereas the fact is that we only need what we need. The daily requirement for most of them is tiny and once we have that, our bodies will tick along just fine. Despite the efforts of many scientists it is difficult to find an example of vitamins behaving therapeutically, that is that an excess of them is better for you in some way. One exception is vitamin B2 (riboflavin), used for treating keratoconus, a rare eye problem affecting the cornea in some people, but this has to be used as eye drops together with ultraviolet light, and vitamin B2 tablets aren't used at all. Another is vitamin B3 (niacin), which can help acne sufferers. Most of us in Western society, who are healthy and eat properly, don't have to worry about vitamins at all.

That said, vitamins are so absolutely fundamental to our biochemistry that it is a wonder the body could survive five minutes without them, and it is not surprising that deficiency will cause disease. These diseases though are not common in the UK, simply because most of us are wealthy enough to get what we need from our diets, but if you are ill, malnourished from whatever cause, or live in countries where diets are limited then you will need to be careful about vitamins.

Each so-called vitamin is in fact a composite of substances in the body that show similar biological activity. They are called by letters of the alphabet (thus vitamin A is a group of compounds called retinols and carotenoids which have similar biological activity), and include pro-vitamins – substances which aren't active themselves but are converted into active substances within the body (beta-carotene is one of these).

Vitamin A is fat-soluble, and this group of substances has two main functions, one to maintain eye health and the other in gene transcription, which enables target genes to be switched on and off and therefore has a role in embryology and immunology. It is a vitamin that is often lacking in populations in Africa – it affects approximately one-third of children under the age of five around the world causing blindness and death. This is because of early weaning and poor diet, such as too much grain and not enough fresh milk and an inadequate intake of fruit and vegetables. You never see dietary vitamin A deficiency in the UK, but you could see it in people who don't absorb their food properly though illness such as cancer or after some abdominal operations. I have never seen a case of vitamin A deficiency. Therefore it isn't a vitamin healthy people in the UK need to take in any shape or form, unless by prescription, and there are dangers in overdosage, because it is fat-soluble. Fat-soluble vitamins are stored in fat and therefore remain in the body for many months. Loads of carrot juice can cause liver damage, hair loss, blurred vision and headaches, and people have died from it. So save your money.

The term **Vitamin B** covers a multitude of substances, all very interesting. The one I had most experience of prescribing was vitamin B6, pyridoxine. For a long time we thought that B6 in high dosage could treat depression and PMT. I can't say that many people I treated with it were helped and eventually using B6 went out of fashion. There has never been any evidence that it works for PMT, and it is not a recommended treatment for any condition now. It has had some success in reducing morning sickness in a few studies, but evidence is mixed.[102] Pyridoxine deficiency is extremely rare even in developing countries where the diet is poor.

Too much B6 can cause neurological problems such as tingling and poor balance. I can't see any reason to buy it now although even I recommended it in the past.

Thiamine, Vitamin B1, on the other hand is something we can easily get deficient in. In the UK by far the most common cause of deficiency is too much alcohol. Associated with an excess of alcohol is often a very poor diet, as people don't eat well when they drink too much, but alcohol excess affects the level of thiamine in the body in many other ways. The result shows up in the brain as nerve cells are particularly dependant on thiamine and there are two common presentations that most doctors in the UK have seen, Wernicke's encephalopathy, and Korsakoff's psychosis. Both these cause serious brain damage and can also cause visual loss.

One of the first patients I treated when I was still a student was a woman in her fifties who had been living on the street and was obviously drinking a lot. She was acutely dehydrated and the first thing my consultant told me to do was to put up an intravenous drip, which contained thiamine and other vitamins. I was very proud that I was able to put up the drip, but then I found I had to do a manual evacuation of faeces because she was so constipated. That means inserting your finger up the rectum and pulling the hard impacted faeces down, not a very pleasant experience for either of us. When she was sorted out and some psychological tests were done she was found to have quite severe memory loss and so the damage had already been done. We never did find out very much of her history as she was unhappy staying in hospital and discharged herself as soon as she felt better. Sadly she probably didn't last long after that.

There is some evidence that people with diabetes can be deficient in thiamine because they lose it in the urine (along with glucose) and this may make kidney complications worse. So some studies recommend extra thiamine[103] for diabetic patients. In developing countries thiamine deficiency causes beriberi, a very serious disease that affects the heart, usually because of a poor diet. People eating brown rice will have plenty of thiamine but when the diet is changed to white rice a high proportion of thiamine is removed in the polishing process, and now that this is known people at risk are advised to eat brown rice.

Riboflavin (B2) is another vitamin that is absolutely critical for the body to be able to make certain important proteins. You can get a deficiency of it if your diet is poor or if you cannot absorb your food properly, but it is always associated with other vitamin deficiencies. The most obvious signs are include cracked and red lips, inflammation of the lining of mouth and tongue, mouth ulcers, cracks at the corners of the mouth. Riboflavin is yellow or yellow-orange in color and is used as a food colouring and to fortify some foods, such as baby foods, breakfast cereals, fruit drinks, vitamin-enriched milk products, and so on.

Niacin (B3) is another essential vitamin. Again a normal diet will give you plenty, and we only see problems with deficiency in developed countries where there is malnutrition from a poor diet or illness. Alcohol may also cause a deficiency of niacin. In poor countries severe deficiency causes pellagra, with symptoms such as diarrhoea, dermatitis, and dementia. It is toxic in high doses, having effects on blood sugar and skin problems amongst others.

Adenosine or adenine (B4) and **Pantothenic acid** (B5) are very important biochemical constituents of the body. However we can probably synthesize them ourselves. That does not stop some people considering they can make money by promoting them though!

Biotin (B7) is a water-soluble substance that is crucial for cell metabolism and is essential for cell growth. Biotin deficiency is rare because, in general, intestinal bacteria produce biotin in excess of the body's daily requirements. There are some people with genetic diseases which affect biotin metabolism but they are very rare and most of us don't have to worry about it.

Inositol (Vitamin B8), again, while an important biochemical constituent, it is probably produced by the cells themselves so is not a vitamin. There is no evidence that it has any effect on anxiety, depression or any of the other problems that it has been used for. There is no known deficiency although again that does not stop some people saying that there might be!

Folic acid (Vitamin B9) is a vitamin that had a huge effect on our practice. Folic acid is a fairly simple molecule that is in itself inactive but is converted into active metabolites (tetrahydrofolate and other derivatives) that are crucial to health and well-being. It is important for cells and tissues that are rapidly dividing, which of course includes cancer cells, so drugs that interfere with folate metabolism are used to treat cancer. There is plenty of folic acid in normal diets and actual deficiency is rare. However, to me, the most important problem with folic acid was its role in embryonic development.

The area in which I practised always had a very high incidence of spina bifida and other foetal neural tube defects; in fact it was nearly the highest in the UK. Spina bifida is a condition when the spinal cord does not develop properly in the foetus. The neural tube, which becomes the spinal cord, normally closes at about 6 weeks gestation, but in some foetuses it never does close. The spinal tissues are therefore exposed, and babies born with this condition would normally die soon after birth because infection would set in and could not be controlled. In any case as the neural tissues had not developed properly, the baby would be paralysed from the lesion down – usually below the waist. In the fifties and sixties neuro-surgeons developed a technique for closing off the exposed neural tissue, and if this was done soon after birth the baby would probably survive.

What wasn't realised at first though was that there was an associated, additional developmental abnormality in many of these babies higher up the spinal cord, and when the lesion in the lower spine was closed off there was an increase in pressure in the cerebrospinal fluid, which also circulates in the brain. The result was backpressure on the brain, and the baby's heads would then swell causing hydrocephalus (water on the brain). This causes severe brain damage to the babies' developing brains. So the result was at 6 weeks, you could have a baby alive, but with paralysis usually from the waist down, urinary and bowel incontinence, and in many cases brain damage. What an awful situation. Over the years in our practice, four babies with severe spina bifida were born, and each child is etched into my brain as I watched them grow up and all the problems they and the parents had.

In one case, the father of the child refused to consent to the operation on the grounds that the quality of life of the child would be too poor. He was overridden by the surgeons who persuaded the mother that it would be best for the child, as the condition was supposed to be 'mild'. The marriage did not last and the mother was left caring for this child who had everything – paralysis, incontinence, and severe mental retardation. The mother was brilliant and did everything for her. But the child died in her late teens of kidney failure – this was a direct result of backpressure on the kidneys due to poor emptying of the bladder.

In fact none of these babies made it into their twenties. Another child, the youngest of a large family where the mother was quite old when he was born, had very severe paralysis although his mental function was almost normal. By the time he was 10 though he had to have both legs amputated because of very poor circulation and he had innumerable operations on his bladder. When he was 11 his mother died of a heart attack (unrelated of course) and care of this child devolved to one of his elder sisters, who again devotedly looked after him, with a lot of help from social services. However it cost her her marriage. The child died of complications from sepsis of the stumps of his legs when he was 15.

The third child was less badly affected, was still confined to a wheelchair, but was mentally normal and was a happy child who went to school and had a reasonable quality of life, but she died at 17 due to recurrent brain infections. Like the others she had had a shunt inserted into the brain to drain off the excess pressure but it got infected more and more often and eventually she developed rip-roaring meningitis, which carried her off.

The fourth child was again quite severely disabled. He left our practice when he was four but I heard later that he had died when he was about seven. What a dreadful illness it could be, though I know that some people with spina bifida have very productive lives and a good prognosis.

Shortly after these children were born, two things happened. One was the discovery of alpha-fetoprotein, the protein that is found in a very high concentration in the amniotic fluid (the fluid which surround the baby) and also in the blood of their mothers where the baby has spina bifida. If this is measured at 18 weeks or so and it is found to be raised, a scan can be done specifically to diagnose spina bifida, and if found the mothers would be offered termination of pregnancy. Not surprisingly most took it. However this is where folic acid came in – it was shortly after this that folic acid deficiency in mothers was found to be a direct cause of neural tube abnormalities, as folic acid is crucial to the development of neural tissue, and even small deficiencies can lead to defects if they occur at a critical stage in pregnancy. Since then all expectant mothers have been prescribed folic acid in just the right dose, from 4 months before they expect to conceive, and this has almost totally prevented spina bifida. There have been no babies born with neural tube abnormalities in our practice since.

Folic acid is also prescribed for people taking certain medications that interfere with its metabolism, such as methotrexate, an anti cancer drug that is also used in several rheumatic diseases. It is also very important for doctors to know not to give folic acid to people with anaemia (it is very important in the synthesis of red blood cells) until they have ruled out pernicious anaemia, as folic acid can treat the anaemia but will also precipitate neural problems such as neuropathy in people who have B12 deficiency as well, as there is a complex interaction between the two vitamins. Folic acid is however reasonably safe in overdosage.

Cobalamin (B12) is another vitamin that causes specific deficiency, this time causing pernicious anaemia, a blood disease which is usually fatal. Everybody is aware that B12 is the vitamin that is found in high concentration in the liver, and the early treatment of pernicious anaemia was to eat over 2 pounds of raw liver a day – what an unpleasant thing to have to do. Nowadays it is given by injection and all GPs will have a few patients on regular, monthly or 3 monthly injections of B12. The interesting thing to me was that some patients seemed to become dependent on it, and were always asking for an injection long before the next one was due. If you then do their serum B12 levels they will be grossly over the maximum recommended level and so you then have to convince patients that they don't need it. I remember many an argument over it, and I still don't know if there is a physiological basis for this or whether it was just another example of the placebo effect – injections being a potent treatment is their own right. It isn't a simple deficiency – the root cause is actually an autoimmune disorder where intrinsic factor produced in the stomach is reduced because the body makes antibodies against it. Intrinsic factor is essential for the absorption of B12 so that people with stomach problems and after gastrectomy will also need regular injections, as it cannot be absorbed from food through the stomach. B12 tablets can be given to people who have B12 deficiency from other causes, as they would be able to absorb it.

Ascorbic acid (Vitamin C) is a simple organic compound which is absolutely essential for many critical biochemical processes including healing processes. It is also an antioxidant protecting the body against oxidative stress. It can be synthesised by most other organisms although some mammals, birds and some fish cannot do so. Humans cannot synthesise it so we have to have it in our diet. Deficiency causes scurvy, which if the deficiency is severe will lead to death within six months. The symptoms include open suppurating wounds and skin rashes. We can store a limited amount of vitamin C so symptoms may be delayed for a time. Scurvy of course was a huge problem on long ship voyages in the 15th to 17th centuries because food stores did not consists of anything fresh and cooking destroys it, and it was a long time before it was realised that vitamin C deficiency was the cause. Scurvy is hardly seen today except in very deprived populations as people only require a very tiny daily dose to enable all biochemical pathways to work perfectly, and this amount will be present in everyone's diet. There is no benefit at all in taking extra. Some people swear by it for preventing colds but if it has an effect it is a very small one even at high doses.

Cholecalciferol (Vitamin D) is a fascinating and very important vitamin. There are two methods of getting vitamin D, through your diet and from the skin, as sunlight catalyses a reaction that produces vitamin D from a cholesterol-based inactive precursor. This second method is by the far the most important and it is the reason why people in northern areas have pale skins. As we know, humans originated in Africa where, as it is near the equator, there is plenty of sunshine and it is easy to get vitamin D through sunlight even when you have a lot of pigment in the skin (to protect the skin from the damaging effects of sunlight). The populations living in Europe and Northern Asia descended from a group of humans who left Africa about 80,000 years ago, and as they migrated northwards their dark skins prevented the conversion of the vitamin D precursor to the active form, and they then began to suffer from the deficiency of vitamin D.

Vitamin D has many functions in the body but it is absolutely critical to the development of strong bones, so people without it suffer from rickets. Children are especially sensitive to the lack as they are laying down bone very rapidly (babies and young children have only cartilage and this is converted into bone by a process using vitamin D as they grow). This means that bones become deformed, with bowlegs being the most obvious sign, but there are manifestations all over the skeleton. In particular the pelvis, being another load-bearing area, can also be severely deformed. This has an immediate effect on childbirth, and mothers who had rickets in childhood often had pelvises which were so misshapen that the baby's head could not pass through at birth. These poor mothers therefore had obstructed labour and in these prehistoric times they and their unborn baby would inevitably die. This then through the process of natural section would mean that their genes would be taken out of the pool and the mothers with lighter skins who did not suffer from rickets would pass on their genes to their children. Over thousands of years this meant that the population as a whole became lighter skinned. A simple vitamin deficiency therefore influences the lightness of your skin.

There will of course be other factors that influenced the development of light skins, such as the amount of ultraviolet light in sunlight at different latitudes, and maybe the interaction with other genes, but vitamin D must be an important factor. The whole concept of race based on skin colour therefore is flawed and it is always so sad to see in countries like Brazil and India that the lighter-skinned people have such an advantage over their darker-skinned peers.

To digress somewhat, recently my husband and I were trying to farm rheas. These are birds of the ratite family, descended from a chicken-sized flightless bird, very much related to the dinosaurs, which lived in Gondwanaland, the continent that broke up into Africa, South America Australia and New Zealand. 50 million or more years ago that primitive bird grew into different species in each continent – Ostrich; Rhea and Darwin's rhea; Emu and Cassowary; Kiwi, Moa and 'Elephant Birds' in each respective area. Anyway, Rheas coming from South America lived in areas which had plenty of sun, and we were trying to farm them in Wales, a very cloudy and sun-deficient place for most of the year. The chicks were easy to hatch and were delightful, with yellow and brown stripes and ran around on their long legs very soon after hatching. But for three successive years a large proportion of the chicks gradually went off their legs and wasted away and died. We had no idea what was causing it although we thought it must be a vitamin or trace element deficiency of some sort.

At first vets to whom took the carcasses for a post mortem seemed equally unsure and several blamed an intestinal infection, Hexamitiasis, which might cause mal-absorption. Eradicating this infection made no difference unfortunately and the poor little chicks were still dying. Eventually it was a specialist vet who came up with the answer – rickets. The hen rheas were unable to get a big enough store of vitamin D to lay down in their eggs in our short sunless summer, and so the chicks very soon ran out of vitamin D to lay down in their long thin legs, which then weren't strong enough to bear their weight, and buckled. It was made worse by the reproductive strategy of rheas. The hen lays a very large number of eggs in a season and uses up a lot of her resources including Vitamin D in doing so, and takes no further part in the rearing. This is done by the male who gathers the eggs in a small nest on the ground and then sits on them for 40 days, and then when hatched, looks after the chicks (well actually it is more that the little chicks are programmed to run after him – there is not much actual looking after going on!) while the female wanders off into the sunset. Many modern women would wonder why this strategy has not been used for other species especially humans!

The strategy has worked very well for rheas for millions of years, but obviously not in Wales. So we made sure that the hens' diet was supplemented with extra vitamin D – and also we discovered that while the adult birds are vegetarians, the chicks are not and a big source of their vitamin intake is from insects, usually found round dung of other animals (Guanacos in South America) and the chicks needed to be outside very quickly to maximise their sun exposure. So despite the lack of sunshine we eventually did go a long way to having healthy rhea chicks.

Back to people then. We now know how important sunlight is in our cloudy islands. Rickets in babies and small children has been seen again in the UK recently after having been eradicated for years in the indigenous population, but dark skinned immigrants, especially those who culturally would expect to cover themselves at all times and do not often go out, are extremely vulnerable. Usually rickets affects babies who are born of mothers who already have osteomalacia, which is the adult form of rickets, and it is important to look out for this, although most doctors would not have come across a case themselves and so would be unlikely to think of it and do the necessary tests. This was the case where a child who was found to have multiple fractures died while he was being investigated. The doctors and social services thought that the parents had caused the fractures and they were arrested for the child's murder. It was only later that pathologists proved conclusively that the child's fractures were caused by rickets, yet the case had to be referred to the family court as well as the criminal court and so it was several months before the parents were allowed to have their second child back. What a terrible time for the parents who had done nothing wrong and were caring and good parents!

However, there is now a lot of publicity and research about vitamin D supplementation for people in the UK, as to whether slightly low levels of vitamin D in the blood – so-called sub-clinical vitamin D: marginal deficiency not amounting to actual osteomalacia or rickets – can be linked with conditions such as falls, cancer, cardiovascular disease, hypertension, immune problems and cognitive problems. Certainly vitamin D has been shown to be involved in various brain functions, since a vitamin D receptor has been found widely distributed in both the foetal and adult brain, and people are looking very hard at the value of vitamin D supplementation in people with dementia.[104] Observational studies have shown a possible link between low vitamin D levels and low cognitive test scores in patients with Alzheimer's disease. However there is no evidence that vitamin D deficiency can cause dementia at the moment, and the link may be an association not a cause.

Multiple sclerosis is a serious disease that shows a marked increase is incidence in populations as you travel northwards, and vitamin D shortfalls have been postulated as one of the causes of this. Currently in Scotland they are debating whether to supplement the diet of the whole population. Recently UK and Canadian scientists identified a mutated gene, which causes reduced levels of vitamin D, in 35 parents of children with Multiple Sclerosis and, in each case, the child inherited the gene.[105] The researchers thought that there was now enough evidence to carry out large-scale studies of vitamin D supplements for preventing multiple sclerosis.

There is some evidence that low levels of vitamin D in the elderly can contribute to an increased risk of falls.[106] Perhaps related to this, elderly women may also have an increased mortality when they have low levels of vitamin D, and elderly people are poor at absorbing calcium. Of course, before the menopause women are protected from osteoporosis by their female hormones. Osteoporosis in women after the menopause is caused by lack of exercise, poor bone mass and heredity, as well as some medical conditions, not vitamin D deficiency, but when doctors treat osteoporosis with any of the many treatments now available, calcium and vitamin D are essential to enable the bones to regenerate. Therefore the doctor treating osteoporosis often prescribes it.

There is no convincing evidence that vitamin D supplementation is necessary in elderly people for any of the other problems that have been linked with vitamin D.

Looking at the literature it seems that low levels of vitamin D are very common. A doctor friend of mine who is quite dark-skinned and lives in a country with lots of sunshine, and has a good diet, says that she is marginally vitamin D deficient, and so are many of the people she tests. One wonders what is going on here, and whether the reference ranges have been properly calculated. After all, the amount of vitamin D will depend greatly on whether it is summer or winter, and many populations may have much lower levels in the winter, yet this has been so for 80,000 years and we seem to have survived. This fact would be critical because as 82% of people in Scotland come out as deficient with the current ranges it won't be long before there is universal supplementation. Then if the reference ranges aren't correct we are going to get a lot of hypervitaminosis D or other side effects of vitamin D supplementation. It is getting to be a fad[107] like many others I experienced during my working life. Many GPs I know are prescribing vitamin D now, but I am sure it won't last. Some studies have shown that vitamin D can contribute to atherosclerosis and so heart disease, and some researchers have even suggested that fortification of so many foods with vitamin D can have had an effect on the increase in heart disease seen after the Second World War.[108] Other effects of too much vitamin D, particularly if you also supplement with calcium, are that the calcium levels in the blood rise and it may be deposited elsewhere on the system where it shouldn't normally be, producing kidney stones and overcalcification in the bones and tissues.

An explanation of my friend's experience would be that in populations where there has been plenty of sunlight over millennia, such as India, the natural blood level of vitamin D is low and it is very difficult to get the levels up to anything near what would be considered normal in Europeans, and if you try you risk giving too much. Another finding recently is that vitamin D levels will rise or fall depending on things like whether there is an infection in the body.[109] So altogether it is highly likely that Nature has got the balance right and supplementation of whole populations and widespread prescribing of vitamin D to healthy people is going to lead to problems in the future.

Tocopherol and similar substances (Vitamin E complex) are fat-soluble and are an important anti-oxidant. Anti-oxidants, as you might think, are molecules that inhibit the oxidation (the process of transferring electrons to an oxidizing agent) of other substances, in the process of so doing they themselves get oxidised. The importance of this lies in the fact that oxidation reactions can produce free radicals (molecules or atoms with unpaired electrons, thus carrying an electric charge) that can cause damage to, or death of a cell. It was thought that this process might be one of the causes of cancer, when the cells are damaged and then go out of control. Although oxidation reactions are crucial for life, they can also be damaging, and all living organisms have developed their own types of anti-oxidants. Anti-oxidants would also play a part in oxidative stress in various human diseases such as cancer and stroke. However, though it was hoped that vitamin E would be something that would improve people's health, and lots of research has been done, there is no evidence that there is any benefit at all from taking excess vitamin E and indeed it may be harmful.

Phytomenadione (Vitamin K) is needed by humans for blood clotting. Older children and adults get most of their vitamin K from bacteria in the gut, and some from their diet but babies are sometimes deficient, because Vitamin K does not cross the placenta to the developing baby, and the gut does not have any bacteria to make vitamin K before birth. After birth, there is little vitamin K in breast milk and breastfed babies can be low in vitamin K for several weeks until the normal gut bacteria start making it. Infant formula has added vitamin K, but even formula-fed babies have very low levels of vitamin K for several days. So newborn babies are routinely given one injection of vitamin K to prevent haemorrhagic disease of the newborn, which used to occur in rare circumstances. Vitamin K is essential for making prothrombin and other clotting factors, which is why severe bleeding can occur without it. It has been used for over 20 years and is extremely safe. It is also essential for bone growth. There are lots of diseases that can cause vitamin K deficiency, from malnutrition, bowel problems such as malabsorption, or liver or biliary diseases that also cause poor absorption, to many other diseases of the blood such as leukaemia, and many drugs cause it. However if you are healthy with a good diet, you are most unlikely to have a problem. It is, however, one of the first things a doctor will try to exclude if you are suffering from any sort of bleeding disorder.

There's also another form of vitamin K, **menaquinone**, known as vitamin K2. I'd never heard of this when I was a GP but recent research suggests it has a role in activating calcium-binding enzymes, thus helping bone synthesis and preventing calcium ending up being deposited where it's not supposed to be, such as in arteries. Some trials (not all) show benefits of supplementation for people with osteoporosis. Certainly if you don't have osteoporosis, you're likely to be able to get all you need from poultry, dairy (especially cheese), and eggs.

By now you will probably have realised that I do not see any need at all for a large industry supplying vitamin supplements to the general public. The whole edifice depends on half-truths, little-understood science and very effective publicity. Until 1985 doctors could prescribe any vitamin for any purpose on the NHS, but in that year a limited list of drugs available on the NHS was brought in, and vitamin pills were excluded except when there was good evidence of actual vitamin deficiency (for instance by measuring the level of the vitamin in the blood). So now doctors will regularly prescribe those vitamins such as thiamine, folic acid, vitamin B12 and vitamin D when specifically needed, and will sometimes prescribe multivitamins in people with poor nutrition due to alcohol, cancer, and other debilitating diseases. No one else needs vitamins, ever. If you think you have a vitamin deficiency, but you don't suffer from severe diseases for which you would be under the care of a doctor anyway, then you almost certainly don't have one, and you should see your doctor about this supposed deficiency and get a proper diagnosis.

Part 6

Diagnosis

Chapter 20
Investigations: how far should a GP investigate patients before referral to a hospital specialist?

Commonly used blood tests – over-investigation – tumour markers – interface between primary and secondary care – effective use of resources

In the UK the GP is the gatekeeper, and his job has been to try to sort out the patient's problem first. But what incentive is there for him to do that? In our area for a long time the most popular GPs were always the ones who didn't try very hard to sort out the problem, and these were the ones who sent half their evening surgeries down to the hospital, either as an emergency or by writing a letter (always marked 'urgent') to Outpatients. This used to drive some hospital doctors mad as very few of these patients needed to be seen at all. From the perspective of those appraising the GP, if they thought this was happening they might mark the doctor down for remedial action. But some patients were usually quite satisfied with this strategy – they got excellent attention from lots of doctors and if there was nothing wrong at the end that was even better. The GPs who tried very hard to solve a patient's problem and then referred late were likely to end up being sued.

Not many GPs send everyone to hospital nowadays of course. It definitely would be negligent if a GP did not do essential blood tests at the very least to see which speciality the patient needed to go to. For instance, for a patient with TATT (tired all the time), a very common condition in general practice, the differential diagnosis is huge but many serious conditions can be ruled out using simple blood tests. A full blood count could indicate anaemia, leukaemia, some cancers, many sorts of infection, including viral infections, some allergies, and clotting problems, by looking in detail at the cells normally found in the blood. The process is entirely automated now with each cell in the blood being measured for size and configuration. If the test shows up an abnormality the lab would make a film of the blood on a slide for a pathology expert to look at, and that will show even more detail about any blood problems. It costs pennies, and is often included in screening people without symptoms at all. There is no reason for GPs to skimp on this test; it can provide crucial information if there is a physical reason for the symptoms and if normal will go a long way to reassuring patient and doctor. Although rare, leukaemia is one illness that every patient and GP will hope is diagnosed immediately, and in most cases all it needs is this one test. When it isn't done, and the leukaemia isn't picked up until it has been there for some time, at the very least treatment is more difficult and the delay can be fatal.

Most laboratories now also do a simple test for non-specific inflammation and this can be a most informative test, giving indications of many autoimmune disorders, general health and infections. We usually used an ESR (erythrocyte sedimentation rate), which measures the rate at which red blood cells settle to the bottom of a tube. It is influenced by many factors, but with many types of inflammation in the blood the amount of certain proteins increases and this causes the red cells to stick together and so fall faster. Fortunately, this test is entirely automated now and is still frequently used, although there are other markers for inflammation such as plasma viscosity and C-reactive protein, again depending on exactly which proteins in the blood have become abnormal.

A very high ESR (over a hundred) in general practice usually means one of three things – polymyalgia rheumatica (a fairly common inflammatory rheumatological disorder) and related conditions, cancer such as multiple myeloma (where the cancer affects the bone marrow), or a severe infection, and the patient is likely to look and feel ill. One patient in her fifties, though, who didn't seem all that ill, had an ESR of 103 and clearly had multiple myeloma indicated by the other tests. She didn't need any further investigation done by me and I admitted her immediately. She did very well, surviving 12 years after bone marrow transplants and chemotherapy. Another patient had polymyalgia rheumatica and this is easy to treat with steroids, so has a much better prognosis. It is very unusual to have levels as high as that though, and most ESR tests that come back abnormal are just above normal and may not mean very much at all. But it is an indicator that something isn't right and of a need for more tests.

Then there is the test for kidney function, urea and electrolytes, which not only indicates if your kidneys are OK (although would not come back abnormal unless your kidneys were failing pretty badly) but also the concentration of sodium, potassium, and other ions in your body, and will give an indication of your general health. It is widely done but is not nearly as useful as the full blood count.

This blood test can't wait around, as if the tube containing the blood doesn't get to the lab quickly the blood will haemolyse (all the red blood cells break up), and this releases a lot of potassium into the blood, invalidating the results. This is a common reason why blood results don't come back and tests have to be repeated.

But then there are other commonly used tests that are less likely to give a positive result unless they are done with at least a small suspicion clinically that they may be abnormal. Endocrine tests for thyroid hormone, or male and female hormones, are done in many situations. The GP would have listed the differential diagnoses and do only the relevant tests but it is a temptation to go on ordering more tests at the same time as a sort of fishing expedition. This is where it gets tricky and some doctors undoubtedly cast the net too wide.

In a recent study of over 7 countries, 61% of doctors said they conducted more investigations than they needed to because of worries about being sued.[110] When in hospital the poor old patient may actually get anaemic from so much blood-taking. 'Diagnostic blood loss' from phlebotomy in patients with acute myocardial infarction (heart attacks) is associated with hospital-acquired anaemia, according to an *Archives of Internal Medicine* study.[111] They suggest reducing the risk for hospital-acquired anaemia by using the smaller children's blood tubes or simply filling adult tubes with less blood! Such anaemia is highly unlikely to happen in general practice of course, although with children it can be a big issue. We do try to keep venepuncture in children to a minimum in general practice.

When considering more complicated tests in primary care there are several issues, such as whether it is beneficial to patients and saves money if GPs do more tests in primary care. The bottom line for doctors should be – can the result of this test change the management of the patient? If it can then even a very expensive test is going to be worthwhile; if it can't, and the next step is going to be the same, then you would have to think very carefully before ordering the test. Also, doctors should develop the habit of considering carefully what the result of a false test result would be – both on the patient, and on the cost of ordering very many more unnecessary investigations. At present this is very low on the list for most doctors, especially hospital doctors.

In the current financial climate there is going to be more pressure for GPs to do more investigations, but many family doctors say they really are too busy to do investigations that are now done in hospitals. What incentive is there for GPs to do more when it is easier, possibly safer, and less likely to end up with the GP being sued, to send patients to hospital? But the fact is that GPs are now extremely well trained and are also very expensive. The average GP principal in 2011 earned just over £100,000 and even young sessional doctors earned over £60,000. People in cash-strapped GP commissioning groups may argue that if GPs merely send most people to hospital without prior investigation then they are not worth the money they are being paid. They are being paid to take responsibility, not to be a tick-box operative – if that is what is needed you can employ a health care assistant with a clipboard. GPs do need to show that they are giving value for money.

The number of tests and investigations that can be done in hospital is huge. With the bill for medical negligence running very high there seems to be every reason for further investigation and not a lot in favour of not doing tests. There is of course a downside. The ease with which doctors can now get tests done and results reported back within a few days means that there is no brake on what is done. There aren't many studies looking in detail at whether investigations done either by GPs or by hospital doctors are necessary. There is no doubt that there is a lot of waste and reduplication of tests, although this is probably improving as waiting times for hospital appointments get shorter. It is still commonplace for all the blood tests done by GPs before referral to be repeated without looking at the results already available. There is also a big variation in the numbers of tests done by different doctors for the same conditions.

One problem is that, although the NHS is one organisation, there have been separate budgets for primary care and secondary care for some time – even before the current trend to introduce market forces. Therefore the bill for GP tests goes to the primary care trust and that for hospitals goes to the hospital trust. But the waiting times are common to both so where there hasn't been enough investment in making the tests available there is a tendency for hospital doctors to deny access to these tests to GPs in primary care. At present most managers are working on the assumption that more should be done in primary care, as this would streamline the system. So a big task is to develop pathways and make sure that every doctor knows which investigations they ought to be doing.

NICE is certainly looking at the problem and now gives guidance on what tests should not be done as well as those which should, and the American College of Physicians has also come up with a list of diagnostic tests that are a waste of money in certain situations, such as serology testing for suspected early Lyme disease and brain natriuretic peptide (BNP) in the initial evaluation of typical heart failure findings – but see *Cardiology* for my opinion on this.

A theme in this book is to discuss the rules by which GPs can be denied access to important investigations. As discussed earlier it is not self-evident that GPs can use all tests which are newly introduced into the Health Service, usually on cost grounds and also on the grounds that GPs do not have the knowledge to use the new tests appropriately. Blood tests, however, are usually available as soon as they are developed, but some will be restricted, the decisions being made by consultant pathologists together with specialists.

Tumour markers are a case in point. They are tests for proteins (usually) that have been developed to follow the progress of some cancers. These proteins are produced by the cancer cells, and as the cells multiply they produce far more of the tumour markers than usual and these build up in the blood and can be measured. Sometimes other changes in metabolism that come with cancer can cause the concentration of certain markers to rise. The well-known markers are prostate specific antigen (PSA), produced normally by the prostate gland but in excess when some of the cells become cancerous, Ca125 for ovarian and uterine cancer, and CEA (carcinoembryonic antigen), another tumour marker which is raised in many sorts of cancers especially bowel cancers. They became widely available about 10 years ago and GPs could ask for them too, and most of us did.

Consider ovarian cancer. Even now ovarian cancer has a very poor prognosis, not because they aren't good methods of treatment – there are – but because diagnosis is hardly ever made early enough.

I certainly remember a sixty year old woman who came back several times with vague symptoms and whom I referred to general surgery. But she waited a long time and eventually the surgeon at operation found advanced ovarian cancer. The oncologists were brilliant and she had over three more years of good quality life. But her symptoms unfortunately were extremely non-specific and very common in women who do not have ovarian cancer – bloating, abdominal swelling, and wanting to pass water frequently, for example. Every GP will see hundreds of women complaining of these in a year, and usually none of them will have ovarian cancer. So GPs will often be castigated by patients groups and consultants for not making the diagnosis early when the patient eventually turns out to have ovarian cancer. Therefore many GPs realised that the tumour marker for ovarian cancer, Ca125, a protein that cancer cells in the ovary will produce in many cases, might be very useful for initial diagnosis as well as for monitoring of treatment. Women who complain of bloating and waterworks problems in whom the GP has no reason to suppose there is anything gynaecologically wrong – for instance periods are normal or an internal examination is normal – can have the test and once in a while the result will be higher than normal, immediately ringing alarm bells. I did exactly this in 2003 and found a woman with a raised Ca125 who did indeed have a gynaecological cancer. She was treated and has done very well.

But then there were questions raised by specialists that GPs were doing too many of these tests and soon guidance came from above that Ca125 should not be used for this purpose. There was a very influential article in the BMJ in 2009 written by a panel of experts. It was a case study of a woman with abdominal swelling, which was investigated by a GP including a Ca125 test. This was high and the GP sent the lady to a gynaecologist, but it was soon found that in fact she had a severe liver problem, cirrhosis, which was causing the swelling, and so she had then had to be referred to a liver specialist. The high Ca125 had been a red herring and so the correct treatment of cirrhosis had been slightly delayed. The consultants then told the GPs exactly what tests should have been done. But they are not GPs and they had no expertise in primary care diagnosis, so this was very patronising. They also said that a retrospective audit had shown that some patients could have been falsely reassured on the basis of negative Ca125 tests, and opined that 'Appropriate requesting therefore means restricting use of tumour marker measurement to patients already known to have the disease.'

Now normally I find the BMJ an enormously helpful and sensible journal, but this I thought this article was very wrong. It all depends on your perspective – a specialist sees nothing but ovarian cancer and is an expert on investigation and treatment on the patients that she sees. I noted that this case study was part of a series on the use of diagnostic tests, but I saw no mention of a GP on the panel. But first a specialist has to get patients referred to them, and a GP who may see one case of ovarian cancer every 10 years and patients with exactly the same symptoms a hundred times a year has an entirely different perspective. Obviously anything that can help narrow down the enormously high number to a more select group will be helpful and I know many GPs ignored this advice. Yes, GPs could be a bit more careful (apparently a sixth of the tests done in one area were on men!) and it is essential to do a full examination and other tests such as scans before referral, but this test and others like it are extremely helpful. So I was very relieved to read that in 2011 NICE had looked at this in detail and finally came up with much more sensible advice, that Ca125 is an investigative test for ovarian cancer, and GPs should be carrying out the test fairly frequently, on the following people:

Women with the following symptoms on a persistent or frequent basis:

- Persistent abdominal distension (women often refer to this as 'bloating')
- Feeling full (early satiety) and/or loss of appetite
- Pelvic or abdominal pain
- Increased urinary urgency and/or frequency.

Although a negative test does not entirely rule out cancer a positive one might save a life. See NICE for the full guidance. It still shouldn't be used in a 'fishing expedition' though, as a false positive is very worrying.

CEA (see above) and CA19.9 tumour markers are other markers that GPs often use. I personally have not found them very helpful, but other GPs I know use them. The well-known test, PSA for prostate cancer, is fully covered in the section on Urology.

Cooperation between specialists and GPs can of course be extremely helpful. Recently a concept of 'shared care' has been developed, where GPs and specialists agree to treat the patients jointly so that, for instance, blood tests can be ordered by the hospital doctor but carried out by the GP. Then the specialist team gives the GP advice to make sure say that the dosage of the medication is altered appropriately according to the results of the test. This is common in Rheumatology and also can be done for routine blood monitoring of warfarin in INR (International Normalised Ratio of the level in the blood) clinics. Warfarin is a drug used to prevent blood clots happening in places in the body where they shouldn't, causing strokes and clots in the lung, and other problems. It is very effective but the concentration of the drug in the blood has to be kept within very strict limits, because if it too high the blood won't clot at all leading to bleeding from places where normally the body's own blood clotting systems would stop it. This can be life-threatening.

When warfarin was first used hospitals set up INR clinics but patients had to have the blood tests very frequently and this was very difficult for them if they lived a long way from the hospital. So GPs started to do them in their surgeries (the pioneering ones first did them themselves) but hospitals soon saw this as an very good method of saving money and asked GPs to do more and more. GPs would usually be slightly out of pocket as they employ the phlebotomists who take the blood. GPs therefore campaigned to get some recompense and it was a bit of a fight. Eventually the GP contract was altered to allow GPs to be paid according to how much of the task they take on, although they don't have to do it if they don't think they have the expertise. Nowadays GPs will also alter the dose of the warfarin taken by the patient according to various computerised algorithms. But it is still a tricky business getting the dose quite right. There are several promising drugs where the level of the drug in the blood is not so crucial. These will be expensive of course but if they are as effective as warfarin then the money saved by not having all these clinics and tests would go towards the cost of the drugs and patients would be very grateful to be spared so much monitoring.

In general patients want to reduce the number of expensive and difficult journeys for tests at the hospital and welcome GPs doing them at their surgeries, so this can be an excellent arrangement. When this is working well there is a written arrangement between GP and hospital so that accountability is clear, and each doctor involved knows exactly what his responsibilities are. It is an extremely efficient way of managing certain long-term conditions.

But where such an arrangement does not exist the GPs find themselves being asked in a hospital letter to do a test, but with no information as to why or what should happen next. If it were easy to ring up the hospital doctor it would be acceptable but this is rarely possible, and in any case takes a lot of time. So GPs are not happy doing tests in their surgeries in these circumstances, but if they do not do them as asked, and send the patient back to the hospital, the patients are annoyed and treatment is delayed. There is a very easy solution to this problem. When the hospital doctor wants the GP to do the test she can write out the form and give it to the patient. The patient the takes the form to the surgery and the nurse or phlebotomist will do the test. But then crucially the result will go back to the hospital doctor, on whose desk it lands so that the next decision is hers, and the GP knows that the patients' care is being continued in a seamless fashion. It is amazing though how each generation of junior doctors in hospital takes a long time to learn this very simple courtesy.

Of course patients need to play their part too. One man has cost the NHS tens of thousands of pounds by faking illnesses – even claiming to be a haemophiliac with AIDS and coughing up fake blood to get a room to himself. Now he has been banned from entering any hospital or other NHS building unless genuinely in need of medical attention[112] This may be an extreme case but Munchausen syndrome where people will fabricate illness for various reasons but often just to get attention is not as uncommon as you might think!

From the USA – A Congressional Budget Office estimates that 'up to 5% of the nation's (the US) gross national product is spent on tests and procedures that do not improve patient outcomes'.[113] It is important to understand that again business interests loom very large here. The industry of developing tests and investigations is very successful and every speciality has been immensely improved by having accurate tests with which to diagnose illnesses, but sometimes at the expense of over-diagnosis and actual patient harm.

Chapter 21
Radiology: screening, ordering tests and issues surrounding private screening services for the 'worried well'

Plain X-rays – barium studies – MRI and CAT scanners – private screening – endoscopies – access for GPs – getting enough radiological equipment.

The growth of radiology as a speciality over the years has been spectacular and many of the big successes in diagnosis of serious disease have been due to developments such as magnetic resonance imaging (MRI) scanners, computed tomography (CAT) scanners, fluoroscopy and so on. GPs in the UK have been able to order plain X-rays, such as X-rays of bones looking for fractures or chest X-rays which are very useful for diagnosing serious disease of the chest, without having to be skilled at actually reading and interpreting them. Consultant radiologists report on all X-rays performed at the request of GPs so that patients can be absolutely sure that the result is accurate. In many hospitals chest X-rays are almost open access – the GP can send the patient down immediately for a chest X-ray without appointment. Most other simple X-rays are done quickly and the patient only has to wait short time, sometimes only hours, and the report is on the GP's desk.

At the present time barium studies for the bowel are available quite quickly, although in the early years of their development there were some restrictions. Nowadays barium meals and barium enemas are not the first investigation for bowel cancer, but they are still used to diagnose other conditions such as diverticulosis. As each new investigation came onstream they tended to be confined to hospitals and GPs had to refer to a specialist in order for them to be performed. But many are available privately, and body scans now are commonly advertised to the general public. They are generally aimed at the 'worried well' and can be CT scans, MRI scans, or other modern technologies.

Whole-body CT scans are a current fad; they are advertised to the general public who have no specific symptoms at all (otherwise they would presumably go to their GP for free) by companies specializing in this, and of course they may pick up serious abnormalities. But this is extremely rare, and most often if anything is found it is a minor abnormality which would never harm the patient. Nevertheless the patient is of course recommended to go to their GP to have it 'checked out'. Usually this means onward referral (as the company is employing 'specialists' and a GP often cannot argue with it), further tests and a merry-go-round of hospital visits, worry and expense to everybody – exactly what a private system would be designed to provide, but not what is needed in a publicly funded system.

I recently saw an advertisement for a private service which provided such scans. The advertisement used an example of a very satisfied patient who had had such a scan and an abdominal aneurysm found which was then treated by the NHS and the patient's life was saved. Now an abdominal aneurysm is one of the conditions that really do need to be picked up early, as an operation before it bursts is far more likely to be successful than in those admitted as an emergency. So this was indeed a success but what it did not say was that the NHS is already implementing selective screening. By 2013, the programme will invite all men for screening during the year they turn 65 while men aged over 65 can self-refer for screening. Men who have an aneurysm detected through screening will be offered treatment or monitoring depending on the size of the aneurysm.

There are also conditions called berry aneurysms in the brain, which may be there from young adulthood on and can cause strokes. (It is said that both Felix Mendelssohn and his sister died from these).[114] These again can be treated if found before they burst. We know that if you are over 50 years, female, or a current cigarette smoker, or you use cocaine, you are more likely to get an intracranial aneurysm. However if you screen asymptomatic patients without risk factors, there don't seem to be any benefits. Because such aneurysms are quite rare, and those that people do have aren't very likely to rupture, together with the potential complications of treating them (which can be quite risky), screening of asymptomatic patients is not a good idea. Even screening of patients with a positive family history of ruptured intracranial aneurysm is controversial. There may be benefits of screening people with one affected first-degree relative[115] (so Mendelssohn might have been saved as his sister died first) but not those with a less definite family history. In fact these people will be offered a scan under most health systems, and certainly will be on the NHS. You need only go and ask your GP.

But the company (obviously) wanted to widen the appeal of the service to a bigger audience, so the headline of the advertisement read something like 'a headache might have really serious causes and any one with a headache needs this service to prevent a stroke'. It then related the case of the person with the abdominal aneurysm. Although everything in this advert is true, it is nevertheless very misleading, as it is well known that the way to prevent strokes is actually to have a healthy lifestyle, keep your cholesterol down and have blood pressure treated well.

If you have plenty of money and nothing else to spend it on then by all means have a private scan but for the greatest good for the greatest number this is not the way forward. If you do not have money to burn, then so long as the NHS continues to be adequately funded people can rest assured that they do not have to spend their hard earned cash on such things.

Definite harm can be done to patients by these scans. There was a patient who had a whole body scan which picked up a small tumour which was very inaccessible. The patient was persuaded (in a private system) to have an operation to remove it, and died of complications.

The risks of over over-investigation in radiology are not negligible. The World Health Organisation classifies X-rays as a carcinogen. The risks are very low for plain X-rays, while the radiation in a barium meal, for instance, is the equivalent of a few years' worth of background radiation and has a 1 in 1000 to 1 in 10,000 chance of causing cancer. CT scans use large doses and increase the risk of developmental problems and cancer. Wikipedia states that 'It is estimated that 0.4% of current cancers in the United States are due to CT scans performed in the past and that this may increase to as high as 1.5-2% with 2007 rates of CT usage.' The problem is not the one investigation you have every now and then but the cumulative effect, especially on the elderly, of so many scans, and we do have to be careful to use such investigations sparingly.

MRI scanning is safer. The reason why my Australian colleagues (see Chapter 1) were able to order MRI scans in children was because so many doctors were asking for CT scans which were more readily available and cheaper, but with a risk of exposing the children to developmental cancers. So the federal government started a scheme which would allow them to ask for MRI scans at a lesser cost. The Australian GPs were by far the happiest and most satisfied GPs at the conference I went to. They had full access to MRI scanning and many other hospital-based radiology tests without the patient having to see a specialist first. They said it worked very well. According to many of my friends who have done GP stints down under, the Australian system is excellent and a joy to work in. It isn't due to any excess of MRI scanners either. In 2010 Australia had 5.6 MRI units per million people, and the UK had 5.9. Austria had over 18 and the US had 31.6![116]I started this book by talking about the shortage of MRI scanning machines. They have been a wonderful invention which will safely diagnose many cancers at an early stage, and many other conditions. GPs in the UK however still cannot order a scan directly, even privately when the patient is insured. The insurers will not pay for it unless asked for by a consultant, who will of course expect to see the patient first. This causes further delays for the patient and the insurance company will have to pay for both the MRI scan and the consultant fee. It doesn't have to be like this.

The question of which doctors should be allowed to order such tests is an important one. MRI scans are expensive and are a direct cost to the NHS. It is different in a private, fee-for-service, system like in the USA or in places on the continent. There, the more MRI scans that are done the better, as the patient pays for them, either directly or through an insurance company. They provide money for the makers of MRI scans, the radiographers who work them, and the radiologists who read them and recommend whether treatment is advisable. In the USA scanners are two a penny and everyone expects a scan for any significant problem. Hence the very high number of scanners.

But in a system with finite resources funded by the taxpayer there must be a way of restricting the use of MRI scans. That system worked essentially by preventing GPs from having access to them. The argument that managers and radiologists would make is that if a MRI scan was needed the patient should see a specialist first. But of course this meant that waiting lists to see the consultant to get a MRI scan built up, and the patient who really needed it suffered. So it just transferred the pressure from one part of the system to another. Indeed the whole problem of waiting lists was in part a manufactured one as GPs had to send the patient to hospital for some conditions because they could not organise the tests themselves.

According to some specialists I spoke to when I was working as a medical manager, GPs were not well trained enough to know when to ask for these tests and therefore would waste precious NHS resources. But that wasn't a fair answer. Early on in the NHS GPs possibly were not well trained enough to use X-rays properly and were too busy to investigate patients themselves. However in the last 20 years or so the standards of training of GPs in the UK have been extremely high and many GPs would like direct access.

In the early days of the NHS there were other agendas. Hospital specialists were guarding their ivory towers and needed to have patients referred to them as early as possible, not only for the benefit of the patient but also to increase their power and prestige. In any system where there are not enough facilities to go round people will fight over them, and the specialists held all the cards. I am quite certain that some patients with severe problems such as cancer or nerve root damage were not diagnosed early enough under that system.

Undoubtedly the best way forward would be for there to be an evidence base behind the rationing, so that GPs would be allowed to ask for a MRI scans under certain circumstances, according to such evidence.

How would GPs perform if they were given access? I did a review of MRI scans done for patients in our practice some years ago, including the 25 per year arranged by us at the private hospital locally (these were ones that the patients paid for out of their own pockets as insurance companies would not do this), and also including ones arranged by the hospital after the patient had waited to see the specialist. The results were interesting. They showed that 80% of the scans arranged by us showed a significant abnormality that warranted further investigation or treatment, compared with only 32% of abnormalities found in scans requested by doctors at the local hospital. So despite the fact that we were dealing with an unsorted group of patients, and that a normal MRI can be very appropriate if it prevents the patient thereby being referred unnecessarily to hospital, we were very accurate, under this very restrictive system, in finding significant abnormalities and certainly would not be misusing public money. Of course people will say this isn't a proper study and of course it wasn't but I have not come across any research showing that GPs are not good at choosing which patients to send for MRI scans.

I also looked at MRI scans done on our patients requested by doctors at larger specialist hospitals, and the rate of abnormalities was 94% – this was expected, as the population they were dealing with were patients who were already known to have problems (they had usually been referred onwards by our local orthopaedic consultants for more specialised care). Interestingly the rate of abnormalities in MRI scans asked for by consultants after private referral by us was only 30%. If a patient is seen in a private clinic and is covered by insurance then there is no brake at all on demand for scans and so theoretically as many could be done as in a private system such as the USA.

I found that of the patients referred by us to a local GP who specialized in physical treatment of back problems (he did manipulation and injections) none was referred on for MRI scans during that period, despite the fact that this doctor had access to MRI scans at the private hospital paid for by the NHS. We were sending the right sort of patient to him and he was happy to manage them without further investigation because he was extremely knowledgeable in his field.

In all cases of course there is a balance to be found between investigating enough patients to be sure that you are not missing anything, and over-investigation.

There was also a big demand for orthopaedic scans, as plain X-rays can be very misleading, especially of the spine. The plain X-rays are often reported on as having various degrees of spondylosis and arthritis, but not many of these changes were significant. One radiologist sensibly would report X-rays not as having so much spondylosis or degeneration but as 'a typical 70-year-old spine'. This was much easier to explain to patients! What GPs and their patients really wanted to know from X-rays of the spine was whether there was any pressure on the nerves coming out of the spinal cords, as these might lead to nerve damage and disability, unless specific treatment was given. But ordinary X-rays did not tell you that. There was a temptation therefore for GPs to ask for MRI scans, which would give this information. But MRI scans for back problems are strongly discouraged. The American College of Physicians has a list of diagnostic tests that are a waste of money and it includes imaging studies for nonspecific low back pain. Therefore GPs, like all doctors, should follow certain very tight guidelines when they ask for such tests. But junior doctors with far less experience than GPs could ask for radiology tests freely once the patient was in hospital.

Knee MRI scans can be particularly useful as they give a lot of detail about cartilage and ligament problems that are not shown up on plain X-ray. We had meetings between GPs and consultants and agreed that local guidelines for knee investigation should say that for knee pain in the under age 20s an X-ray is the best choice. You are looking for fairly simple conditions here, and a straight X-ray should be sufficient. However there are still pockets of areas where GPs are sometimes denied access, against evidence. For instance, there is evidence that for patients with osteoarthritis of the knees, a standing rather than lying X-ray is the best test. This is because it is then evident when there is a diminution of joint space, a hallmark of osteoarthritis. When patients are lying down this is not necessarily obvious and a patient may be said to have no problem when they in fact have marked arthritis of the knee. Yet in our area all knee X-rays are done with the patient lying down, against current guidelines. When GPs pointed this out to radiologists, they said that the extra time and effort in getting standing X-rays, which might be more difficult in the elderly population in question, would be too expensive. They preferred to re–X-ray the patient when they got to clinic, usually many months later, ignoring the fact that as some patients would have been erroneously said not to have arthritis, they would never have got to outpatients. So although initially agreeing with the GPs, the consultants and managers nevertheless managed to prevent GPs getting the investigation that best evidence at the time said they should get.

For people with knee pain between the ages of 20 to 55, MRI scans are much better than straight X-rays as MRI scans pick up cartilage problems (cartilage does not show on X-rays, only bones do). For the over 60s though, an X-ray is again the best primary investigation for knee pain. X-rays will readily show arthritis which is very common in this group and an MRI scan can be done if the radiologist feels more detail is needed. An MRI scan can show up so many abnormalities that it is difficult to know what to treat. However there are wide variations in recommendations from different sources.

In the future, with GP commissioning, it should be possible for GPs to have direct access to MRI for knees and shoulders under strict guidelines. Most areas already have access to MRI scans for back pain when there are risk factors for pressure on the nerves from the spinal cord. Usually GPs would need to update themselves regularly in their Continual Professional Development (CPD) learning to improve their skills in interpreting MRIs, and this should relieve the load on orthopaedic clinics.

It is possible that advances in technology and increasingly sensitive testing are now driving over-diagnosis of many conditions. One such is thyroid cancer. The number of people diagnosed with thyroid cancer has risen two and a half times from 1975 to 2005, because of improvements in techniques of ultrasound scans and fine needle biopsy, yet the death rate has remained constant and quite low, and extremely low in younger people. Although treatment is very successful it seems unlikely that this is the whole story. Early in 2002 I had a young patient, a girl in her late teens, who was diagnosed and treated for thyroid cancer. Everything went well, but she was a very anxious girl, and soon after she had a bout of very severe depression, which the psychiatrist thought was related to the stress of the diagnosis. She took an overdose but fortunately recovered. Now I wonder whether she may have been one of those who would never have had any problems with the thyroid cancer, as it seems that many of these 'extra' cases would never have caused problems. Or perhaps she would have had depression anyway. It shows how difficult it is when tests pick up a diagnosis that has to be treated.

MRI scans are safer than plain X-rays but require careful interpretation so that non significant unusual appearances are not investigated further causing worry and distress to the patient and cost to the Health Service. Of course in a fully private system this would not be an issue – the more investigations done the better and the patient is always of the opinion that 'better safe than sorry'. For ultrasound scans the risks are lower as they use sound waves not radiation, and these are an investigation of choice in the areas where they are useful – obstetrics, gynaecology and abdominal scans for gallstones for instance. But in the past GPs were often restricted in their access to abdominal ultrasound.

Another important set of investigations is endoscopy. This means looking inside a patient with an endoscope and it may be a colonoscope, into the bowel, a gastroscope into the stomach or a hysteroscope looking into the womb. Endoscopies, like MRI scans, are extremely useful. Radiologists, surgeons and gastrointestinal specialists will all do them in different hospital departments. These days nurses also do them very competently, having gone on special courses to learn how to do them. This will immediately increase the number that can be performed. In some places GPs can do them too, and it would be very useful to do these in large practices and very convenient for patients.

The hope is that with the power to commission going to GPs under the current reforms to the NHS, GPs themselves will be able ensure that such important investigations are done in primary care wherever possible. This may well increase the need for more training of GPs, but GPs are highly paid and there is a real need to use their extensive training to the full. There might not be a huge increase in the number of investigations being done anyway as many of these would have been done by the hospital anyway. In the past also two MRI or CAT scans may have been done – one by the GP and then by the specialist, so that those duplicates could be avoided.

I am sure that if GPs had got full commissioning powers at time when the overall cake was increasing as in the last 5 years, this would have happened. But now in times of shortage of money I am not sure that this will happen, as short-term imperatives will lead to axing of good services and very little development of improvements, whoever is doing the commissioning.

It so also imperative to make the services more efficient, and there have been advances in the MRI services. Now they are done at any time of the day including early mornings and late evenings, using the expensive plant of the scanner as efficiently as possible. Previously the MRI scanner was only operational during strict office hours, which was a big waste of expensive equipment.

There may be a problem in the future with the procurement of radiological equipment.[117] There were significant investments made during 2000–2007 in England, but from 2007–2008, the capital funding system for trusts changed, with capital expenditure now being funded from trust revenue and loans. Trusts now take financing decisions for delivering services for machines (whether purchasing, leasing or managed equipment services), and have to recover the costs of financing through the revenue they generate from commissioners, while acting as a provider in an increasingly competitive market. There are many concerns that the expertise for doing this just isn't there yet, and it will take time during which mistakes will be made. It really is an area in which it is vital to diagnose many problems quickly and I very much hope that the UK does not fall behind again.

Part 7

GPs and their patients

Chapter 22
Accessing health care: making the best use of GP time

Managing demand in GP surgeries – using other members of the primary care team effectively – practice organisation – workload – home visiting – complaints – out-of-hours care – other business models

My patients were a great source of interest to me, and I thoroughly enjoyed most consultations, exhausting though they could be. It is very satisfying to be able to help people sort out things that were bothering them, though of course serious illness was always worrying for me as well as the patient. Many patients became friends and I really missed them after I retired. Over the years though the relationship changed, especially when our job emphasised lifestyle and prevention. Telling a patient to stop smoking every time you see him can put barriers up. And then when the 'consumer' model and 'patient choice' became paramount it could be very difficult to adapt. There had always been patients who demanded a lot of us, making appointments very regularly when there didn't seem to be any particular need, and that could be difficult unless you could address the underlying reason for the frequent consultations. This was what we were exhorted to do as good GPs – but it wasn't always possible to get the patient to oblige with a satisfying underlying reason after which the consultations should theoretically have become less frequent.

One of my patients, a woman in her mid-thirties, made appointments twice or three times a week after she registered from another practice, and was clocking up an enormous amount of medical time with numerous complaints, some of which were bizarre, until we were able to get a grip – but it had become a habit and the patient found it very difficult to cope without the twice weekly 'fix'. She was also seeing a very large number of specialists at the hospital, one appropriately as she had a neurological problem, but others were totally unnecessary. Once we told the hospital specialists about her behaviour in primary care, they were able to reassess her case more realistically. She was certainly an exception, but quite often we were all left with the impression that many people led very boring lives and a visit to the doctor was an interesting event – you could talk to somebody of high standing who was very knowledgeable, about yourself – the most interesting topic of all to most of us! And it was free!

We know that in general most acute problems get better on their own and only if a symptom does not do so in 3–4 days is it worth going to the doctor. We always used to laugh at patients who complained that they couldn't get an appointment until a few days time, and then when they finally did get one, they complained that the problem had gone, as if they didn't understand that any appointment would then have been a waste of their and the doctor's time, and risked their taking treatment that would have been at best useless and at worst cause them harm from side effects. Of course in some cases it is better if the patient does come early, and fortunately with the greater level of education most people now know to come to see a doctor straight away, that day or the next, for 'red flag' symptoms like breast lumps and rectal bleeding. But other things are not so clear-cut and it can be difficult for the patient to know when to insist on a same day appointment.

After the NHS was established, most GPs put some barriers between the patient and getting an appointment to see the doctor. When I first started in practice, the method was usually to allow long waits to develop in the waiting room (there was an apocryphal story of the doctor who made the wait even worse by sawing off 2 inches from the front two legs of the surgery chairs); long waits would inevitably happen if every patient who wanted to be seen on that day actually came in. This was always unacceptable to busy people and benefitted only those with plenty of time on their hands and nothing better to do – not the sort of patient we wanted to reward at all. So then GPs tried to stick as rigidly as possible to appointment times, which meant that very few people waited longer than, say, half an hour. But this meant that at the end of the session – and no doctor can consult for longer than 3 hours without becoming a gibbering idiot – there would still be patients left to see who had not been able to get an appointment. Some practices allowed waiting times to get an appointment of up to a month, except for an 'emergency' which of course was impossible to define precisely.

So, with the new emphasis on quick access to a GPs surgery from 2000, there were new tricks to reduce demand – telling people appointments were full now but if they phoned in again in an hour they might be fitted in, asking people to phone very early e.g. at 8 am, and so on. Another well-publicised method was not to make advance appointments at all, so that though you could easily get an appointment for that day or the next you could no longer book up 2 weeks in advance. In reality none of these addressed the problem of relative scarcity of doctor slots, which could only be managed by having more doctors (not a feasible solution given the cost to the NHS of each GP).

There are more intelligent solutions. One good solution involves subsidiarity – a fascinating word that means that everything should be done at the most appropriate particular level of complexity. Thus those simple tasks that could be done by a worker with only the lowest level training should be done by them and no one else, leaving the nurses and doctors to concentrate on the things that only they could do. In this way British patients could get the best of all worlds, and waiting times to see GPs could remain low. But not all practices managed this, because of course employing more ancillary staff could be expensive, and most of the money comes straight out of the doctor's profits (the NHS at one time subsidised such expenses but that has been abolished now). It would be much cheaper to allow waits to build up and not to employ extra staff. Another solution was also for the doctors to work longer hours themselves, and some GPs do indeed work very long hours, but there is great variation between practices. From the workload study done in 2006, full-time GPs (i.e. who worked eight or more sessions) worked an average 44.4 hours per week, excluding work outside their practice and out-of-hours work,[118] and that is surely enough. More recently I have seen a figure of 41 hours. Each session is nominally 3.5 hours, but there is a lot of paperwork and management done on top of that.

However what sort of a service the patient gets also depends on the size and organisation of a practice, and how many of the GPs are actually working. Many doctors work outside the practice, as there is lots of other work that GPs can do, such as medical politics, training young GPs, work in prisons and for private companies. Most of that sort of work is paid for separately on top of NHS fees. 'Back fill' – someone has to do the work in the practice when the GP is doing something else – is usually done by locums or sessional doctors, but if these arrangements break down (and they quite often do) there may be too few doctors in the practice to get through the patient load, so that the patients may not get the full value of the money the NHS was paying out for their care. There is a columnist who writes for doctors about life in his inner city practice, and time after time the appalling workload he describes is actually because there are too few doctors actually working in the surgery on that day despite there being enough doctors employed in the practice. In any case locums are rarely able to fully replace a full-time permanent doctor, as there is a lot of work they can't do, putting further pressure on the full-time doctors and their patients. I have known of cases where doctors in small practices who know each other very well (for example two close friends or a husband and wife team), agree for only one of them to be consulting at any one time, in order for both of them to do other work, and this can reduce the actual time available for patients. With the new reforms in England this is only going to get worse, as GPs are required to join commissioning groups and spend more time on management. I personally don't see how this problem can be solved in times of austerity.

An additional pressure is that the average length of surgery consultations with GPs has increased from 8.4 minutes in 1992/3 to 11.7 minutes in 2006/7[119] and is undoubtedly more than that now. This is a great improvement and reflects the increasing complexity of the work that GPs do, including a lot of work on chronic disease management that was previously done in hospital outpatients. There is considerable pressure from GP leaders to increase the resources so that GPs could allocate 15 minutes to each appointment. The drawback to that would be that if a patient failed to turn up it would be a waste of the doctor's time. At the moment the DNA (did not attend) rate in many areas is just about right, so that you can catch up with the essential paperwork between patients!

Of course it is very difficult to generalise as to whether you are getting value from your doctor. Populations do not all have the same health needs, and rich areas may have a consultation rate much lower than those deprived areas where there is a lot of long-term illness. Practices with a high number of elderly patients, such as in south coast resort towns, also have a much higher than usual workload, and this is not fully taken into account by the payment system. Patient consultation rates for GPs vary tremendously, but overall patients visited their doctor five times a year in the UK in 2009. In other countries the rate may be much higher – in Spain it is nearly eight times a year – so British patients are quite considerate of their doctors. Certainly if you find yourself always having difficulty getting an appointment, or waiting a long time in the surgery when the doctor over-runs continually, then you should think of changing surgeries. On the other hand you may find that a particular GP is always overrunning precisely because she is a very good GP and gives an excellent service to the patient, and it may well then be worth the wait. The alternative might be waiting no time at all to see a GP with no people skills and not much interest in your problem (who probably shouldn't be a GP, but that is another story).

Although the average patient only consults 5 times a year this hides a huge variation. Like many other occupations and situations, 30% of the patients account for 90% of the work. These may be the very sick, the terminally ill, or the ones who just don't cope very well. There is a lot of pressure on GPs to do more and more complex work as mentioned above, and shifting work from hospitals into general practice has been the goal of health service managers for many years, but as there are never any more resources (staff, or money for staff and equipment) to go with it, GPs often resist, sometimes with patients becoming the piggy in the middle. But there is no doubt in my mind that if a service can be supplied in primary care it should be.

Examples of services that are now done in primary care are investigations such as blood tests requested by specialists in hospital, to save the patient an extra visit to the hospital, injections prescribed by hospital doctors, 'shared care' schemes where GP and consultant share the monitoring and prescribing medications with known side effects, and services such as treating skin lesions and family planning. Services such as physiotherapy, psychological and counselling services, podiatry and dietetics are all services that should be available outside large hospitals in convenient venues such as cottage hospitals and community health centres as well as the doctor's surgery.

For most people in the UK, the bottom line is that the service has to be there when they really need it and should be paid for by their taxes, not by the patient. The NHS has stuck to this principle by and large since its inception, prescription charges in England being the big exception. The services themselves of course have changed out of all recognition, and so has the way they are accessed, as people change how they use the services over time.

Home visiting is one service that has altered. This was common before the NHS started and in its early years, for very practical reasons. Before the Second World War the doctor may have been the only person who had a car, there were no telephones, and calling the doctor may have been a difficult task with people having to walk to ask the doctor to come. Home visiting was enshrined in the NHS at first with both GPs and Consultants required to visit patients at home. Consultants were required to visit a patient's home if asked by a GP to join them on a domiciliary visit (DV). GP and consultant were supposed to visit together and the consultant would be paid a reasonable fee for attending, while the GP was not. Even in my early days as GP it was rare for GP and consultant to attend together but DVs were common and the source of a lot of extra income for some specialities – geriatrics and psychiatry for example. Nowadays though it must be fairly rare to do them.

The GP's contract put an onus on the GP to decide to visit where it was necessary, although she was not compelled to do a visit if she deemed it unnecessary. But if in retrospect the patient was not able to get the treatment that they really needed because they were unable to travel to the surgery, and subsequently made a complaint, the doctor would be brought before a Service Committee to decide if the GP had made the right decision. This was a body chaired by a layperson and included at least one doctor, but certainly in my time of sitting on such committees, it was dominated by laypeople. It was therefore very necessary for the doctor on the panel to make an excellent case in the doctor's defence if the complaint were to be dismissed. If the doctor was found guilty i.e. he had made the wrong decision he was found 'in breach of contract' and could be fined or suspended. The complaint would then go before the GMC, which could punish the doctor further. Only GPs who were full principals i.e. had an NHS list of patients, were liable to this procedure. If a locum or assistant had treated the patient, the doctor employing him was put before the committee and the punishment would apply to her, not the locum.

All quite right too, one would say (if one wasn't the GP facing such a committee, which was extremely stressful). However, rather out of the blue in 1990, this changed. The Service Committee hearings were disbanded and patients were now supposed to complain to the practice itself. Practices had to set up a process whereby the complaint was looked into within set timescales, and the emphasis was on looking at the events together, with the patient and doctor attending meetings to resolve the issue. Only if the patient was still dissatisfied at the end of this procedure would the complaint go to the local health organisation, where panels of lay and medical people were set up to look at the complaint. I do remember a patient, who had to be considered a 'vexatious' patient on any definition, who had complained many times about every doctor she had ever seen, making a complaint about me. The complaint centred on the fact that I had disclosed, in her presence, to the social worker who was supporting her, that she had in fact had a similar problem previously and it had been dealt with by the social services. She was very angry because she had not told them this and thought she could get more money out of the system. My heart sank when I saw the complaint, as whatever the merits of the case it always meant that a committee hearing had to be convened and these were lengthy tedious and involved a lot of preparation. I was delighted when the practice manager told me that the new rules had come into effect the previous month. The patient withdrew the complaint when she heard that.

It turned the dynamic completely, so that the patient had a much reduced chance of 'punishing' the doctor for his or her perceived misdeeds. The practice in-house procedure can be daunting for the patient who now has to do more of the paperwork, although a patient's representative from the local Community Health Council (organisations set up in 1974 to provide a voice for patients) and the public would always be available. Now the Community Health Councils have been abolished in England, (without consultation in 2003) although they are still maintained in Wales and Scotland. Therefore many patients' groups have pushed for a return to the old system.

Why did it change? I think the dominant feeling was that there ought to be a consensual way of solving these disputes, rather than the very adversarial approach used previously. It must also have been quite expensive to have the local health organisation arrange so many tribunals, and it must have been a relief for them to put all these administrative costs on the practices (without any extra pay of course). But the existence of the service committee hearing had been a very powerful tool for patients to 'keep their GP in order' especially about home visiting. It perpetuated a perception by many patients that a doctor 'had' to do a home visit if asked. Certainly in my early years there was no question of triaging the calls at all – all a patient had to do was to put a call in the book before 10 am for a routine visit, or ask for an urgent visit at any time of day or night.

This was of course very onerous for GPs, and even as general practice was developing apace from 1966 to 1990 with new premises under the cost–rent scheme, the old system of doctors going round with a bag in all hours to see patients in their own homes, often for very trivial complaints, prevailed.

As most people had by then got telephones and many had cars, it became more and more unnecessary for doctors to do so many home visits. It was also quite unsafe, as medical care had developed to such an extent that to treat most emergencies properly would need sophisticated equipment. Even for less urgent problems it was often very difficult to examine patients in their own homes, often with poor lighting, usually with the TV on, the dog barking and the rest of the family coming and going. Ever since then I have had an aversion to noisy dogs! There was no respect for the professionalism of the doctor under these circumstances, but we all did many unnecessary house visits, increasingly unwillingly, well into the 1990's. However the house visit was the bedrock of the old relationship between GP and patient, which has largely been lost now. The bond cemented between doctor and patient when the doctor had visited and understood the life style of the patient and could put it into context; the bond in the few cases where there really was an emergency was a very strong one.

The real problem with home visits, especially out of hours, was that the service was overused and often abused, often being used by people wanting to be reassured in their own homes that they weren't ill – if they thought they were really ill they would go to hospital. So, as it was impossible for most GPs to be on call 24/7 for their own patients themselves, deputising services were set up. These were profit-making services and the way they were set up meant that there was an incentive for the doctors employed by the deputising services to do a call physically rather than give advice over the phone. This led to the expectation that a doctor had to come when called, and even those areas where the doctors did the calls themselves in a rota or cooperative it was difficult to give telephone advice or see the patient at a better-equipped facility.

Things change though and British general practice has managed the transition well, so that even if there is no longer the old bond between a single doctor who knew everything about a patient and often was a real friend, there is still a trust between most patients and their GPs, which is very beneficial to the healing process. Where this does not exist primary care loses a lot of its value. Patients now rightly have much more say in how services are run and can use web sites to flag up poor services.

Home visiting still has its place, for instance for bed-bound elderly patients, although in many cases the community nurse may also be involved. Those who regularly go to the hairdresser though should not expect a visit! Visits to care homes are in effect home visits and these are a big part of modern-day general practice. The main reason for home visits is of course palliative or terminal care, and in most areas these are still done by the doctor, although in some areas specialist nurses, Macmillan nurses or community nurses will do them on their own or in conjunction with the doctor. These are an integral part of modern primary care, as in survey after survey patients say they would prefer to die at home rather than go to hospital, yet still in some areas only a minority of patients achieves this aim. In the UK all usual palliative care is provided in this way together with local hospices and their out-reach clinics. Palliative care specialists are a tertiary service for those people with difficult-to-control symptoms and are invaluable.

Contrast this with the USA, where most care for people with terminal illnesses is provided by oncologists, surgeons, radiologists or medical specialists, without a strong primary care team to help the patient through their illness. In New York the number of futile treatments is very high[120] and so the average spending during their last year of life is huge.[121] This is bad for patient and very costly for the country's health system. In the USA therefore there is a real need for more palliative care to be given earlier in the patient's illness, by primary care nurses and GPs. The fact is that oncologists will offer more and more futile treatments if they are available and if the patient – or more often the relatives – push for them. In the USA this may be more the rule than the exception.

Out-of-hours care, defined as any medical care required between the hours of 6:30 pm and 8 am, used to be the responsibility of a doctor with a patient list. If you accepted a patient on to your list you would have to agree to visit them at home on a 24-hour basis, so that meant that the patient had to live a distance from the surgery that was practical for the doctor to drive to. This still applies to daytime home visits and so the present Government's wish to get rid of patient lists and allow a patient to register with any GP, for instance one near their place of work, is fraught with difficulties. Most GPs at present are against the idea, except possibly those GPs in areas where there are few residential streets and lots of industrial or office units, who might welcome the extra work. The patient list is a fundamental part of British general practice and it seems a pity to lose it. Many other countries would like to have such a system, as it makes accurate GP records much easier, compared with systems where patients can go to different GPs whenever they wish.

So what are the disadvantages of having to register with one practice? The main complaint of patients' groups is that patients who work some distance away from home cannot easily access their GP during working hours. It may be a real problem for some patients living in metropolitan areas but GPs estimate that less than 5% of patients will actually take advantage of this, presumably to enable them to visit a doctor in the lunch break or before or immediately after work. As out-of-hours care is now separate, and most GPs do not work weekends, there does not seem to be a substantial reason to object to this. Another objection, however, is that if a patient is ill at home and then needs GP care, then the GP won't have the records. However usually in these cases the original GP will have retained the computerized records from when the patient was registered there, and the patient can be seen as a Temporary Resident (TR). The system of TR allows any patient to be seen by a NHS GP anywhere in the country and this does cover almost all cases. The only proviso is that a patient must have a valid address in the area he is staying, so this does rule out being seen on day trips (although it is easy to bend the rules here).

Some people may object to not having the freedom to go to any doctor of their choice depending on their condition, the underlying assumption being that some practices are better at dealing with some complaints than others. While this is theoretically true, I can't think of many reasons why a patient might want to see a doctor in one practice for one thing and another in another practice for other things. Even if the patient could get the information on a GP's particular skills, it would soon go out of date.

The change in 2004, when GPs were allowed to opt out of both out-of-hours care and Saturday morning surgeries, for a very small reduction in pay, was a great surprise to many doctors and led to some bad feeling especially when GPs also got a rather large pay rise. Many of us expected out-of-hours care to be modified, as it had been a long time since most GPs had actually looked after their own lists of patients out of hours, but few expected it to be removed altogether, and now there is a push in some areas for GPs to do at least Saturday or Sunday mornings. GPs can earn extra money if they do, although the costs of opening up the surgery with reception cover are quite high. It would certainly help with continuity of care.

The present system, with GPs being required to make sure patients have good access to their services and essential home visiting is safeguarded, is considered fair. In most surveys, GPs perform well in providing adequate numbers of appointments for GPs, nurse practitioners, practice nurses, and other staff, and a doctor not doing this will be noticed. It does mean that patients may have to be diverted from a doctor to other professionals where appropriate, and this must be done in a considerate way.

In major conurbations of course the previous (Labour) government brought in walk-in centres and Darzi centres. These provide direct competition with established GPs and we did wonder why. British general practice is very accessible compared with that in most other countries and these did seem to duplicate services. Now that we are in a time of austerity the less successful of these are being quietly closed. Many GPs felt that they pandered to wants versus needs, fuelling ever increasing 24/7 demands, and potentially undermining decades of patient education about the natural history of viral illnesses. From a consumer point of view of course you may want professional healthcare advice rather than using your own resources or taking advice from friends or the Internet. But immediate advice for usually self-limiting problems does cost money and perhaps these consumer 'rights' might be limited in favour of activities more likely to improve health outcomes. Of course the private sector wants a foot in the door, but these could remain just that – a private add-on extra. GPs are flexible, affordable, adaptable and dependable, and in most countries the value of a portal system of primary care is recognised. There is no evidence that outsourcing to walk-in centres, shared business services, the cherry-picking of elective procedures, and other health care activities will be cost effective. But GPs can't compete with big corporations under the NHS procurement process or EU tender rules, so that there is a big risk that in England the whole system will be fragmented.

That doesn't mean to say that GP services can't be improved, but in my view they should remain the bedrock of primary care in the UK. GPs in many areas are improving access, continuity of care, and long-term outcomes, and doing it more cheaply than establishing new centres. If they are not then the Government's initiatives to promote competition should improve standards, and most GPs accept this.

Other improvements that are needed are things like encouraging local GPs to register more transient patients, who have been disadvantaged under the previous system. Basically you have to have a permanent address to be registered as a patient on a GPs list, and unless this is changed, another way of organising their care needs to be found. Some of the people concerned are amongst the most disadvantaged in the country and they need a very flexible service. So governments and health boards have sometimes set up special systems to do this with new money, but in some areas GPs could do it for less.

Another very important way of improving access to healthcare is to use the services of other members of the primary care team. Most people know by now that many eye problems are better dealt with by optometrists (see Chapter 25), that pharmacists are an invaluable and underused facility, and that practice and community nurses are able to treat many everyday conditions, and of course mostly do all the chronic disease management within practices.

The ultimate political reason for improving access to GP services is of course a managerial one – to help reduce accident and emergency (A&E) attendances, as these are the really expensive bits of medical care. The new reforms will put more power in the hands of GPs, and we hope they will be able to make these improvements. I think most of us agree with this. But there is no need at all to change the system to do it – a lot of these improvements are happening now with practice based commissioning. Introducing market forces only works up to a point. It remains to be seen what will be the effect of the Health and Social Care Act now that it is operational.

Chapter 23
Doctors' attitudes: safeguarding patients

*Shipman – revalidation – Patients Association report – patients choosing doctors –
removing patients from lists – doctors' activity*

Most GP practices nowadays contain more than two doctors. Single-handed practice has been under a cloud ever since Harold Shipman used the privilege of running his own practice with public money to patronise and then callously and deliberately murder his patients. We hope this was a one-off criminal activity, but there is no doubt that there haven't been enough safeguards in the past to protect patients. It was only because Shipman was able to escape the normal interaction with his colleagues by going into single-handed practice that he could get away with it for so long. People trusted doctors. The enormity of it all was brought home to me in a book about Shipman[122], where it mentioned that his killing could have started as early as 1969 when he was a houseman – first year in hospital training. I was a houseman at the same time and I well remember the strain of doing a full day's work then a night on call when I would be woken up several times to attend to often very sick patients, then do another full day on top. The worst would be 48-hour stretches at the weekend when I would be desperate for some sleep. From looking at the times of the deaths that happened when Shipman was on call during those days it seemed that from the very start of his work, there were increased rates of deaths of patients on the wards that he covered. He always did an evening ward round just before going to bed, (this was said to be very good practice – not all of us managed it) and it seems possible that he then identified the patients he thought might have a problem in the night, so killed them in advance to prevent him losing sleep. It shows that trust in your doctor is the first and foremost thing a patient needs, and that this trust must be continually earned and safeguarded.

So now single handed doctors – doctors who work entirely on their own without any interaction with colleagues on a day-to-day basis – should be confined to very rural areas, and even there safeguards should be built in. Many of the recommendations from Dame Janet Smith, the Chairwoman of the Shipman

Enquiry, on regulation of doctors have been enacted, including enabling the public to see whether a doctor has been disciplined by the General Medical Council (GMC) (Shipman had been before the GMC but he was allowed to continue to practice), ensuring that doctors who have a history of drug abuse (as Shipman had) are scrutinised effectively, and checks for abnormally high death rates at GP practices. This last seems very much a case of shutting the stable door after the horse has bolted. Who ever would believe before Shipman that a doctor would do this? It is also a difficult one because a practice with a nursing home containing very sick patients who are expected to die soon will show up in these checks, and also practices with a high elderly population will have high death rates. Still, although it is by no means a simple check, it can be done.

Following this case the GMC has been completely changed and now consists of 24 members, 12 lay and 12 medical, all appointed by the Appointments Commission, and though the Chair at the moment can be a doctor, he or she does not have to be medically qualified. Its main function is to protect patients, and the times when it seemed only to be concerned about doctors who had affairs with patients are long gone.

The main plank of Dame Janet Smith's recommendations, revalidation for all doctors as is done in many other countries so that doctors have to prove regularly that they are up to date, has at the time of writing not been fully implemented. The first 'cycle' of revalidation, in which every licensed doctor will revalidate for the first time, started in early December 2012 and will end in March 2016. Doctors are now being regularly appraised, so that they have to bring a portfolio of their work annually to be scrutinised by other doctors, and in many areas this works well. But it is not designed to weed out poorly performing doctors – it is meant to be formative and supportive. So at the moment medical managers find it very difficult to use it to remove doctors who are not up to scratch. Revalidation is supposed to work by appointing a 'responsible officer' who will make a recommendation that the doctor is up to date and safe to practice, and if the officer is good at her job she will be able to remove poorly performing doctors. In my experience most doctors try to comply with such checks and will bend over backwards to make sure their practice improves when questioned, but I am quite sure that Dr Shipman would have used every lever he had to pull the wool over people's eyes. After all, he falsified his day-to-day data, took steps to silence any criticism by force of personality, and lied time and time again, so I am not sure that this revalidation would prevent another Shipman in itself. Only the realization in the general public and the authorities that there are rogues out there and not all doctors can be trusted will help to prevent another tragedy like that. That is very sad.

The average size of a GP practice is now about four, so that all patients should have a choice of doctor within the practice. Patients used to be assigned to individual doctor's lists and often had a regular ongoing relationship with that doctor, and this still happens in some cases even though the payment system now no longer reflects this. People with an ongoing complaint, or a multiplicity of problems that require regular attendances, usually do prefer to see the same doctor every time but this is becoming more difficult to manage. The average of four hides the fact that some practices are now very large with seven or more full time doctors, and this does mean that it may be difficult to see the same doctor every time.

A recent report from the Patients' Association (PA) has highlighted many shortcomings of GPs.[123] The General Medical Council's figures show a 23% increase in complaints about doctors, 47% of which relate to GP's, and the PA survey showed that

- 39.3% of respondents rated their GP's communication skills at five out of ten or less;
- Only six out of ten patients believe their GP treats them with compassion;
- 80% of patients said they wanted to be more involved in their care;
- nearly one in four of patients who raised concerns with their GP felt that they responded poorly;
- 26% of calls to their Helpline relate to communication in Primary Care;
- 12% relate to concerns about referrals from the Primary Care to the Acute Care Sector;
- 10% relate to patients being removed from their GP's list after making a complaint.

So all is not well with primary care, at a time when it will need to concentrate as never before on improvements which will be needed to take on the coming changes in the NHS in England.

The big problem that I see is communication between GP and patient, which obviously has had to change markedly over the years, from the system that I first practiced in, where you saw the same patient over many years, got to know them well and ordinary human decency made the relationship work. Now with the higher turnover of more mobile patients, multi-ethnic communities and the increasing complexity of medical care so that each patient is managed within a practice by many different people, especially specialist nurses and healthcare workers, this is all getting very diluted so that the prized one to one relationship is becoming eroded. This is what is making communication so difficult. GP computer systems in general are excellent, much better than in hospitals, but even with these it is sometimes difficult to keep track of what is happening to patients, and this exposes some of the problems when two people, the patient and doctor, have to have the same understanding of the pathway of care. The important thing here, which the PA has underlined, is that patient feedback is essential to give a detailed account of where the pinch points are. We must put structures in place to capture the feedback and act on it.

For instance, one problem we noted was that of marking the results from pathology as they came through. We, the doctors, would mark them 'normal' or 'see doctor'. Of course just because they were normal didn't mean they shouldn't see the doctor, but some patients assumed that even if they already had a follow-up appointment they didn't need to see the doctor again if the test was normal. After a patient didn't come in and eventually was found to have an infection we had to change what the receptionist told the patient to make sure they still kept their next appointment.

Obviously the PA is right when it says that communication skills should be taught better in the training of all doctors, but in my view there are some people who will never have the relevant skills however carefully they are taught. We had a trainee once who managed to upset patients time after time. He was arrogant, self-opinionated and had no idea his patients weren't agreeing with him. He had weird medical ideas too: he didn't believe in physiotherapy, for instance, and told everyone to do exercises he had made up (which didn't work, or so the patients said). He also had very odd ideas about diet on which he would lecture patients on obsessively. The year he was with us several patients left our list because of his hectoring style. Despite having a long series of remedial interviews he didn't change and at the end of his year his trainer had to decide whether to sign him up or not. It was difficult as actually despite his manner he diagnosed and treated the patients perfectly adequately, and his knowledge base was sound. But his trainer decided she had to fail him, which was a disaster for his career and there were endless repercussions. I don't know whether he ever got another medical job – I expect he did as there are plenty of jobs that can be done with a medical training which don't involve patient contact, but I have come across fully trained doctors in practice like that and I don't know how they got through. The BMA says that these are skills that can be learned, but some people undoubtedly find it easier than others. It is all the more difficult if the doctor is not from the UK. Not only are there cultural expectations that might be different in the two countries but also the very reason for moving to another system may be because the doctor hadn't really got on in his or her country of origin. Revalidation is supposed to help here, but I am not so sure that it will.

The PA writes that patients need to be in control of their care and their views need to be taken into account, and of course that is true. Patients want a lot more information from their GP than they used to and have a right to be guided through the care that they can expect. Patient and doctor have to work together to get the best result from the NHS, and with the reforms not only do GPs have to help the individual patient in front of them but they must also consciously seek to improve care by commissioning the best services. In a way this is good, because so often in the past GPs have known very well what services would im- prove patient care but not been listened to. Still, there is a conflict – what the patient in front of them wants and needs may not be possible given the needs of all the other patients in the commissioning group. The decision used to be taken far away by managers in a different organisation but now it is coming ever nearer to home.

In most practices there is a choice whether to go to a doctor or nurse. Nurses have expanded their role tremendously in the last ten years and now take on ever- increasing responsibility for direct patient care, and the running of the practice. There are differences of course in their training and in their outlook but there is a lot of overlap. Nurses in many practices are the first port of call and it is easier to make an appointment with the nurse than the doctor. They often have longer ap- pointments and have a more educative role. They are becoming specialists in the field of treatment of chronic diseases such as asthma, hypertension and diabetes and are often prescribers in their own right. But a nurse without the qualification to prescribe has to waste his time hanging around outside the doctor's room to get her to sign the prescription he has written. (Well, that is a bit bending over backwards in the gender balance issue as, though there are more female doctors than male ones in general practice now, I have only met one male practice nurse in my career.) Nurses are beginning to act more autonomously and get their own patients following, and the patient can make a choice knowing that the nurse will treat most things effectively and will hand over to the doctor for some conditions where appropriate.

So, assuming a doctor is what is wanted, what sort of patients might go to which sort of doctor? What are patients looking for when they choose a doctor for an important consultation? (We are assuming that most patients would not mind whom they saw for straightforward matters such as a strained muscle or acute infection).

Well, what sorts of doctor are there? There are obviously ones who have an excellent manner with patients and these doctors are invariably popular. But even these paragons have to get through a surgery and so won't be able to give much more time than a consultation needs. Doctors themselves do not usually choose their patients so it is up to the patient to make the choice. They may choose doctors who are similar types to them – female patients often like female doctors, male patients may prefer male doctors, for instance. Patients do tend to cluster around doctors of much the same age – at least, older doctors often have a following of patients who have grown up with them over the years. No-nonsense types may like no-nonsense doctors – 'just get on with it doc'. The anxious patient may value a doctor who explains more and empathises more. Patients may like a doctor who is computer-literate, who gives lots of links to useful websites, and uses email for simple questions. Some people definitely do not, and may resent the time the doctor spend in a consultation looking at the screen. But do patients choose doctors for their behaviour such as whether they are more likely to prescribe antibiotics, for instance, or refer to hospital? Would patients even know which doctors do what?

There isn't a lot of evidence about why some doctors refer or prescribe far more than others. Do female doctors refer more than male doctors for instance? The evidence is that they don't – there is no difference in average referral rates between doctors of different genders. There was one practice of six doctors where there was one very high-referring doctor, who was male, and another very low referring doctor who was female. The high-referring doctor referred 15 times as many patients compared with the low-referring doctor. They were 'outliers' in a practice where all the other doctors in the practice had referral rates that clustered around the average. Now if we assume that they both saw a similar mix of patients, that is a huge difference, and these differences can be maintained month after month, year after year. It would be difficult to see how a difference in the two doctors' mix of patients could account for this, as it is the patient who chooses the doctor not the other way round. There might be small difference with one doctor seeing more 'quickies' – patients with short-term acute, non serious illnesses – than the other, but this isn't sustainable for long because the other doctors would complain, as they are the easy consultations.

So what would account for this sort of difference, and what do patients make of it? They are sure to notice, as we know they exchange stories of what happens in consultations. After all, this difference must mean that a patient who goes to one doctor with a condition will be referred to hospital while another identical patient will not be referred. Who is right?

It might be thought that there is an age difference, with older doctors referring less because they have more experience and are more confident in following up people to see how the illness unfolds instead of rushing in to refer to specialists. There did seem some evidence of this amongst the doctors I was working with but it seemed to affect only those doctors who trained before about 1980. Before that time the training of GPs was very much towards being self-confident and managing conditions themselves, but after that date the training became more thorough and doctors were more aware of guidelines. So as the older doctors retired average referral rates went up, but for doctors trained after that, doctors seemed not to have a difference in average referral rates in their different age groups. There are some very obvious exceptions where older doctors refer much more. This may be more a matter of mindset and custom and practice. And it remains to be seen what will affect this. Younger doctors are most likely to find to easier to change their referral behaviour.

It was certainly true in our studies that young doctors in training ('registrars'), referred more and that this reflected their inexperience. Recently there has been a trend for the supervising GP (each young doctor will have one supervising doctor – their trainer – who should be aware of how the doctor is referring) to actively vet the referrals and this should be a good thing. While some patients might not mind too much, it is a complete waste of their time to be referred to hospital unnecessarily. Hopefully this process would ensure that registrars refer only patients who need specialist opinion.

However, locum GPs – doctors who worked in lots of different practice to fill in for sickness or other absences – also had higher rates of referral. This reflects the fact that they may not be able to follow the patient up so easily and so to play safe, they might have to refer earlier than other permanent doctors might, and this is entirely understandable. The biggest variation came from sessional doctors, especially those doing only one or two sessions a week. This mostly reflects the variability of small numbers as referral depends to some extent on what walks in through the door, but it also reflects inability to follow patients up. Locums face similar problems. This should be addressed by practices under clinical governance so that a regular partner who can follow these patients up could mentor such doctors.

Personality factors are also important as some doctors tend to be less confident in managing patients and encouraging self-management by patients and some are more anxious about medico-legal problems if they do not refer.

There may be practice factors at work here too – practices which are smaller and very cohesive, where the doctors share their cases with each other and discuss them regularly, seem to have fewer 'outlier doctors' and so a narrower spread. The practice mentioned above did have a lot of communication between the doctors, but they tended to keep their own ideas on how to manage patients and never changed their patterns of behaviour over many years. This was not the only practice where this happened of course. There were many others in the area that also had a huge spread of referral rates.

So the reasons for this huge difference in activity must be personal to each doctor. They must lie in the realms of training, personality, beliefs in their own knowledge, individual experiences, willingness to deal with uncertainty, and attitudes, both political and sociological.

I think that patients on the whole accept this sort of situation, at least at the moment. They may be aware that there are differences and are prepared often to shop around for the doctor who will do what they want. It is a patient's choice of course. So for example, a patient who has been to the same doctor several times with, say, back pain which is not getting any better, may choose to go to another doctor in the practice who referred someone they know, in the hopes that perhaps there may be a better treatment out there that the doctor will recognise and so refer on. And of course with a fifteen-fold differences such a patient must be right in thinking that at least sometimes this is a possibility. Sometimes a doctor may not be aware there is a new treatment available, or not diagnose the condition properly, and this must be very bad for patient care. Conversely I was always aware that doctors who referred most of their patients very quickly would get very few complaints and would never make a bad mistake – but at the expense of wasting patients' time and clogging up outpatient departments unnecessarily. The truth probably is somewhere in the middle and most doctors now are more comfortable knowing that their activity rates of referral, prescribing and investigating are within the norm for that area.

But for patient safety as well as for efficiency of the system there should really be some consensus on what sort of conditions should be referred and which can be managed in primary care, and that was what we tried to do with our peer review system.

It is interesting to try to look at some of the personality and attitudinal factors that affect a doctor's referral and prescribing habits. I once sent round a rather complicated questionnaire to doctors I was working with. Most completed it, and the results were very interesting. The numbers were not large enough to be formally significant but it did give us some idea about doctors' attitudes and how they managed their patients. I gave them statements such as the following, and doctors were asked to rate them on a scale of 1 to 5, with 1 signifying complete agreement and 5 indicating complete disagreement.

- Doctors should generally do what the patient wants if it is not actually harmful.
- GPs should refer patients they cannot help even if the hospital sector is unlikely to help much either.
- A doctor's role should mainly be to inform patients of the choices available to them.

There were 32 questions in all.

I then scored them in a rather unscientific way, which is why one can't read too much into it. I am sure more people are doing research on this and will be able to present more accurate information, but the gist of what I found was that, as you might imagine, most GPs clustered in the middle, but there were indeed clear groups of 'outlier' doctors.

High referrers

Doctors who had a high activity level seemed to be less sure of themselves and less likely to believe that a diagnosis was correct without exhaustive tests. This applied even to the more academic doctors who were more knowledgeable than other doctors but this knowledge sometimes seemed to confuse them. Other doctors in this category were less likely to believe in the evidence base behind their decisions, or sometimes were not aware of the evidence.

They were certainly less able to deal with uncertainty. They tended to worry about their patients especially about being sued or having a complaint against them. They were sometimes perceived as being more caring, 'nothing but the best for my patient', which might mean referring a patient again and again for more second opinions.

There were no doctors in our groups whom I would categorise as lazy, though some did seem to take the easy option at time.

Low Referrers

These doctors by contrast tended to be didactic, more confident, tolerated uncertainty well, and did not worry over much about complaints, believing that these could happen to any doctor at any time and would have to be dealt with properly when they happened.

On the whole these doctors quite liked guidelines and were strong on knowledge of the evidence base, but were happy to override it at times. They tended to be quick and businesslike in their dealings with patients although many were also considered to be empathetic and had good consultation skills. In no way would they be considered to be 'bad doctors' by patients – these doctors had a good reputation locally.

There were doctors who caused concern because they were not referring patients who would benefit from referral. The point of the project was to encourage sharing of knowledge and ways of working, and the referral rates of the lower referring doctors increased during the year, although by a smaller amount than the highest referrers reduced theirs.

We identified a few doctors who were referring far fewer patients than their colleagues. In each case the practice took the opportunity to discuss the findings with the doctor. In one case they did not find any cause for concern as it related to the number of patients that the doctor saw per session, which was considerably fewer than other doctors in the practice saw (the other doctors were aware of this and she was paid less as a result). In others though there was some cause for concern, and one decided to retire. Another left mainstream medical practice, although we don't know whether this was cause and effect. It seems that the fact that we were looking at referral rates in detail made doctors aware that maybe their ways of working were outside the norm, and adjustments were made.

As for views on society and medical politics, there was a strong tendency for the GPs who were happy with the hospital sector, and trusted the specialists to get it right, to have high referral rates. These GPs tended to feel that the secondary care sector was there to take all the difficult problems, and was at bottom more important. Such doctors could be reluctant to continue to manage patients in primary care, and some were also quite resistant to managers interfering with their rights to refer to anyone they chose. They were also against any sort of rationing and were especially resistant to the idea that they should take any responsibility for rationing care. They thought that politicians should admit to doing the rationing and should make it clear to patients what could or could not be treated. It is clear that a few doctors are actively opposed to any thought of responsibility for reducing demand, seeing that as something for the politicians and patients themselves, and for hospitals to work more efficiently.

Low referrers on the other hand felt they were being realistic when they referred less often, and also were preventing harm to patients from too much intervention when they acted as a gatekeeper rather than a sign-post for entry into hospital care. They were less negative to managers and would often join in with attempts by managers to make the system more efficient and save some costs. Some felt that the emphasis on what medicine and treatments could achieve was grossly overplayed, by the media, by the specialists themselves, and by commercial interests, and it was the GPs job to insert some balance and perspective into a consultation.

Some doctors indicated that they were very unhappy with the way the hospital sector had allowed very long waiting lists for many years, and felt all the blame for poor performance lay squarely in the hospital sector, but this view covered the whole spectrum of GPs referring habits.

From all this, we can see that it is very difficult to get it right. I think it is clear that it would help to have much more standardisation of referral patterns, which together with the problems of implementing guidelines in primary care, means that commissioning groups and planners have a lot of work ahead to ensure a safe and effective service for all patients.

This does not apply only to referral to hospital; it also applies to how GPs investigate their patients. So far there has been very little published work on how GPs use the tests available to them, and how safe and efficient they are. From my experience, doctors who are high referrers may often investigate their patients more too, although one would have thought that doctors who investigate their patients thoroughly would then be able to manage them in primary care.

From a patient's point of view then, the advice I would give is that if you know a doctor is outside the norm – either referring or investigating much more or less than other doctors – then I would avoid them for complex problems. Such doctors may be very considerate and nice but they are definitely putting their patients and the system as a whole at risk.

Defensive medicine

Defensive medicine is something that we barely thought about when I first started in practice. Patients had much lower expectations and usually were reluctant to complain if the relationship between them and the doctor was good, or they thought the doctor had done their best. It was much later when the rate of complaints and the practice of suing doctors through the courts became so common, that doctors routinely altered their behaviour to play safe in case patients sued.

In a recent study where 3000 doctors from seven countries were surveyed by the Medical Protection Society (MPS),[124]

- **73%** said they practised defensively to avoid complaints or claims;
- **77%** said they practised more defensively now than in the past;
- **78%** noticed their colleagues practising defensively, e.g. ordering more tests than were medically necessary;
- **41%** had chosen to stop dealing with certain conditions/performing specific procedures to avoid complaints and claims;
- **37%** changed prescribing habits;
- **61%** conducted more investigations.

One study estimated that defensive medicine adds 5–9% to overall health costs for some countries,[125] and a large part of the health budget has to be set aside to cover successful claims.

There is of course a difference between making a complaint against a doctor and suing through the courts, and there are many people who will sue because they are advised to do so through the no-win no-fee system. Yet many people still do not complain or sue when things go wrong, and when things went wrong in my practice we all found that an apology and an assurance that everything possible would be done to help ensure that such a thing would not happen again was enough.

Patients' organisations say that a patient is likely to risk being struck off the doctor's list if they make a formal complaint; that is, when they are still not satisfied after going through the practice's in-house system. In the report of the Patients Association[123] it was noted that 4.4% of respondents said they had been removed from their GP's list after making a complaint. While I can sympathise with the patients affected, I know that in a situation when I have been dealing with continuing, often complex, medical problems direct with a patient who manifestly thinks I made a mistake, I found it very difficult to be objective. Obviously if I thought I had made a mistake I would apologise, and if there was doubt I would try to achieve a better understanding with the patient about what went wrong. But in these cases all that will have been gone through within the practice's own complaints system, so if the patient takes it further, then trust between the two of us has broken down. And without trust GPs try to look behind every decision

– what will the patient do if I say this? What would other doctors do? I don't think it is possible to give good care under these circumstances. What tends to happen then is that the patient decamps to another doctor within the same practice, and this is by far the best solution. Maybe the second doctor even would think the patient is right, as the complaint goes through the system, and support the patient, or would quietly keep her own counsel. The problem arises when there is no other doctor in the practice who is willing to take the patient on, and in a way it is a tribute to the practices that it is as low as 4.4%. I think the Patients Association would really like to ban the facility of removing patients from a list altogether, and I feel this really would not be in the patients' best interest. In my experience a patient is usually removed from a practice after a long history of mistrust and disagreement, and it is probably inevitable. That said, every practice should follow the recommendations set out in this report and consider very carefully whether there is an alternative.

Most patients who are removed by a practice without their consent, for whatever reason – because they move house, the administrative boundaries change, or some other reason (for instance, it is often policy that practice staff should not be registered at the practice they work in) – find an acceptable new GP without problems. There is a minority of patients however who have been removed from several GP practices previously and now find themselves unable to find a doctor to take them on. These are usually patients who have big problems. Sometimes they have a personality disorder; sometimes they have challenging views or ways of life; but obviously they are very much in need of NHS care. So there is a system of allocation by which such patients will be found a practice. The new doctor will be informed that this patient is coming and it is then in the interests of both sides to arrive at a means of working together. In my experience it is surprising how often this succeeds, with both sides wanting a new start and to be free of the bad feeling in the previous practice, and all goes well. I remember a patient though who made life very difficult for the practice, especially the dispenser, by coming in and demanding narcotic drugs daily, (they were prescribed under a special system that was supervised by the police). Once she phoned up saying that she was abroad at an important meeting and she had to have her next supply the next day when she arrived home. The message was passed on and the doctors pushed through her request urgently (even though it wasn't actually due) and it was dispensed. When one of the receptionists heard about this she said 'Oh no, she wasn't abroad, I saw her in the phone box in town yesterday!' All efforts at controlling the situation failed and she eventually landed on a three-month rota where each doctor had to have her on their list for three months and then could move her on. But they only did that if there were continuing problems and once she lasted a year. Eventually she became genuinely ill with an unrelated condition, and was subsequently a model patient, staying on one doctor's list until she died.

Fortunately, clinical governance, complaints, and patient safety have improved out of all recognition in the last twenty years. There are systems by which poor practice can be reported, and near-miss events are usually scrutinised to see if lessons can be learned.

Whistleblowers still run the risk of losing their jobs, however, and there is more to be done to make sure that managers do not victimize doctors, and that doctors do not protect each other. And many people think that the system we have now would not have identified Shipman any earlier, so every one has to be vigilant.

Part 8

The interface between primary care and hospital specialities

Appropriate referral and cost minimisation

Chapter 24
Dermatology and human evolution

Removal of skin lesions – diagnosis of skin cancer – GP minor surgery – skin allergies – subcutaneous fat and the aquatic ape theory

Many people I chat to think that everyone should be able to have any skin lump or bump removed without charge by the NHS. Any lump or bump which lasts for more than a week or so is called a 'lesion' and can be a cyst, a wart, a solid lump and of course cancer of the skin. Rashes by definition come and go. Here in lies a problem, as it is not always obvious what is a cancer at first. The other problem is that all skin lesions are on the skin and therefore may be obvious to both the owner and other people. This means that some may be unsightly and therefore cosmetically worrying even if harmless.

Historically, in the UK almost everyone who had a skin lesion that bothered them would have it removed, although pre-NHS and for a while afterwards some people would be reluctant to go to hospital for such things and would go around carrying sometimes very large lesions on their faces or other conspicuous place, sometimes to the detriment of their health. Even recently I had a very elderly patient whose wife 'wouldn't let him' have treatment for a growing lesion on his ear, which was obviously a cancer, yet no amount of persuasion would get him to go to hospital. Eventually he had to go for treatment because it was bleeding uncontrollably, but it was too late to save his life. We had made innumerable appointments and even got the surgeon to agree to see him immediately if he turned up (when he arrived at the surgery we would take him there) but it was to no avail, and you can't force people to have treatment. But that is extremely unusual. Mostly people come with lesions that have been there only a short time, and, as is their right, they want to know immediately whether it is cancer and to have treatment straight away. This has to be a priority for all dermatology departments.

Our local consultant dermatologist once told us that the incidence of malignant melanoma in our part of Wales was the highest in Europe, possibly because of the predominant skin type (Celtic fair skin) and the modern tendency to go on short holidays to places where the sun is very strong. This was a legacy from the time when the risks of malignant melanoma were not fully realised, and few people used strong enough sun cream – indeed full sun protection was not available at that time.

Fortunately now it is often not necessary to remove a lesion just to find out if it is cancer. Dermatology units now use dermatoscopes – a sort of 3-D magnifying glass – to diagnose cancer, and they can be extremely accurate. It is often possible for an experienced dermatologist to tell from high-resolution pictures emailed to them or by tele-medicine whether the patient needs to be seen in clinic.

However, it usually falls to the GP to give an initial opinion as to whether a lesion might or might not be cancer and of course all GPs err on the side of caution and will refer anything at all suspicious, and it is then the job of the hospital to see them quickly. One good thing to point out to counteract all the hype about skin cancer is that the death rate has remained steady for many years despite a huge increase in diagnosis. We hope this is a result of early diagnosis and good treatment – but it may also suggest a certain level of overdiagnosis too.

But of course 99% of skin lesions are not cancer and will never become cancer. Some may be infectious and get better with antibiotics or on their own (pimples, carbuncles, abscesses) but most just stay there, be they cyst, fibroma, lipoma, or whatever. Some have effects on function – for instance a large lump on a finger, or a cyst on an eyelid interfering with sight, but a high proportion is at most a nuisance. Some may irritate such as a spot under a bra strap, and some may be cosmetically noticeable and a cause for concern. Some are just there and the patient would like them to not be there. But can, and should, these lesions be removed on the NHS?

Up to about 1990, if a patient wanted a lesion removed the GP would normally refer to hospital without further questioning. The letter would be sent and the patient put on a waiting list to have it looked at. Then if it was thought necessary to remove it (which it was for most of them), the patient was put on to another list to wait for it to be removed. However, with increasing sophistication of patient understanding of disease, the adverts telling people they might have malignant melanoma so they must go to have everything checked out, the drive for perfection, especially cosmetically, the aging of the population, and the relentless march of market forces, demand began to outstrip the supply of hospital staff to see these patients quickly and waiting lists began to grow. Waiting lists were not at first seen as anyone's problem apart from the patient's. The GP's work was done when they sent the letter, and although they could and did write more letters to expedite appointments, they had no power to insist on urgent treatment if the hospital did not agree. Waiting lists in dermatology in 2002–2003, if the condition was marked routine by the GP, might be 2 to 3 years. It was amazing in retrospect how long this situation went on for.

As part of the drive to reduce these waiting lists, we could see that it was impossible to guarantee that everyone could have every lesion removed whenever they wanted. But this wasn't a message the public, and therefore the politicians, wanted to hear. So at first they tried to shift the problem. In 2004 GPs were paid for the first time to take on minor surgery (as it was called) i.e. removal of certain lumps and bumps. In return for a fee for each treatment (fee for service), GPs undertook to equip the surgery to a certain standard, get themselves trained and undergo regular supervision, and employ and train staff such as nurses to assist. They had to buy in their equipment, suturing material, scalpels and other instruments and keep them all sterilized to high standards. All this cost quite a lot of money and depending on how many lesions were treated the GP might or may not make a profit, in other words have money to pay himself for doing the surgery. Most GPs in bigger practices undertook the task with enthusiasm as most had had previous training to do the work and were keen to improve their skills.

However there was always a pressure, once the system was set up, to do as many treatments as possible to recoup the initial investment, so the costs tended to rise. At that time the list included warts, and so immediately hospital dermatology departments withdrew from treating warts and verrucas, and this became the GP's responsibility. Warts of course are harmless and in the end go on their own. They are caused by viruses, and whether they come or go depends on the balance between the virus's strength and the patient's immune defences. Verrucas, though more painful and often quite large, will also go eventually. Treatment however is not trouble-free, and GPs had to buy in liquid nitrogen, which could be dangerous when transported and had to be used at one session. In one area a van 'blew up' when carrying it which caused a lot of fuss. Nevertheless it meant that most people who wanted warts treated could have them done in the GP's surgery. Nowadays people can buy preparations which can freeze warts, but they can't be prescribed so people have to pay the full cost.

This reduced the load of the hospitals quite considerably. However it is no cheaper for the NHS for GPs to do the minor surgery than for it to be done in hospital, and so recently many areas have drawn up a list of lesions that should not normally be treated called NNF (Not Normally Funded). Any lesion that was considered cosmetic only was deemed outside the NHS and hospitals started to send these patients back to the GP. GPs being the patient's advocate of course and so wanting to get their patients treated, started to 'game' the system by never putting the word cosmetic in the letter, and stressing other problems the patient had – itching or enlarging or whatever. And if the patient's letter got through the screening process and the patient arrived in clinic the surgeon was often happy to do it – that was after all what they were trained to do. So the NNF system was not always adhered to and some patients got treated and some didn't. This was especially true of patients with cosmetic lesions on the face. If the GP made enough of a case that the patient was very distressed then this might ensure treatment, but then health boards got tougher and might demand psychiatric evaluation. Sometimes the GP bowed to patient pressure and would treat such lesions but the trouble was that few GPs are trained in cosmetic surgery and the results may not be as good as if a plastic surgeon did it, and the GP might be sued. Once I treated a lesion on the face of a young man who was about to get married. The lump was a small haemangioma which bled easily and, though benign, was an awful nuisance to him. The operation went fine and the man was delighted but if his wife hadn't been pleased with it I might have been sued!

With the drive to give only cost-effective treatment on the NHS, the lists of lesions that can be done are more rigorously enforced. People who have lesions that are not considered to need treatment are now advised to leave them alone or go private. Some patients do not like this but otherwise the likelihood is that waiting times will rise again and some patients with unrecognized early cancer will not get treated. This happened once to a patient I know who had a very small spot in the middle of an area on her leg with poor blood supply. She was referred straight away but not seen in good time and had to have a much larger piece of skin removed than otherwise would have been the case, with a lot of discomfort.

Sometimes it is not possible to ensure that everyone with lesions that turn out to be cancer are seen straight away, but everyone tries his or her best. Lots of areas have systems whereby GPs take good quality digital photos of the lesions and send them electronically to the dermatologist, who can then give an opinion on whether the patient needs to be seen. Sometimes in rural areas they even have tele-dermatology where the GP shows the picture of the lesion and can talk to the dermatologist over a video link, and they can discuss the treatment of the lesions together, usually with the patient there as well. These arrangements have been found in trials to be very effective. Tele-dermatology is practised very widely in Australia where of course the distances patients would have to travel are immense, and cancer of the skin is extremely common; the doctors I spoke to highly recommended it.

Chronic skin diseases like eczema, psoriasis, and acne are common problems in young children. The treatment is often prolonged and hard to keep to, and so some practices have trained nurses who can give detailed advice on how much cream or ointment to apply when and what problems to look out for. The nurses get very skilled and are sometimes able to prescribe themselves, if they have attended a special course to become accredited prescribers. This is again a big help to providing a good service for skin problems within the practice.

As detailed in Chapter 14, very few practices do patch testing for allergies now because of the risk of an anaphylactic reaction, and in general, dermatology departments discourage referrals for allergic rashes, debility, or food allergies. Locally they tend to investigate only for contact dermatitis. Severe allergies should be referred to an allergy specialist, but they are in short supply. Hyperhidrosis (excessive sweating) can be a very severe problem for patients and can be treated with Botox (a neurotoxin secreted by a bacteria which inhibits sweating). But in many areas this is not available, as it hasn't been funded. This is certainly something patients ought to be able to get from the NHS. Hirsutism (excess hair) can be a great problem and can be referred to dermatology, but sometimes gynaecology (for women) or endocrinology departments will also investigate excessive hair growth.

Dermatology was one of the specialities in which GPs used to train to become GPs with a Special Interest, aka GPSIs (known colloquially in the trade as Gypsies). This idea was very popular at one time with managers who thought that this would be a cheaper option – train GPs to a higher standard than usual so that they can see more simpler lesions in the practice and thus save money. So schemes were set up where GPs spent some time in dermatology departments treating patients under the direct supervision of a dermatologist, and at the end of the training the GPs then sat an exam. There was also a requirement for the dermatologist to continue to assess the GP as she worked in the practice. It was a very successful scheme in one way as patients were very happy to have their lesions treated in the practice by a GP and the doctors enjoyed the variety. But it has gone out of favour recently as managers have added up the total costs, and re-alised that in fact GPs are more, not less, expensive than the hospital. What they hadn't taken into account was that in most large dermatology departments a lot of the routine 'cutting' is done by doctors in training or nurses, not by consult-ants. As GPs are as well paid as consultants this meant that the GP scheme was more expensive. So it proves you do have to look at the full picture before trying out innovative schemes.

Talking of cutting and stitching, one thing that has always interested me about skin cuts (if you aren't interested in paleontology you can skip this bit, but it does have implications for modern medicine) is that almost any large cut in humans has to be stitched; you can just see the wound gaping and you know that it isn't going to heal easily. If the two edges of the wound are next to each other the wound heals in a trice, but this is rare, and if they are not, the healing process is very different. Instead of quick healing, the wound has to granulate up from the bottom with a big scab. This eventually comes off leaving a red area, which then slowly heals, from the edges, taking weeks to cover the area completely. So what used to happen in pre-historic times? Any sizable cuts weren't going to heal; they would get infected as well and take a very long time to close up. But I don't think prehistoric hominids went around with sterilized needles, stitch scissors and fine catgut as thread!

This was brought home to me when our cat, a half-wild moggie who regularly used to get into fights with the farm cats next door, sustained a dreadful wound just below the neck. It looked awful, and we resolved to take it to the vet. But when we tried to get the cat into the basket it went beserk and we couldn't catch it. We were very busy, so decided to take it the next day. But somehow we seemed to forget about it, the cat wasn't complaining and other priorities intervened.

Amazingly after a week this huge wound seemed to just close up. When the day came for the next appointment with the vet we looked at it and found it had almost healed up. Why was that? A human would have needed at least 6 or seven stitches.

The explanation which appeals to me is the aquatic ape theory, first promulgated by a scientist, Sir Alister Harvey, an English marine biologist. Back in the nineties, Elaine Morgan, a writer for television, popularized the theory by writing some very interesting books on the subject. The theory postulates that back in the Pliocene age, a prehistoric ape-like primate lived in coastal areas and spent such a lot of time on the beach (it was very hot in Africa at that time) and in the water that it became semi aquatic. Now if you haven't read Elaine Morgan's books you would find this a bit bizarre especially as you won't find this theory in any of the official anthropological or paleontological accounts. But it has happened that during evolution several species, including elephants, have gone through an aquatic phase and come out of it again.

Anyway, the theory is that this small ape-like primate spent a lot of time swimming, raising its young on beaches and learnt to dive and adapted to life in a very human like way – sunning itself on the beach, eating crustaceans on the beach, and catching and eating fish. Rather a nice lifestyle most humans would think. During this time, the orthodox theory goes, other primate ape-like species were running around the savannah and learning to walk and somehow managing to lose their hair. Also undoubtedly they were eaten by predators in a big way, as they couldn't really have been very good at walking and running on their hind legs. Elaine Morgan thinks these species went extinct rather than going on to rule the world, and I agree. Other primates rather sensibly carried on in the woods and trees and became the apes. So what happened to the skin of these prehistoric primates that went to the sea-shore? They lost their hair, as wet hair is no insulator and doesn't protect against anything. They developed sub-cutaneous fat in order to keep an even temperature (fat is a very good insulator), and the body became very streamlined just like other aquatic mammals. They became very good divers. Just think of an Olympic diver – the beauty of the symmetry and grace of the clean lines as it cleaves the water – would a gorilla do that? The results were that they became very good at wading (practising walking on two legs so as to keep their heads above water) so started the process of becoming bi-pedal. They became good divers because they could now control their breathing, as people can today, as can all diving birds and mammals (such as dolphins, and seals), and so they could learn to speak. Eventually, so the theory goes, the seas around them dried up and they migrated back to the land, now more bipedal than they were and more importantly, able to speak and communicate.

They now had a totally different type of skin from almost every other mammal. Instead of thin skin, with a lot of hair and very little subcutaneous fat, they now were hairless, with all the difficulties that that entailed in keeping warm, were exposed to the sun and overheating, and the subcutaneous fat under the skin now made a wound gape when cut. Also the long cut, which if you were horizontal in the water would be longitudinal, would fit with the dermatome (natural lines of the skin), whereas horizontal cuts, which were more likely to happen if you are upright, would gape more. There was nothing we could do about it except put up with it, until we learned to stitch. It is what Elaine Morgan called 'a scar of evolution',[126] just like all those back problems we get because we now walk upright.

So remember the dolphins in Chapter 10? Yes, they are mammals. They are sea-going mammals that have taken the process of going aquatic a lot further than our species ever did. They are also very intelligent. But they also get insulin resistance to help them deal with famine – but can even turn it off if there is too much food around! Researchers are now looking at the genes behind this mechanism in order to see if they can come up with something that can turn insulin resistance off again, thus solving our propensity to develop type 2 diabetes very readily.

Also remember our lack of urge to get salt when we don't have enough of it, causing dehydration in small children due to loss of salt, solved by giving one teaspoon of salt and one of sugar to children in the developing world, and the stokers who 'forgot' to load up on salt when they were sweating a lot? All this is understandable if we were in an environment where salt was everywhere!

If this primate existed its fossilized bones would now be under the sea, but if its descendants later went back to the land, beachcombing their way round the world when the climate changed and land became more hospitable, they would now be in a position to dominate the earth – able to speak, communicate, walk on two legs and free the arms to make tools. But they now had to do something in order to cover the skin when they got cold, to get more pigment to protect against the sun, and could no longer be so sure that their wounds would heal so well. They also could develop diabetes in times of plenty.

There isn't any other explanation for us losing our hair that makes sense. Scientists don't seem even to try to answer this question. But our skin does seem to be adapted to water, and our ability to sweat and so lose salt very easily is also explained by this theory.

If you would like to learn more, look it up. (Google 'Aquatic Ape Theory' and read the book 'The scars of evolution'). It is a great read. It appeals to me as a doctor because it explains things about the soft tissues of our bodies that can't be explained in any other way. But as soft tissues don't fossilize we can never get any evidence about them from paleontology, and so sadly, the theory, though never disproved, is ignored. Scientists still routinely talk of 'the Savannah Theory' despite the awkward fact that the savannah did not appear in Africa until well **after** the period in which fossilized hominid bones have been found, which show that they were already way on the way to becoming bipedal.

Chapter 25
Eye Problems

Importance of Optometrists – front-of-eye problems – macular degeneration and its treatment – legal case – cataract pathways.

Our eyes are vastly important. Most people feel that seeing clearly is of the utmost importance to their lifestyle and are motivated to do whatever is necessary to maintain good vision, from childhood to old age. Blindness is also feared greatly because of its implications for independence, which does make for a high emotional component in some ophthalmology conditions that everyone must understand.

For everyday conditions, when you have a problem with your vision you have a choice; you can go to your optician, or to your GP, or for some things like hay fever straight to your local pharmacy for advice. Usually if you can't see clearly but have no other symptoms you would go to an optician, but for pain, discomfort or more serious problems with vision you would go to your GP. However things have been changing recently, and opticians are becoming more and more the eyecare professional of first contact for many eye problems.

Historically opticians were regulated by the Optical Council, and as the term optician implies, they were concerned with the physics of getting your eyesight just right with lenses. Although many were aware of how to recognise problems of eye health and general health, because conditions such as diabetes and blood pressure can easily be spotted by looking into the back of the eye with an ophthalmoscope, opticians did not consider that this was their field and would always refer on to a GP whenever an abnormality was found. This was done on a special form, GOS 18. However as the training for opticians became more complex, it altered to include a great deal on the pathology of the eye i.e. what can go wrong, how to recognise it and how to treat it. The opticians called themselves optometrists to reflect the change in emphasis, and began to campaign for their training to be better used by the NHS.

This then grew into one of the biggest turf wars in medicine, not with GPs, who were very happy to let optometrists do more (sadly, GP training typically only includes 1 or 2 weeks in hospital ophthalmology and most of their eye knowledge comes from their training year in general practice itself) but with ophthalmologists, many of whom were horrified. The medical mafia was at work, and ophthalmologists were much happier to take referrals from GPs and write back to them than to optometrists, and many refused to involve them directly for years. I knew this was a problem all over the country, not just in our area, because a manager who had just come from a post in the London area said it was just the same there. So the infamous form GOS 18 was used as the vehicle for communication between optometrists and ophthalmologists with the hapless GP being the postman – unfortunately a postman who had to read each letter carefully to make sure no action was needed on their part, which was really quite rare. What GPs would prefer if they were themselves not directly involved with the care of the patient, would be for the relevant communication about each patient to be directly from optometrists to ophthalmologists and back, with themselves receiving a copy that would inform them if they were required to take action.

It got very angry at times. I remember a meeting with GPs, optometrists and ophthalmologists all present (a very rare event), which developed into a harangue from ophthalmologists, some of whom said that they would never allow optometrists to do some of the work that had historically been done by the hospital because they could never be sure that they had adequate training. An optometrist patiently explained that they had had at least 4 years of comprehensive training, some of it under the supervision of local ophthalmologists themselves. In fact the conditions that can better be managed in the high street optometrists are legion, from initiating referral to one-stop cataract services and being responsible for the post-op check, to glaucoma monitoring in the community, and many others. Optometrists are now the first port of call for many people with any eye problem, and in most areas the optometrists can now investigate and treat themselves, refer on to the GP or direct to ophthalmology. Optometrists with their excellent skills and facilities in ophthalmoscopy (looking into the back of the eye) are very good at diagnosing some brain tumours for example.

This has been helped by schemes in Scotland and Wales that allow people to have a full examination by high street optometrists for any eye problem at no cost to the patient. The NHS pays the optometrist for this initial eye examination for people who come in directly to optometrists as first port of call, and there are other schemes that involve them in diabetes care, pre and post cataract care and glaucoma monitoring.

So now if you think you have a cataract, you would first be advised to make an appointment with your optometrist, who will also almost certainly be the one who picks it up if you are unaware of a problem. The optometrists is also the one who is able to diagnose if you are likely to develop glaucoma, and can follow up people at risk regularly to check their intra-ocular pressures without being out of pocket. Optometrists can help deal with optical causes of headaches and will correctly diagnose the visual disturbances due to migraine aura that can be very frightening for patients when they have them for the first time. Also they can often diagnose brain tumours as well as or better than GPs.

For better or for worse ophthalmologists are primarily surgeons, and there are very few purely medical ophthalmologists who do not operate at all. So the result of many referrals to a hospital is surgery. Also ophthalmologists have one big advantage over other specialities in that they can see most things that go on the eye directly or with modern equipment, unlike other surgeons who have to find out what is happening by more indirect methods such as scans. The result is that ophthalmologists aren't on the whole very interested in the patients' story, the history of the problem nor in how the patient feels about their eye problems because they know they will get the answer as soon as they examine the patient. Maybe this does not matter if the problem can be cured quickly but in my experience ophthalmologists tend not to be very good at talking or listening to patients, so the GP and the optometrist have to interpret what the ophthalmologist has to say more than in other specialities.

This reminds me of a patient with a complicated series of problems with his eye, who saw various ophthalmologists and received many different diagnoses. He was a GP himself and found it very difficult to work. After many consultations an operation was done, which truth to tell didn't work very well and eventually, rather in desperation, the consultant gave him large doses of steroid drops which finally sorted the problem out. Probably if the steroid drops had been given first an operation might not have been necessary but communication was very poor in those very busy eye departments. But the reason why steroids were not tried beforehand was that steroids can have very nasty effects in some people and so there are very clear guidelines about using steroid drops in ophthalmology. They are always initiated by consultants and never normally by GPs because they can increase the intra-ocular pressure and cause glaucoma. They can also cause blindness when used for a painful red eye when the cause is a viral keratitis, as steroids will cause the infection to spread.

Another pitfall in general practice is using atropine (an anti-cholinergic, which is a transmitter substance important in many parts of the nervous system) drops to dilate the pupil. This is never done these days (there are much better shorter-acting drops which work) but I remember a patient when I first started as a GP and knew very little about eyes. She was in her seventies and came in rather stoically saying that she had become blind in one eye a few days previously. She had been treated with atropine eye drops by another doctor but I wasn't really sure what was going on. I referred her to the hospital but only after she was seen was I told that she had had acute glaucoma from the atropine drops, because she had a narrow angle to the front of her eye and the drops had caused the pressure to rise inside the eye, causing damage to the optic nerve. Sadly the damage had been done immediately and nothing I could have done would have helped but it certainly taught me never to use atropine or steroid eye drops in general practice without full investigation. It is also dangerous to prescribe tablets that act in a similar way to atropine, such as hyoscine used in travel sickness pills, as they can precipitate glaucoma in susceptible people.

So called 'front-of-eye problems' – styes, blepharitis, dry eye and lid problems – are often diagnosed by optometrists, although the patient will then need to go to the GP, who can prescribe. Optometrists in some areas can prescribe on the NHS from a limited list but many can't, so GPs will do so. Otherwise the patient would have to pay for their medications. Blepharitis is by the way one of these chronic sink diseases that can cause a lot of discomfort and pain and will be ignored by many eye specialists, but GPs are often good at dealing with it, sometimes in conjunction with a good optometrist. Dry eyes are a common complaint in older people and this can easily be managed in primary care either by a GP or an optometrist.

If you have an acute red eye you can also go to the optometrist directly, as they can use a slit lamp to accurately diagnose a problem with the inner eye or the cornea. GPs don't have these very useful diagnostic tools, at one time found only in hospitals. If anything serious is found of course the optometrist will refer straight to the hospital.

Age-related macular degeneration (ARMD) is now a most important disease to be picked up in primary care, and optometrists are very well placed to do so in routine check ups. Many have digital cameras, which can pick up the first signs of so-called 'wet' macular degeneration – the treatable kind. Wet ARMD is the more severe form of macular degeneration where, as part of the degeneration of the retina (the macula is the extra sensitive part of the retina that we rely on for our fine vision) extra blood vessels grow into the macula and cause bleeding which destroys the cells necessary to pick up the incoming light. Ten years back it was common for patients with macular degeneration to be put at the back of the queue on the waiting list for years, so in spite of the fact they were going blind they had to wait to see a specialist. Now it is seen as imperative that patients are seen quickly, because the 'wet' form (about 10% of cases of macular degeneration) can be easily treated and blindness prevented if caught early. The treatment is by intra-ocular injections of Lucentis, a new and effective treatment that has been fully funded in order to prevent blindness. I have written about this story in Chapter 16. So if an elderly person notes that straight lines appear wiggly or there are other distortions it is best to make an appointment to see the optometrist straightaway.

The diagnosis of wet macular degeneration was the only case I had where I was sued. It was in 1997, when the only treatment for wet ARMD was laser therapy, and indeed it was suitable only for a minority of people with the wet form, as the main focus of the degeneration had to be slightly to the outside the main centre of the macular area, the part which is essential for fine vision. It worked by destroying the new vessels that were forming in the macula but it destroyed other tissues too, so that it could even make vision worse before stabilizing the condition so that no further sight loss would occur, leaving you hopefully with some useful vision. Laser therapy for ARMD was therefore very limited in its effectiveness and could also lead to scarring of the macula and additional vision loss.

The gentleman in question was a patient in his 70s, a retired engineer, who had been on my list for some time and I knew him well, as he was a neighbour of mine. He had bought a run down cottage and had intended to renovate it and then sell it at a profit. He didn't have much of a pension and didn't have any savings and the money would have been very useful. However he was very unlucky in that he borrowed heavily from the bank to finance the rebuilding but then hit a downturn in the housing market just as he needed to sell it. Interest rates were very high and he faced financial ruin. Eventually the bank bought the house at a knock-down price but it left enough for him to be able to move into a smaller house some distance away. This was my undoing, as he did not notify our practice of his change of address and telephone number, and assumed he could still stay on my list even though his new address was well outside our practice area and we would never have let him stay on. Just at this time he developed further trouble with his vision. He had had wet ARMD diagnosed 5 years previously in his right eye, and had been offered treatment with lasers then but had declined when he learnt of the risks. When, as usually happens, he developed the same problem in the other eye there was a delay in getting him seen at the hospital (the GOS 18 form did not get to the right department), and the hospital also delayed treatment, because they thought he was out of their area too. I think it was at this point the patient decided to try to sue the health service. He kept careful records of every contact with the hospital, which in truth did not respond very quickly (the consultant I spoke to at the time told me that in his opinion the treatment was useless), and certainly by the time he was seen it was decided after investigation that his condition was not suitable for treatment with lasers. Whether there would have been any benefit if he had been treated straight away was then a matter for the legal teams and both the hospital and my solicitors were involved in a long legal case which ended after 2 years with the patient getting a settlement of £20,000 plus costs divided equally against me and the hospital.

I am recounting this case in detail as it demonstrates not only how things can go wrong because of a series of mishaps, but also that perceptions of the value of treatment can alter so much. Nowadays it is unthinkable that someone would get recompense because they didn't get laser therapy for ARMD. In fact it hardly ever helped, and nobody gets this treatment now because the new treatment does work and everyone from GP to optometrist to the man in the street knows that it works. Any delay in getting treatment now would indeed be grounds for considerable compensation and rightly so. (And also of course if the optometrist had sent the letter direct to the hospital there would have been no case against me).

However, the patient got a little nest egg, which made his later years more bearable, and I don't think any one would begrudge him the money except that of course most people don't get any compensation for illness. Perhaps there should be a no-fault compensation scheme, thus preventing the huge legal costs involved. However the sad thing is that because so many don't sue when things go wrong, to offer compensation in all such cases would cost much more, even including the legal costs, and that is why it is not usually done – except in New Zealand. There they have a successful no-fault compensation scheme.

For people with the more common dry type of ARMD there is still very little effective treatment. Just recently however eye surgeons have been promoting a type of surgery which would deflect the light rays from the damaged macular reason to a less damaged part of the retina, using implanted lenses. It is called the IOL-VIP system (it stands for Intra Ocular Lens for Visually Impaired People). It is a very ingenious solution but has not yet caught on widely. It would only be suitable for severe forms because the damaged macular area is, in its healthy state, much more sensitive to light discrimination than other parts of the retina and so it is unlikely that people would get back sufficient detailed vision for reading and fine discrimination back. However anything that helps is to be welcomed.

The availability of treatment for wet ARMD has certainly increased the workload and referrals to ophthalmology, now fortunately most often from optometrists rather than GPs. With any new treatment there will be a need for education to make sure the right people are targeted. Patients previously diagnosed with the commoner kind of macular degeneration, the dry sort, which is still mostly untreatable, may hope that they can benefit and ask for another opinion from a consultant on their suitability for Lucentis, but would probably accept a referral to optometrists instead.

So most people with deteriorating vision can go to an optometrist first, in Wales and Scotland at least, where optometrists are paid for assessing acute eye problems. If there is a problem which needs to be referred to hospital the optometrist can now do this directly without having to go through the GP with all the possible delays that this might cause. If the optometrist can solve the problem himself the patient is very satisfied (sometimes all that is needed is a good pair of glasses) and if not, ophthalmologists will get a much more detailed referral letter. It is obvious though that the clinical pathway between GP, optometrist and ophthalmic doctors can be quite complex and confusing. We collected data on referrals from GP and optometrist to hospital and to each other, and this was crucial in looking at the appropriate pathways for referrals, to prevent optometrist referrals to primary care being routed to secondary care mistakenly. In many cases the GP needs to see the patient himself to decide on further action, such as for headaches, and migraine aura.

In most areas now there is a well-defined Cataract Pathway. Optometrists identifying a cataract or suspected glaucoma account for 60%–80% of referrals, and follow a well-defined protocol so minimising delay for the patient. There is a high conversion rate to operation i.e. most patients referred turn out to need to have their cataracts operated on. But sometimes GPs or opticians do not properly assess the need for an operation prior to referral, and ask the ophthalmologist to make that assessment. They should, prior to referral, perform an assessment and consider the impact on daily living (e.g. driving, reading) and whether the patient is willing to undergo an operation and aware of risks and benefits. That said, cataracts are so readily and successfully treated without problems that it is rare for patients not to agree for it to be done. All referrals are reviewed by local clinics, which directly list patients for operation in the local hospital so that the patient is first seen in the hospital clinic on the day of operation. In some areas, a predefined letter has been adopted by all practices to assist in this process. This streamlines the system and ensures that there is no delay for patients. Also the cataract post-operative check can be transferred to optometrists, thus saving valuable outpatient slots in hospital. In this way some of the load can be taken off ophthalmologists, who are very busy 'saving eyes'.

There are a few cosmetic procedures usually done in hospital eye departments, by consultants specialising in oculoplastic work. Oculoplastic procedures are, as you might expect, a form of plastic surgery round the eyes and are often done mostly for cosmetic reasons such as blepharoplasty, ptosis (droopy eyelids when these interfere with sight), and accidents, which involve the tissues round the eyes. It is extremely specialised work and can make an amazing difference for people with burns of the face.

GPs often refer conditions such as chalazions (styes) and cysts on the eyelids quickly, but in general such problems need not be referred unless present for more than three months, as many resolve before this time. Oculoplastic surgeons also deal with eyelid problems, but xanthelasma, those yellowish lesions found round the eyes of some older people which are a marker for high cholesterol in the blood, are nevertheless harmless in themselves and many areas are now refusing to fund them (they are on the 'Not Normally Funded' list). The same applies to blepharoplasty, the removal of bags over and under the eyes. These have to be done privately if at all.

There have been other new developments in the treatment if eye disorders. Keratoconus is a degenerative condition that usually involves both eyes. It affects the shape of the eyeball and causes blurred vision and light sensitivity. Wearing spectacles or contact lenses can help some people who have this condition. Photochemical corneal collagen cross-linkage is an outpatient procedure. First a local anaesthetic is given in the form of eye drops. Then riboflavin (vitamin B2) drops are applied to the eye, and it is exposed to ultraviolet light. This procedure aims to stabilize the outer coating of the eyeball, called the cornea, with the intention of preventing further changes to its shape.

For a long time now orthoptists, who specialize in the balance of the eyes, have dealt with squints both for children and adults, within the ophthalmic department.

In this way long waits to be seen by eye specialists can be avoided, which should be good news for the many more people in older age group who are going to need these incredibly successful procedures, which will allow many more people to keep their sight as long as possible.

Chapter 26
Urology

Erectile dysfunction

I, along with many others, had never heard of erectile dysfunction until the mid nineties. We called it impotence, and not many people consulted us about it. It was, and is, an embarrassing problem that caused a lot of distress but was rarely brought up in a consultation even if the consultation was about relationships or even family planning. There were no specific treatments that worked. Gradually though treatments became available and the first really useful one was delightfully named Muse, a mechanical method of getting an erection, although the reality of using gadgets to get one's erection was far from delightful. Nevertheless urologists could prescribe it and so when the problem was distressing enough we referred cases to them. This all changed of course when effective treatment came in.

In the early nineties Pfizer was researching a new drug for angina which worked by opening up the coronary arteries, but hit a big snag when they were doing phase 3 trials in many different countries. It had quite severe side effects and could cause sudden cardiac death in people with angina. The company was then advised to recall the batches of the drug that were being used for the trial, and messages went out to the researchers in the various countries to send them back to the company. After a while though it became obvious that the drugs were not being returned, and some months after the end of the trial Pfizer was becoming worried about what had happened to them in view of the fact that the drug had such serious side effects. It transpired that they were not being returned because men had found the tablets very useful indeed for an annoying little problem that affected them from time to time, and so the tablets were being syphoned off so to speak. Pharmaceutical experts were intrigued and looked into it further. They saw the potential of the drug and spent the next year or so premarketing the drug – 'raising awareness' of the condition called erectile dysfunction – obviously a term not so loaded with negative connotations as impotence, and there was a huge publicity campaign aimed at the general public as well as doctors.

When Viagra came on stream of course it was a blockbuster and a game changer. As soon as it was licenced men were not only being told there was treatment but also they were being advised to go to their doctors to get it. This put health organisations all over the world in great difficulty. It was expensive – that is about £16 per tablet – at that time, and if the floodgates were opened for men to get it on prescription the cost would be huge. Even men without much of a problem would want it, in unlimited supplies. It couldn't go on sale without a prescription at first anyway because it could kill if a man with angina took it. So the problem was hurriedly looked at and in the UK a compromise was reached. Anyone who had a medical condition causing impotence such as diabetes, spinal cord lesions or cancer and its treatment, could get it on prescription. It would then be free for people over 65 or who had diabetes, but otherwise the patient paid the prescription fee (as the other conditions weren't on the list for free prescription if you were under 65). They were limited to 8 tablets a month for cost reasons – I don't think there has ever been any evidence that having sex more often than twice a week is bad for you! People without any of these medical conditions – the vast majority, usually where there was no obvious cause for impotence – had to pay for it unless they could prove severe psychological distress as a result of their condition. That was of course a get-out clause, and GPs were then on the firing line.

I certainly got many requests from young men to prescribe it and sometimes did if in my judgment they were suffering sufficiently! It all depended of course on how well the man presented his case and whether he seemed a responsible person. Drug addicts and alcoholics would need their primary problem dealt with first, and we were often aware of men who would sell the tablets on. There soon of course developed a flourishing on-line market in Viagra, which at least had the merit of bringing prices down, but men who genuinely had no money spare could get quite desperate after they found it did indeed work. So most of us GPs, being sympathetic sort of guys, did prescribe it for 'psychological' reasons. Sometime we referred on to urology but it didn't solve the man's problem or ours, as they then languished on waiting lists for a very long time. Urologists weren't very keen to see them quickly. So cash-strapped health organisations then said that GPs couldn't prescribe it unless the man had been seen by a hospital specialist and that included the men with medical reasons for their impotence of course. Waiting lists for urology then soared, and as managers were by now getting targets for people to be seen under 18 weeks from referral to treatment, that again posed a problem. So in many areas the pathway is that the patient has first to be seen by a psychologist to prove 'psychological distress' and only then can be referred to urology where the specialist will give the go-ahead, and prescribe the drug.

Such roundabout and confusing restrictions of prescribing in the UK come directly from the fact that the NHS has to supply any treatment needed under NHS rules – that is at reduced price or free. Lifestyle drugs such as Viagra, and also to a lesser extent drugs like Tagamet, which can prevent the normal problems with digestion that you will get if you overeat, hadn't been thought of when the NHS was started. Presumably the reforms going through Parliament at the moment will get rid of this anomaly and allow lifestyle drugs to be excluded from normal medical care. Some GPs of course will prescribe without authorisation if they think it is the right thing to do, and so long as they don't reach the attention of the pharmaceutical advisors of the primary care trusts (PCTs) and Health Boards too frequently they might get away with it.

Overactive bladder

Overactive bladder (OAB) is a condition that GPs will see often. It affects men and women of all ages, although it is more prevalent in older people and in women overall. However cystitis, which is a bacterial infection of the bladder, is much more common, and this has to be properly diagnosed and excluded before the possibility of an overactive bladder is considered. The infection (urinary tract infection or UTI) isn't always confined to the bladder and may ascend to the kidneys causing damage, and so must be taken seriously. Most practices have a system where a patient can bring in a specimen of urine and have it tested without necessarily seeing a doctor every time, and an appropriate antibiotic can be given straight away. This is important, as cystitis can be extremely painful and upsetting. If it is mild the patients can treat themselves with cranberry juice, as there is evidence that it works, but recurrent cystitis can be a problem. Only if an infection is excluded can a GP consider the possibility of overactive bladder, which has almost identical symptoms to cystitis – having to go to pass water frequently and immediately otherwise you feel you will wet yourself (urgency), pain when passing urine and immediately you finish, and having to get up at night to pass water.

For a long time we doctors were unaware of the existence of OAB and for many patients frequently being told that there was no infection therefore there was no treatment must have been very frustrating. I once took over a patient from another GP, and on going through her notes I found there were 56 normal bacterial reports from the pathology lab, and no abnormal ones at all. The receptionists had got into the habit of telling her to bring a specimen in and sending it off to the lab, while she waited for an appointment to see the doctor. What a waste of her time, the lab's time, and our staff's time. The doctor had obviously missed what the reception staff were doing and probably didn't even look at the result, as he was well aware she didn't have an infection and indeed she may have forgotten about it by the time she saw the doctor (she was certainly a very frequent attender). It is a great improvement for patients that this sometimes very distressing condition can now be recognised and treated. It may well be a problem of spasm of smooth muscles, akin to IBS and dysmenorrhea, which may be due to abnormalities of the functioning of the nerves to smooth muscle. This is why, as in IBS, bladder problems can be made worse by stress.

People seem to react to stressful situations in ways which form a pattern in that individual so that some patients will get headaches (spasm of the muscles around the scalp); some low back pain (spasms of the muscles there), some IBS, and some gynaecological pain (pelvic pain syndrome). Some lucky people don't suffer any of these. It would be good if we can find out what is the actual mechanism behind these related conditions. In fact we now know that OAB syndrome is common and is associated with symptoms that can have a significant impact on a patient's quality of life. Up to 9 million people aged 40 years or over suffer from symptoms of OAB, and about 5 million will need help or treatment from a healthcare professional. However, the embarrassing nature of OAB means that the problem is likely to be under-reported, and that many people will suffer in silence. Both men and women can suffer from this condition, although it is commoner in women.

There are some medical conditions, such as stroke and multiple sclerosis, that can cause similar symptoms as they can result in the little muscle controlling the passing of urine (the detrusor muscle) being overactive because the central nerve supply has been affected. Diabetes can cause these problems due to small vessel damage to the nerves, also the menopause in women because of lack of oestrogen resulting in thin tissues. Prostate problems in men can also cause similar symptoms.

So if a patient has urinary symptoms such as frequency (going to pass water very frequently), urgency (discomfort making you feel you have to empty your bladder now), or nocturia (getting up at night more than once to pass water), then these conditions above have to be excluded first. If the cause is none of these then the problem is diagnosed as OAB and NICE suggests cutting down on caffeine and/or alcohol, moderating your fluid intake (drinking too much or not enough fluids can worsen symptoms) and then trying bladder training. This aims to re-programme the nerves to the bladder by getting people to hold on for longer and longer before going. The trigone area of the bladder (an area at the back of the bladder) has a plexus of nerves inside it which can get over stimulated when the urine collects on top of it, and accustoming the area to having more fluid on top of it can help. The reason why getting up in the night is such a problem is that when lying down the trigone area gets more stimulation as it is now horizontal and this makes people wake up – there is usually very little fluid in the bladder at night because the kidneys are good at concentrating the urine overnight, but what there is is right over the trigone area. Bladder training should continue for a minimum of six weeks.

If a patient still has to go to pass water frequently, then drugs which calm down the excessive stimulation of the nerves to the bladder can be prescribed. However such drugs do have side effects such as dry mouth, constipation and dizziness. Overactive bladder can cause a great deal of anxiety and stress, and patients need to have their concerns handled sensitively. Nowadays many urology departments have developed special clinics run by nurses which will deal with OAB and also with recurrent bladder infections from whatever cause. They also deal with incontinence (the leaking of urine when you are not actually intending to pass water), which is of cause another common problem, often more serious.

There are many different treatments, some of them surgical, as in women incontinence can also be caused by a vaginal prolapse, and both OAB and weakening of the vaginal muscles can co-exist. The aim of these clinics is to make sure that patients can get treatment quickly without waiting a long time to see a specialist. GPs see a lot of patients with all these conditions as well and need only refer the more problematic cases.

Bedwetting

Children's bedwetting and daytime wetting are also problems which GPs see often and treatment is usually by a sort of behaviour modification programme which is carried out by health visitors or nurses working in the practice or in the Paediatric department of the hospital. Treatment with drugs (heavily promoted to GPs) can also help.

Urine analysis

Blood in the urine is a very frightening symptom and should normally be referred to an urologist. GPs will usually test for an infection first as this is by far the commonest reasons for blood in the urine. If there is no infection it is said that people under 50 should be referred to a nephrologist, as kidney problems are more likely than bladder problems, while over 50s should be referred to an urologist as bladder problems and especially bladder cancer can occur at this age. However, with the advent of accurate strip tests with which to test the urine, many people are found to have blood in the urine on this test without any other problems. This is called microscopic haematuria. The problem is often one of faulty or over-accurate tests but specialists think such patients should be investigated. This can be carried too far though.

A recent journal article concluded that if a patient does not have hypertension (high blood pressure), protein in the urine (proteinuria – normally there should be no protein in the urine but many conditions can cause it to leak out through the kidneys), or abnormal kidney function then it may not be helpful to investigate a patient under 40.[127] The fact that such patients are inappropriately (and often invasively) investigated ignores the high frequency of the condition, the very low pick-up rate of significant disease, the possible complications, and the opportunity cost of such resource allocation. Many nephrologists now routinely return such referrals to primary care.

Prostate

Prostate problems, such as the very common benign prostatic hypertrophy (BPH), where the prostate just grows too big as men get older, used to have to be treated by an operation, originally quite a big operation where the prostate was reduced in size surgically. Nowadays there are very good drugs, such as finasteride, which over time can reduce the size of the prostate, and GPs can prescribe these without having to refer to a specialist, unless the treatment is not successful after at least three months trial. (Before the development of these drugs, a herb, Saw Palmetto, was widely used for treating lower urinary tract symptoms attributed to benign prostatic hyperplasia, but recent trials showed that this herb was no more effective than placebo). If the patient is put on medication for BPH, it can be continued for many months, and NICE recommends that yearly prostate-specific antigen (PSA) tests be done to exclude cancer of the prostate.

Prostate-specific antigen tests were developed in the 90s and measure the level of a tumour marker, a specific protein made in the prostate gland, in the blood. The level will be raised in most men with prostate cancer. There is considerable controversy over when to ask for this test, and indeed whether men should be screened regularly to try to reduce the death rate from prostate cancer. The actual level in the blood depends on how old the man is; for instance, in men aged 40–49 it should be under 2.5 ng/ml, and between 70 and 79 years it should be under 6.5 ng/ml, as the normal level rises with age. There is no age-specific range published for men over 80 years old, as the necessary research has not been done in men of that age, so we just do not know what is a normal PSA in men over 80.

However it is well known that there is no way of finding out exactly how tumours diagnosed as a result of these raised PSA tests will behave and herein lies the problem. There is no doubt that prostate cancer can kill. In younger men, from 40 to 60, it can be a very serious disease indeed and can spread outside the prostate very quickly. But as men get older more and more of them will show signs of cancer in their prostate glands, yet fewer and fewer of them will get any signs or symptoms of cancer. About 80% of men who die of other causes will have evidence of cancer in their prostates, which has been unrecognized and is not doing anything harmful to its owner.

So as with breast cancer, patients and their doctors are in great difficulty. If you screen for these cancers in all men using a PSA test (and in women using mammography screening), you will find many people who appear to have cancer, but there is no way of knowing whether the cancers will ever cause problems in that person's lifetime. No tests are perfect, and there will always be false negatives where the person does have cancer though it doesn't show in the test, and false positives where the test is positive but the person turns out after further investigation not to have cancer after all. If you screen men in the younger age groups you will find very few cancers but those you do find will need treatment. But for those very few to be diagnosed early you will have to cause a lot of anxiety to those men with false positive tests, maybe do unnecessary treatment with bad side effects, and spend a lot of money on the screening. So far in the UK the evidence on screening, according to principles set up by the relevant scientific authority, is not sufficient to prove that PSA testing would do more good than harm. In the USA it used to be recommended that men over forty have a yearly PSA measurement, but this has never been the practice in the UK, and in May 2012, the U.S. Preventive Services Task Force (USPSTF) changed its advice and recommended against routine screening for prostate cancer.

But the situation is different for each individual and there is nothing to stop any person going to his doctor and asking for a test, and the guidance given to GPs in the UK is that the test can be done after fully-informed discussion between patient and well-informed GP (and after doing a rectal examination, which is where the doctor examines the prostate through the back passage). So all GPs should discuss this in detail with their patient so that he understands the limitations of the test and the likely outcomes if positive.

There is of course all the difference in the world between testing every man between certain ages, and testing those who have a reason for asking for it such as a family history, and those who have symptoms that might be related (though most prostate cancer is entirely symptomless). I used to agree to do the test very readily in men up to the age of 75 to 80, and of course I used it for diagnostic purposes. Several times I included a PSA test in a battery of tests I was doing for men in their seventies who were obviously ill, when it wasn't clear what the cause was. In two cases the PSA came up sky high giving me the diagnosis – metastatic prostate cancer, which was then successfully treated – and the men still died of something else! There were often reasons why a man would need one done, for instance if someone else in the family had it, or if men had some waterworks symptoms. After 70 I used to think that the benefit of doing the test depended much more on the man's health and whether he was likely to die of anything else rather than on the level of the PSA. If a man has a life expectancy of less than 10 years, because he has already got other problems such as heart disease for example, then I would really discourage doing it.

If the PSA test result comes back in a borderline range or slightly above the normal guidelines, and other reasons for the rise such as a urinary infection have been excluded, I believe it may be better for the GP to repeat the test a few times before referring to the consultant. Then if the level is rising over several months or years, then referral can be made. In any case the urologist will usually do this before recommending any more diagnostic tests (so called watchful waiting). However it is sometimes difficult not to refer straight away – once the patient knows that his risk of cancer has increased it is difficult not to refer, if only to prevent being sued.

The definitive diagnostic tool is a prostate biopsy, and if it is positive it will give a grading as to how aggressive this cancer is. Fortunately, treatment of prostate cancer is excellent and if the consultant thinks it is necessary there are several options, such as surgical treatment and radiotherapy as well as 'active surveillance', which is much as the same as 'watchful waiting' except that you now know that the cancer is there. So consultants in urology now spend a great deal of time discussing the pros and cons of treatment – surgical treatment carries the risk of urinary incontinence, and this and hormone treatment both carry a high risk of impotence, and all this treatment may not even be necessary. It is indeed very difficult to choose the best path and we urgently need better tests that would tell us whether this cancer is likely to cause trouble in a man's lifetime.

A new study of men with early prostate cancer found no difference in death rates whether they received surgery or no treatment.[128] It followed up 731 men from 1994 for twelve years and showed that of those who had had surgery to remove the prostate gland, there was only a non- significant increase in survival (3%) compared with those who did not have the operation. Considering that 50% of men who had had the operation had impotence directly related to the operation, and 10% had permanent urinary incontinence, it seems that surgery may not be the best option for many. There were difficulties with the study in that that they did not recruit as many men as they wanted, so the study may not have been adequately powered, and also the men were in the older age bracket, so it does not really help those men in their forties, fifties and early sixties, especially those with aggressive tumours proven by biopsy, who need to know what the best treatment is.

Surgeons are trying very hard to improve the complication rate using very expensive techniques, sometimes involving robots, but there is not so far any evidence that the complication rate with the these is any better, although the recovery may be quicker. Active surveillance or sometimes radiotherapy, which has a much lower complication rate, may be a much better option.

However, when a cancer is found only when the cancer has already spread, treatment can still be very effective. In the two cases above, the men were both given chemotherapy and one had radiotherapy as well, and both survived with treatment for between 5 and 10 years and died of something else, in one case a stroke and in the other general deterioration of old age.

This whole subject is an example of how important it is to be wary of screening campaigns, and also not to let enthusiasm for surgery drive men and women into thinking that the only thing you can do with a cancer is to take it out. Now that we are diagnosing so many more tumours, we do need to realise that treatments other than surgery, and even no treatment at all, may be better.

Chapter 27
Neurology

Severe neurological diseases and their diagnosis – headaches – specialist nurses.

Severe neurological diseases

Neurology is the speciality that deals with the nervous system – not the 'nerves' that you get when you are anxious, which is a feeling, not a problem with a specific nerve, but the nervous system as a whole. It consists of the brain, the spinal cord and the nerves coming from them with long tendrils covered with myelin sheaths. Everyone knows that this speciality covers some of the most disabling and frightening conditions known – multiple sclerosis (MS), Parkinson's disease (PD), and motor neurone disease (MND). Add brain tumours, which are treated by neurosurgeons but diagnosed and managed by neurologists, and you have a nasty set of diseases.

Despite many advances recently it remains the case that they are all incurable and some are untreatable with anything effective. Often symptoms are insidious and non-specific so that it is easy to think you have one. Some of them – MS and some forms of MND – occur mainly in young people so it is small wonder that people can be convinced, usually wrongly, that they have a disabling neurological disease. But it is difficult for GPs to diagnose neurological diseases in their early stages precisely because the symptoms are non-specific and sometimes depend not in the symptoms themselves but on the pattern over time.

Officially, MS can be diagnosed only when you have had at least two demyelinating lesions in the brain or spinal cord separated in time and space. A demyelinating lesion is a where the myelin sheath, the covering round the nerve become damaged by the disease process, and can cause many symptoms depending where the affected nerve is. So the first problem you present with to your GP is likely to be misdiagnosed as something else, and only after you have developed more symptoms due to separate bits of damage to a nerve can it be clear that there is something more serious going on. Similarly, MND can present with very nebulous symptoms – sometimes just weakness – and sometimes the patient does not think it is serious at first.

So diagnosis, especially in a speciality when there is no cure, can be sensitive as well as difficult. While a GP may suspect there may be something more serious going on, it seems very unfair to tell a patient of your suspicions straight away if you are likely to be provide wrong. But it is necessary to do it.

One patient I remember very well. She was a nurse, who was working part time as she had a young family, and I had seen her frequently with her children's ailments. One day she came to me complaining of weakness and pins and needles. She told me she had had it before and it was definitely 'nerves' – her husband wasn't supportive with the children and she found it hard to keep things together in the house. She wanted Valium. I talked to her for a bit about her life and how to manage things better, and I didn't give her Valium but gave her something else (a mild antidepressant I think). Stupidly I did not examine her. She seemed satisfied and went away. About ten days later my partner was called to the house, as she was extremely unsteady. He examined her and found clear signs of demyelination, and he was very critical of me, correctly, for not diagnosing it earlier. It transpired though, that the patient knew she had a neurological problem and the previous episode some years ago had been quite serious. She had self-diagnosed MS and decided she wasn't going to tell anybody – including me. She was hoping not to have to tell anybody especially her husband. I felt very bad about it, but she continued to see me rather than the partner who had made the correct diagnosis. Sometimes people don't always tell you everything!

Another nurse (I don't think it is commoner amongst nurses but they are particular challenging because they know more than the average person) was very worried as she had a severe back problem and we thought the pain and weakness in her leg was due to that. Soon though there were unequivocal signs in her legs which meant that there was a severe problem here, and when the specialist ruled out a back problem MS seemed a possibility. It took some time though before she saw a neurologist, who made the diagnosis. Nowadays MRI scans will make the diagnosis a lot quicker, as if there is a reasonable suspicion an MRI scan will show whether there have been previous lesions and this can clinch the diagnosis. I eventually confirmed the diagnosis to her on a home visit, and she took it very well and positively, even writing a book about her experience, which she gave to her friends and relatives.

The GP's job is not only to listen to the history but also to make a full examination, as once there has been nerve damage there are likely to be physical signs. In the case of the first woman, my partner had found signs of spasticity (increased tone meaning that her leg was stiff to move and her reflexes were brisk) and this was a definite signs that immediate referral was indicated. So it is clear that a GP has to have a high index of suspicion whenever people complain of weakness, pins and needles and other vague complaints and can be a difficult decision when to refer. Once you have suggested referral of course most patients will be very worried and find the waiting time to see a specialist very unsettling.

But in most cases you don't find anything like that and the symptoms can be due to many other conditions, most of which will go on their own. For instance, there is a condition called meralgia paraesthetica, which is a trapped nerve in the thigh, causing a burning or stinging sensation in the distribution of the nerve over the front of the thigh. Though definitely neurological, it is due to compression of the nerve by seat belts, tight trousers, obesity, or pregnancy, and can complicate conditions such as diabetes mellitus and alcoholism, where nerve damage can occur. Once you have examined the patient and there is no problem in the abdomen that could cause it, the patient can be reassured that it is not MS, and simple methods of treatment and time will sort it out.

Headaches

Symptoms like headaches can also be very worrying. Everyone gets headaches from time to time, and there are so many different sorts that a GP needs to take a proper history of where the pain is, when it comes, what are the precipitating factors and whether it is associated with other symptoms, to find out the cause. However it is nearly always possible to get an idea of the probable cause in a first consultation. The two most common sorts are tension headache and vascular headache. Tension headaches are like a band round the head, and can be caused by neck problems, and tension in the muscles round the head. Vascular headaches are throbbing, and typically caused by migraine. The brain itself has no pain receptors so the pain comes from structures round the brain. Headaches are always troubling and may be very severe indeed. Cluster headaches, a specific sort of migraine, and the thunderbolt headache of a subarachnoid haemorrhage (a form of stroke) are the most well known. Trigeminal neuralgia a nerve pain in the face is also a very nasty sort.

So in order to try to be sure of recognising the sort of headache that might be really serious GPs have to look for 'red flag' symptoms – those where the patient should be referred without delay. One of these is 'the worst headache you have ever felt in your life'. This may be due to a subarachnoid haemorrhage, a burst blood vessel in the brain, which causes bleeding into the tissues around the brain, and will need immediate treatment by a neurosurgeon. Another red flag is a post-ejaculation headache – a severe headache coming on soon after having sex, which may again be due to a stroke. (That is a very nasty thought.) Early morning wakening headaches, if new and persistent, can be a sign of a brain tumour and really any entirely new and progressive headache can be serious.

But most headaches are not due to anything serious, though they can be very debilitating. I certainly saw many patients with very bad headaches and nothing seemed to help, though ibuprofen and the triptans for migraine were very helpful, but one should beware the analgesic-induced headache or medication overuse headache. This is a chronic headache which is actually due to the medication itself. People will start taking paracetamol, ibuprofen, triptans or stronger tablets for their headache, which relieve it for a while, but later it wears off and the patient gets a rebound headache. People will then take more medication and soon the headache from being a simple tension or migraine type headache transforms into a chronic daily headache. Wikipedia says that this is the third most common type of headache. Although only 1–2% of the population will suffer from it, it is a great problem worldwide. The main difficulty is that patients cannot believe that the painkillers are the cause. In any case even if they do agree to withdraw the medication there is nearly always a recurrence of sometimes even worse headaches. Sometimes inpatient therapy is needed to treat the patient and it is a big source of disability. The aim will be to get the patient on to something that will prevent the headaches which is not a painkiller, for instance a migraine prophylactic, or a beta blocker (which is commonly used for anxiety) or amitryptiline, that most useful of drugs, in small dosage. Certainly people need to know that taking painkilling medication for headaches can be a bad thing, and can be advised to try other things.

Headaches and migraine were by far the highest reason for referral to neurology, yet neurologists don't have magic answers. Patients should try the usual things first, working with their GPs to find out what is best for them. If they do have to be referred, GPs should ensure that details of medication already tried, the doses used and for how long they have been tried, are supplied in the referral letter.

Sometimes even if it seems clear that the cause of the headache is not a brain tumour the patient would like to be referred. The result is, in our survey at least, that most patients referred in neurology are the 'worried well', adults in their 30s and 40s rather than the elderly who are the ones who mostly suffer from neurological diseases.

Neurology referrals have been increasing year on year, which must be due to patient expectation of prompt investigation and GP unease about missing something, as there has not been an increase in the incidence or prevalence of neurological diseases. Most diseases in neurology do in fact occur in the elderly, certainly over 65, and it was a surprise that many of our referrals to neurology were much younger – the peak age was 45. Very few of them had a serious neurological problem, and the reason seems to because serious and frightening neurological conditions such as multiple sclerosis and brain tumours can occur in younger people. Many of these referrals for people in their 40s and 50s were therefore also of the 'worried well' and although some of these may not have needed referral, in many cases they may still have to be investigated. What is interesting though is that this cohort will be decreasing in the next 10 to 20 years, and even if the numbers of referrals of the over 70s doubles there may still be no great increase, and there could even be a decrease for purely demographic reasons.

There aren't any easy alternatives to referral either, although some areas have headache or migraine clinics. There aren't any community-based services other than those developed by the neurologists. It would of course reduce waiting lists to see a consultant if GPs could ask for MRI scans themselves, as many patients would be spared the agonising wait to see a specialist. I have said a lot about this at the beginning of the book and also in Chapter 21. But sometimes MRIs can show up odd lesions which are very difficult to sort out and these would need referral to a specialist, yet few would cause any harm to the patient. However I had one patient who was dissatisfied after seeing a neurologist who had not done an MRI scan, and she was still convinced she had a brain tumour. The proper thing to have done was to have spent time with her to find out any underlying problem, or re-refer her back to the neurologist but in the end she paid for a private MRI scan, which was normal. After that she was entirely satisfied and I didn't see her again for some time. This behaviour may reflect a public perception from TV shows and the media generally that such scans are (or should be) much more available than they are.

One development recently that has been enormously helpful for some patients has been the training of specialized nurse practitioners for chronic neurological diseases, for MS, PD and MND. They know a lot about the problems of living with such diseases and will visit regularly.

Falls and dizziness

Falls and funny turns can be due to many different conditions, from cardiovascular to ear, nose and throat (ENT) problems, and in some areas there are specialised falls clinics. Falls in the elderly are a very common indeed and can be real problem, resulting in hospital admissions and fractures and loss of independence. Many areas are looking at falls and their prevention in great detail. Dizziness is a common symptom, and just recently I attended a talk about a booklet for treatment of Meniere's disease and other conditions causing dizziness. It is based on re-programming the vestibular system by shaking your head! Now that may be a simple idea that works in some people, where otherwise there is nothing except drugs which don't work very well.

Epilepsy in adults is seen in neurology clinics, and will need specialist management. A good description of a first fit by an observer is crucial. Mobile phone videos welcomed!

When I looked at our referrals for an audit once I discovered with chagrin that a patient I had referred to neurology actually needed to see an urologist! The patient had turned up in clinic and the neurologist had to spend some time with him before realizing that he was in the wrong department. He said it quite often happened, and GPs need to take care if dictating to secretaries!

Chapter 28
Rheumatology

Rheumatoid arthritis – incidence and treatment – PMR – hypermobility – osteoporosis

Rheumatoid arthritis

Rheumatoid Arthritis (RA) is an autoimmune disorder where the body makes antibodies to its own tissues, and we don't really know the reason why. It is a serious, life-threatening, painful and debilitating disease and in the past people with a diagnosis of RA would be certain to have a prolonged and painful illness, which would lead to severe joint damage and probably early death.

The treatment of crippling diseases in rheumatology has improved enormously in recent years with the development of new drugs, the monoclonal antibodies (their names all have a suffix '-mab' on the end to reflect this). In arthritis the damage to the joints comes from inflammatory substances, in particular anti-tumour necrosis factor (TNF), in the synovium, the lining of the joint. TNF is a relatively recent discovery; it promotes the inflammatory response, which causes many of the clinical problems associated with autoimmune disorders. Fortunately new TNF inhibitors have now been developed which are at the cutting edge of modern pharmacological treatments and are a great success story (albeit another very expensive one). Monoclonal antibodies targeting these substances suppress inflammation and produced rapid symptomatic improvement. So for the first time there are drugs available which actually modify the disease and prevent it getting worse, unlike the painkillers and anti-inflammatory drugs used previously, which merely helped the symptoms. These drugs are known by the acronym DMARD, Disease-Modifying Anti-Rheumatic Drugs. Oddly enough a herb from the Amazon rainforest, Cat's Claw Vine, has also been found to inhibit TNF and also has been used to treat arthritis. However there are only small trials to indicate that it actually works in patients.[129]

Joints are the main organs damaged by RA but other tissues are affected as well; so that there are lots of other symptoms such as eye problems, skin problems and gastrointestinal symptoms to add to the patient's woes. I do remember a patient in her early fifties who had it terribly badly and all her joints were crippled within a few years, and she was anaemic from gastric bleeding because of the painkillers she took. At first the surgeons tried to operate on some of the worst affected joints, her hips and hands, but the operations failed and eventually the surgeon threw up his hands in despair and said to her daughter – 'I can't do anything else for your mother. I will have to let you take her home and nurse her.' Which she did devotedly for the next few years until she died – of a gastric haemorrhage. In those days daughters often did that: she had brought up her family and never had a job. Nowadays the daughter would have had to give up her job and would have a hard time financially, even with a carer's allowance.

The new drugs are very expensive indeed – up to £15,000 to £18,000 a year – but can be very effective if started early in the course of the disease to prevent permanent damage to joints and other tissues. So it is now extremely important to diagnose rheumatoid arthritis early. However, joint pains are common, and very few patients in a GP's surgery are likely to have RA when they first come to a doctor with such symptoms. The doctor must be careful to identify that one patient, and refer him quickly to hospital. There are some very good blood tests that might indicate that a patient with joint pains has RA, and GPs do them very freely, but they are not foolproof. Rheumatoid arthritis diagnosis is clinical; that is, it can be diagnosed solely on history and examination – so if patient has morning stiffness lasting for at least 30 minutes, and has swollen joints in the hand (more than three) which hurt when you squeeze them, then they might have RA. If symptoms are not so clear-cut then GPs are advised to refer if they still have symptoms after 6 to 8 weeks even if the tests are negative. Early RA is often very responsive to non-steroidal anti-inflammatory drugs (NSAIDs) such as ibuprofen, which are simple and cheap drugs and indeed a good response is suggestive of the condition. So GPs are advised not to delay diagnosis because a patient responds well to NSAID treatment.

There are however conditions that mimic RA. Viral or reactive polyarthropathy (poly means lots and arthropathy means a disease of the joints), can be severe but settles within 3 months, and it would be important to make sure people aren't treated with powerful drugs when they don't need them. Obviously some people may have to be referred early, but there would be no need to refer a patient who has got better in that time. Because there are fewer rheumatologists in the UK per head of population than in most of Europe, this is a speciality where it is very important to send the right patient early, but not to send the patients who don't need to go, as this just makes it impossible for those who need treatment to get it early enough. There are lots of blood tests that can help: there are simple ones such as RA Latex antibodies, and many other new markers that can tell the GP what sort of rheumatological problem the patient might have, and so whether they need to refer. There is good advice from NICE for both osteoarthritis and rheumatoid arthritis.

However, it seems that maybe doctors, GPs and rheumatologists are now making the diagnosis of RA more often, and certainly the incidence of RA is now rising considerably, especially in women, while it previously had been steady for many years. This rise in RA follows a 4-decade period of decline, and the study authors speculate that environmental factors such as cigarette smoking, vitamin D deficiency, and lower dose synthetic estrogens in oral contraceptives may be the source of the increase. An alternative explanation might be that the availability of good new and expensive drugs has increased the demand for treatment by increasing the number of people diagnosed. You can see how this happens – a doctor wants to be absolutely sure that he has done everything possible to prevent disability. But all drugs have side effects, and over-medicalisation and over treatment can be very bad for patients.

Once RA has been diagnosed then GPs usually are involved in sharing care with the rheumatologist to ensure that their time is used best, and GPs will do the blood test monitoring and check patients regularly. With this treatment patients with RA are assured of a much better outcome with much less deformity than previously.

Polymyalgia rheumatica

Many other common rheumatology conditions can be diagnosed in general practice. Probably the commonest is polymyalgia rheumatica (PMR), which occurs in people older than their mid-fifties and usually in their seventies and eighties. It affects muscles rather than joints and causes severe muscle pains, usually in the shoulders, arms and thighs. There is a very characteristic presentation when patients (usually women) first notice a problem when they can't easily comb their hair because their arms and shoulders are too painful. The diagnosis is easy too, as the ESR test (as described in the investigations section) is nearly always raised to quite a high level. If so, then an oral steroid, such as prednisolone, is the treatment and this should work within a couple of days. Usually the patient is over the moon as all the symptoms go completely. The starting dose of 15 mg can then be tailed off to a low level but most patients need to stay on a low dose for years. The textbooks say that it burns itself out in 2 years, but I have to say that that has not been my experience. People have their ups and downs and it is difficult to get off the steroids altogether. At doses under 5 mg prednisolone is reasonably safe, but if the dose has to be higher because otherwise the disease returns then there are other drugs that can be used by specialists. In general typical PMR is usually treated in primary care, and GPs will refer on if there are problems in weaning people off steroids later on.

Occasionally the tests are negative and one retired farmer in his eighties complained of very characteristic symptoms for many months yet the ESR was always normal. After some time I did give him the prednisolone and it worked wonderfully well. However I don't think the disease was true PMR as he was able to stop the tablets very quickly, though the symptoms did come back several times afterwards.

There is a more serious related disease called temporal arteritis and this causes pains over the temporal region in the head, and pains in the jaws. In this disease the ESR is usually very much higher and there is a risk of blindness so these patients should be referred to a rheumatologist immediately, however it is quite rare and quite difficult to diagnose.

Hypermobility

Hypermobility is another important rheumatological condition that has been around for ages, but unfortunately it passed me by until the late nineties. I certainly didn't get told about it in my training and knew nothing about it until a patient, a health service manager in her thirties, came to me complaining about pain in her knees. There was nothing to find on examination and blood tests were normal. I treated her with ibuprofen, a simple NSAID and referred her to physiotherapy, but she was less than impressed. She told me that her mother had had exactly the same symptoms and she was sure there was something that needed a diagnosis. So I referred her to our local rheumatologist, not thinking there would be anything to be gained from it. She waited a very long time (despite being a NHS manager!) but in the end she got a life-changing diagnosis from a locum who had been brought in to tackle the waiting list. She was diagnosed as having symptomatic hypermobility syndrome (HMS) and she was quite convinced, correctly, that this answered all her concerns. It was definitely a wake-up call for me!

Hypermobile joints, which have the ability to move beyond their normal range of motion, are common and are often just a talking point. Can you put your hands flat on the floor with your knees straight? Can you bend your left thumb back on to the front of your forearm? and can you bend your right little finger at 90 degrees, towards the back of the hand? Some people can, most people can't. But in some people all or most of their joints are hypermobile.

Having a few hypermobile joints isn't unusual, and in many people with many joints affected, joint hypermobility isn't a problem and requires no treatment. Doctors refer to this as benign hypermobility syndrome. It is common in children and decreases with age. In childhood this can be an advantage in certain sports and they can excel in them. But in some people, hypermobility causes joint pain and a higher incidence of dislocations, sprains and secondary osteoarthritis. Over the years, unfortunately, the fact that the joints can move way out of their normal range leads to stress on the ligaments that provide joint stability, which become loose and weak.

The main reason to distinguish these conditions from 'normal' wear and tear is that on the whole patients with HMS respond very poorly to operations and invasive investigations. The muscles and joints don't heal well because the underlying problem is an inherited connective tissue disorder, thought to be caused by faulty tissues such as collagen, and the skin can also be very stretchy and heal badly. So what are definitely not needed here are multiple investigations such as arthroscopies and joint operations; they are unlikely to help and may make things worse. The treatment of choice is physiotherapy, but because these patients' joints are already fully mobile they do *not* need stretching exercises, and the physiotherapist must know to concentrate on balance and stability. Sometimes patients seem to be very unfit because their muscles are weak and sometimes they have poor posture, but the physiotherapist must be aware of this. Flat feet, chronic spinal disc problems with back and neck pain, are also common. I can now identify people with hypermobility in the street – but of course they may not have any symptoms at all!

The diagnosis of symptomatic hypermobility can easily be made in primary care. There are two scales (questionnaires) used. The Beighton score consists of a series of nine questions (the sort mentioned above) – e.g. 'Can you bend your right elbow backwards?' which identify how many joints are affected (out of 10). If you score four or more, you probably have joint hypermobility. Most people score less than two. If you also have symptoms, such as joint pain, you may have joint hypermobility syndrome and to diagnose this the Brighton criteria (yes, it is very confusing to have two different scores with very similar names) is used. This adds to the Beighton score by asking how long you have had problems like joint pain or back pain (has to be over three months to diagnose HMS) or whether you have ever had a dislocated joint or partial dislocation in more than one joint, or in the same joint more than once. So the GP will take these two scores and work out whether you have symptomatic HMS, but will also check that nothing else is causing the problems. Rheumatoid arthritis has to be ruled out early of course.

The form of the syndrome which includes other manifestations of connective tissue disorders, such as gastro-intestinal problems, autonomic disorders (such as a tendency to faint or intermittent fast pulse), and easy bruising, is called Ehlers–Danlos Syndrome – Hypermobility type. This is fortunately pretty rare. It is said that there is an association with some features of fibromyalgia and that some patients are more anxious than usual. That has not been my experience however and most people tend to be very positive in outlook.

Osteoporosis

Another condition that is generally classified as rheumatological is osteoporosis, and this is an extremely common condition. One in three women and one in twelve men over the age of 50 will suffer an osteoporotic fracture, and these fractures are painful and disabling. Hip fractures used to be a common cause of death, with 50% of people who had suffered one being dead within a year.

Even now with effective treatment 20% of people will die; usually, it is fair to say, because they are old and may have many other problems. It doesn't follow that preventing fractures will prevent death, but immobility after fractures may well hasten it.

All fractures are painful, but osteoporotic spinal fractures are extremely painful and the pain is poorly controlled by ordinary painkillers. I certainly saw women in agony for weeks, yet there was little we could do before modern drugs were available. Colles fractures, the very common wrist fractures, are also often a result of thinning of the bones, but fortunately heal quite quickly.

The risk factors for osteoporosis are well known – lack of exercise, smoking and family history are the main causes but there are medications that also cause it (such as long-term steroids) and other diseases. Of course oestrogens, the female hormones that women lose when they pass the menopause, are well known to protect against osteoporosis, so that after it women are more likely to develop the disease than men. Calcium is important as it is incorporated into bones, so an adequate intake is also essential. Lack of exercise is a real problem, not only in the elderly but also more particularly in the young. The reason is that peak bone mass – that is the heaviest your bones become – is dependent on the amount of exercise you take, and if you don't take much exercise when young your peak bone mass will be lower. As the threshold for developing fractures is fairly constant then the more bone mass you have in your prime then the more you can lose before having symptoms. Women over the age of 60 who have never exercised much and who are lightly built therefore are prime candidates, especially if there is a family history and if they have ever smoked. Men can get it too, though it tends to start later.

So to prevent osteoporosis, you shouldn't smoke, you should take plenty of exercise, should aim for a dietary intake of 1,000 mg calcium per day, and choose your parents wisely!

For elderly people who are fit you will only need to have tests for osteoporosis done if you have risk factors or if you have had a fracture that might have been due to fragile bones. The investigation of choice is a dexa scan. This tells us exactly how much bone has been lost in several places (spine and hip usually). Dexa scans can be requested by GPs, and in some areas radiologists and rheumatologists will give a full diagnosis with recommendations for further treatment back to the GP, so that the patient does not have to go to the rheumatology clinic unless they have established osteoporosis. The diagnosis most often made by a dexa scan is osteopenia, where there is thinning of the bones but not enough to cause symptoms. Osteopenia and Osteoporosis are mostly managed by GPs and they are big business at the moment. They fulfil all the requirements for a bombardment of GPs from above – a good evidence base, lots of profit in many sorts of drugs, lots of public concern – and are something that is going to get much worse as the population ages.

It is well known that oestrogens will treat osteoporosis very effectively, but, because of the increased risk of cancer, oestrogens are not recommended unless in special circumstances. Now drugs called bisphosphonates are recommended, and these reduce the risk of osteoporotic fracture in those who have had previous fractures. However, it is said that they do not reduce fracture risk in those with osteoporosis who have not previously had a fracture. They are a class of drugs that prevent the loss of bone mass, by inhibiting the digestion of bone that happens normally, thereby slowing bone loss. They have quite severe gastric side effects, causing gastric inflammation and erosions of the oesophagus. The recommended way of avoiding these side effects is to take a tablet only once a week and to stay upright for at least 30 minutes after taking them. Even so, they can be hard to take, and sometimes it is necessary to take a tablet which counteracts the acidity (PPI) to protect the stomach at the same time. There are more and more drugs being developed and NICE is kept busy recommending which of these new drugs should be used on which patients. There is no doubt that established osteoporosis, where patients are getting repeated fractures, has to be treated as vigorously as possible, but again it is a bandwagon as more and more me-too drugs are licensed.

Fibromyalgia has been considered in a separate section. Patients are often referred to rheumatology, but specialists can't do much for them, except offer a specialist diagnosis, written information and occasionally to refer to chronic pain services. Sometimes a rheumatology department will set up a specialist multidisciplinary service run by physiotherapists, but as fibromyalgia and ME groups are often against physical exercises even when appropriately graded, they haven't been very successful, and in times of austerity are unlikely to be financed.

Chapter 29
Respiratory disorders

Asthma – athletes – causes – over and under diagnosis – COPD – improvements in treatment

Asthma

Asthma is a serious disease. When I was doing a paediatric job in the early 70s many children were admitted with severe asthma, and one little girl, aged two, was admitted almost every other week. Her asthma was extremely difficult to control with the medications we had then – oxygen, humidity, steroids and bronchodilators – and she was never free from wheeze. Then she came in with an even more severe attack and nothing we did could save her. She died while being closely monitored by nursing and medical staff. Her parents of course were distraught and we felt quite helpless.

Asthma is due to an allergic inflammation which blocks up the tiny airways in the lungs. This has very little effect on breathing in but greatly reduces the amount you can breathe out, and this causes the wheeze. Eventually the airways become so blocked that a patient goes into respiratory failure and can die. Incidentally, people suffering from anxiety have the opposite problem – they feel they can't get enough air in due to adrenaline's effect on the respiratory rate, so it should be easy to distinguish between people complaining of shortness of breath who have asthma and, on the other hand, those who are anxious. These latter patients can be reassured that they do not have asthma though it is sometimes difficult to persuade them as hyperventilation (over-breathing) is equally as frightening as asthma. However, in people who have both, the asthma unsurprisingly makes them very anxious and they may hyperventilate, so then it isn't easy to sort out what is happening. One elderly anxious lady who lived on her own used to call the ambulance practically every week, because she thought she had asthma. For this reason it was difficult for the GPs to reassure her. She didn't have asthma and eventually had to go into residential care, where she was looked after and became much less anxious. It isn't only elderly people who get anxious of course, and at all ages to feel short of breath is very frightening.

Treatment nowadays, especially for children, has improved but some still die. There was a peak of asthma deaths in 1966[130] with two thousand people in the UK dying, and of those about eighty were children. Then the number of asthma deaths halved and by 1976 there were just over a thousand deaths. But then it started climbing again, going right back up again to two thousand but with only 1% of them being children – twenty. No-one knows why. At present deaths from asthma are falling but they are still higher than they were in 1976. More people are developing asthma than they were in the 1970s as the prevalence also rose from the mid sixties to the late eighties, and this was true in most Western countries. In the USA between 2001 and 2009 the number of people with asthma shot up to 12.3%, according to a recent report.[131] Lifetime asthma prevalence is still reported as 24% in children aged 9 to 12 years in the UK. Most deaths now occur in the older age groups and many people die of asthma in their forties or fifties.

A lung specialist told me recently that hardly anything has happened therapeutically in thoracic medicine in 30 years, compared to cardiology or even psychiatry. Yet from a GP perspective that is very difficult to believe. The treatment of asthma, we thought, had been revolutionised by the development of aerosol inhalers, which could deliver steroids and bronchodilators directly to the lungs, instead of having to go through the blood system after taking tablets. Home nebulisers seemed a fantastic innovation enabling us to quickly give big doses of active medications direct to the lungs via a machine. Pharmaceutical companies worked very hard to perfect the delivery systems of inhalers to improve treatment, and if you had asked me, I would have said it was very successful. All inhalers were very expensive, although there weren't any big breakthrough of drugs for them to deliver, with steroids and bronchodilators still being the mainstay of treatment even now. But maybe the improved treatment wasn't keeping pace with the higher incidence and severity of asthma.

The idea was that if you could keep asthma at bay with low-dose steroids through inhalers as preventatives, then patients would have fewer exacerbations. People with asthma had to use their inhalers regularly and asthma checks were introduced in general practices. The main measurement of asthma is with peak flow meters, which measures the peak amount of air you can breathe out. But sometimes asthma sufferers can be unpredictable, and I remember well a patient who appeared in our surgery one afternoon, severely short of breath and going blue (cyanosed). The nurse saw him in the waiting room and whisked him to the treatment room, where we gave intravenous steroids, oxygen and nebulized bronchodilators. He improved in the next thirty minutes and then all of a sudden he ripped off the mask, said he was better, and just went. We never even knew his name – he wasn't our patient but had seen the surgery sign and just come in. In fact that man could easily have died. I have no idea whether he did use his inhalers regularly but it was obvious that the attack had come upon him very quickly indeed.

There are many theories about why asthma is such a problem in the developed world. Air pollution from cars, factories, and power plants is one possibility as there are several components that are linked to asthma, including ozone, formed when pollution reacts with oxygen and sunlight. Also sulphur dioxide, emitted from coal- and oil-fired power plants, reacts with nitrogen oxides, released from tailpipes and power plants, as well as from indoor gas stoves. Particulate matter, tiny particles of soot and other contaminants that can lodge deep in the lungs, are produced by a variety of combustion sources including diesel vehicles and coal-fired power plants. But the biggest cause of asthma is likely to be tobacco smoke, and there is a lot of solid evidence behind this.[132] Of course smoking rates are now reducing but children who are exposed to smoke are very likely to develop asthma and children are spending more time indoors than they used to. Genetic factors also play a big part as a child with one asthmatic parent has a one-in-three chance of developing it. If a child has two parents with asthma, the chances are seven out of ten that the child will have asthma. Dust mites and moulds are another cause of asthma and other allergies.

Asthma is common in the normal population, but it's also very common among elite athletes, for example, it was said that more than one in five of the members of Team GB was affected by the condition.[133] It has been said that it might be because some athletes want to justify using drugs (β agonists), to improve their performance. But this is unlikely, as no definite evidence of increased performance with these drugs have ever been found. (It has also been said that there is no evidence that any of the drugs used by athletes for this purpose actually do so, but presumably there must have been some effect!) Current explanations focus more on the effects of intense exertion, and cold air, as obviously the rate of flow of air in and out is much more than in those who don't take so much exercise. The exposure to allergens and particulate matter, for instance chlorine in swimming pools, is therefore much larger. In addition athletes undergo a very detailed diagnostic evaluation and so any tendency to asthma will be discovered. It's interesting that there's a dose-response relation: higher-level athletes have a higher prevalence of asthma. More curiously, and still unexplained, is the fact that athletes with asthma are more likely to win than those without!

Asthma can also be over-diagnosed. I had a patient who was a very keen cyclist who competed at a national level. On one occasion he had a cold and asked for, and got, a bronchodilator to try. He was supposed to come back for full evaluation, but never did, and according to our records carried on using the inhaler for three months then stopped. He then applied for the Army, and put down that he had used an inhaler. They immediately wrote back and said that they could not consider him because he had asthma. The lad was distraught, as he really wanted to join, and asked us to write to the selection board. We did, but they would not change their minds. The rules were that if he had ever been prescribed an inhaler he couldn't be considered. This seemed very unfair to us. It is essential to make a clear-cut diagnosis of whether someone has asthma or not in order to treat them properly, and sometimes we do give an inhaler to see what effects it has on the peak flow rate, as part of the diagnostic work up. But it is important only to make the diagnosis when you are absolutely sure.

Overdiagnosis is common according to one Canadian study.[134] 30% of people diagnosed with asthma may not have it, and 67% do not need treatment. That is a lot of expensive inhalers wasted. At the same time, many people with asthma are not diagnosed and many of those who know they have asthma don't take all the preventive medication they should.

Chronic obstructive pulmonary disease

Chronic obstructive pulmonary disease (COPD), which used to be called chronic bronchitis, is now at epidemic levels, because of the smoking rates of 30 years ago. Unfortunately people who have smoked tend to have many different diseases as they get older, and people in their fifties and sixties can get very frail as a result, as frail as people in their eighties who did not smoke. Treatment has not been revolutionised, and there is no cure, but people are living longer with it because of the widespread use of oxygen. It is a very debilitating condition and very frightening indeed, resulting often in multiple admission to hospital. It is one of the conditions that many doctors and managers think can be managed at home much more often than it is, but even though home treatment with antibiotics, sometimes intravenously, nebulisers oxygen and steroids, is perfectly possible, it is such a distressing and frightening condition that people often do go to hospital.

The variation in admission rates in different areas though is huge (from 124.7 to 646.5 per 100 000 population for PCTs)[135] and it is clear that people in deprived areas are more likely to be admitted. There are many possible reasons for this, one of which may be that more people in deprived areas continue to smoke even when they have COPD, they may have less family support, or they get less preventative care and effective treatment from their GPs. If that is so it should certainly be important to look into that. The only thing that definitely reduces hospital admission is flu vaccination and this is something that all GPs will look at carefully as it is included in the QOF.

Palliative care is important too, as the final weeks can be very distressing. Care at home can be wonderful though, and one man I knew died at home with his wife looking after him throughout, although they did not call the doctor or the ambulance when he was obviously dying. Some neighbours criticized the wife for this but she told me that that what was he wanted and I am sure it was much better for both of them.

For other lung conditions, including the very unpleasant allergic types of diseases such as farmer's lung, asbestosis, interstitial lung disease and certain types of lung cancer (non-small cell), there haven't been any great improvements in treatment. Infections are largely treated much the same as 30 years ago. Your chance of dying from pneumoccocal septicaemia is no different. It is dictated by what happens in the first 24 hours and is even uninfluenced by antibiotics. Even treatment in intensive care overall hasn't led to large improvements in survival from 30 years ago, although the treatment of respiratory sleep disorders is better.

In fact reducing smoking rates and the banning of asbestos have done more in 30 years than anything to improve people's lung health.

Part 9

The interface between primary care, hospitals/ care homes and social care

Cost implications and dilemmas for the GP

Chapter 30
Care of the elderly

Establishment of care homes – care in the community – patients at home – delayed transfers of care – going, going, gone – integrated care pilots – dementia.

A big change came over the care we gave to the elderly in the early 1980s. This was when the emphasis changed from local authority homes for the elderly and community hospital care, all provided by the state, but which was in very short supply, to care in private care homes – nursing and residential homes – provided by the private sector and paid for by social services on a means tested basis. It was of course a change made necessary for the burgeoning numbers of frail elderly folk who did not have family to look after them in their own homes. Not only were people living longer, but also the increasing tendency for women to work outside the home made it difficult for them also to look after their elderly parents. Men of course had never looked after their parents in any numbers. So in our locality an enterprising couple, he a nurse and she a business woman (an unusual way round) set up first one small home which then grew quickly to a very large home, and then, as they saw what a great opportunity this was, opened four more. Needless to say the people who filled them weren't usually patients of ours, but people drawn from the whole area and further afield, such was the pent up need for such a service.

We GPs were taken aback. Yes, each of these patients would attract the usual capitation fee of (then) £15 or so for a year's care, (remember the capitation fee assumed that each patient had average needs, and that the healthy who never attended would compensate for the few who were ill and needed a lot of medical care), but these were all people who were ill or at least had a need for help with activities for daily living. Some of them were very ill indeed. In addition they never came to the surgery, as transport costs would have to be paid by somebody, so we always had to go to them. This was a great increase in work for very little extra resource in a very short time. We estimated that 100 care home residents would need at least 12 hours per month of GP attention if they had 2 visits of 15 minutes each per month. That wasn't a huge amount of time to spend on patients who often came with lots of medication to sort out, who needed full examinations and also sometimes a full memory check. I think we did make representations to the BMA and the health authorities but got nowhere. The rules were there, these patients were 'in the community' now, and therefore we had no choice but to do the best we could. Occasionally the authorities agreed to increase the number of GPs in a practice to recognise the extra work.

At first patients who were paying privately for their care in the homes thought that they were entitled to private care from their GPs and it took some time before it was generally accepted that we could not give that level of care. So we got on with it. Sometimes the care homes would pay a bit extra (recouped from the patient) to give us more time with the patients, but usually we rationalised things, with most of the patients who came from elsewhere being registered with the same practice to minimise travelling (they did have a right to a doctor of their choice if they wished but most agreed), and worked out systems to be able to give as much care as we could. It got worse when local long-term psychiatric hospitals closed and more EMI homes (for elderly mentally infirm patients, who mostly had Alzheimer's disease) opened, as these patients could take even more time to sort out.

Over the years the numbers of patients stabilised, and usually it was possible to look after them without having to send them into hospital frequently. There are three main types of care homes: residential, for people who need help with everyday living but not nursing care; nursing homes, where people are more ill and often have complex problems; and the EMI homes for those with Alzheimer's and other mental problems. As time went on though we found that people who had been in long-stay beds in hospital, or even in acute beds in hospital, were being transferred to nursing homes. These homes were funded to provide trained nurses who were very helpful to the GPs in doing blood tests and small procedures (even though there was never a dedicated treatment room). This I thought was much better for them and the care we could give them was much more appropriate as we could take the patients' views into account as to what treatment they wanted. Gradually people in residential homes became more like those who had been in nursing homes, and they sometimes needed a lot of nursing care as well as more complex medical care, and our district nurses were very busy looking after them. Finally, people who had been in residential homes were now encouraged to stay in their own homes, and that included people with very complex needs.

Recently the NHS agreed to pay GPs extra to give really quality care and this has been very welcome. Looking after patients in care homes has become an important part of a GP's day-to-day life. Although many people will not agree, I think that on the whole care homes are well run (they certainly now have to reach quite high standards of care, unlike at the start when the entrepreneurs made a lot of money out of the system) and we really could not do without them. But they are of course very expensive, and cash-strapped authorities sometimes try to limit the number of people they are prepared to support. There is an ongoing political discussion on how much people should have to contribute to their own care when they have to stay for a long time. But looking after people in their own homes, while the ideal for many, can be fraught with difficulties. Here are some of the people I have looked after in the practice.

A man aged 74, an ex-soldier who was known to be an alcoholic, lived in sheltered accommodation, which meant there was supposed to be a warden, but when the live-in warden retired the hours were reduced to one person coming in for two hours in the morning. This man had early liver failure, which resulted in problems with his oesophagus, in which blood vessels were swollen (varices) from the backpressure from the liver. This regularly caused him to vomit huge amounts of blood, which needed emergency treatment. He also had persistent diarrhoea with malnutrition and also heart arrhythmias. So he was regularly admitted to hospital, roughly every two months, but he would discharge himself as soon as possible because he couldn't get alcohol in hospital (he got it delivered by a local store when he was in the flat). He sometimes got into a terrible state, and once I visited him to find that he had been too weak to get to the toilet when he had very bad diarrhea, and the flat was covered with faeces, mixed in with empty bottles and spilt booze. Public health people were called but he was perfectly rational and insisted on staying at home, and so he did, but he regularly had to be admitted to an intensive day care bed where he was transfused with blood, rehydrated, fed and then given tender loving care. He refused to go to day care because he knew he would be nagged about his drinking, so he got more expensive regular visits from various professionals.

There was also a ninety-two year old woman who had moderately severe heart failure and widespread skin rashes on her legs, which were much worse when her legs were swollen. She lived with her son who did his best, but she argued with him all the time. She could walk only with difficulty. The district nurse visited frequently to dress the weeping sores on her legs and of course we GPs visited often to try to optimize her medication. She regularly got stroppy and refused to go to bed at night and stayed the night in her chair, so the swelling of her ankles got even worse. She had a low sodium level (hyponatraemia) from diuretics, and things regularly got so bad that both she and her son begged for admission. She usually stayed for weeks in hospital, as her heart failure was difficult to control. Although more regular visits from nurses, regular blood tests, care by community geriatrician, and more social care might have helped, it was essential to get access to respite beds, when she could go to give both her and her son a rest from each other.

Another patient was an 85-year-old woman who had had recent successful heart surgery, but also had severe rheumatoid problems, and then she started to get 'funny turns'. She was very anxious and thought that hospital was the only place where she could get treated. So she called doctors as an emergency and went in out of hours. She needed more day care with community physician input regularly.

Another 94-year old woman with mild occasional irregular heartbeat and possible angina (though not proved) and otherwise quite fit, lived in an ideal bungalow near town, and her son looked in regularly. However suddenly she started getting very anxious whenever left alone and had regular 'hysterical' attacks, during which she lay on the floor and called the neighbours in by knocking against the wall, and they called the GP. She was fully investigated in hospital but nothing was ever found, and she was discharged quickly every time. Talking to her, I found that she wanted to go into a nursing home, but needed funding (actually she owned her own home but her son expected to get that when she died), and the social services would not agree to fund her. They suggested admission to a psychiatric hospital when it happened next. So this was done but the psychiatrists promptly discharged her with a diagnosis of 'anxiety' and the pattern repeated itself. After several more acute admissions to hospital, the social worker got the message and finally arranged nursing home care, even though she didn't really fit the needs protocol. I suppose eventually the house will have to be sold to help pay the bills.

A seventy-year-old man suffered from very severe irregular heartbeat, which went so fast that it put him into heart failure (severe paroxysmal arrhythmia). It happened once every month or so and he had to be admitted every time, as his condition needed an intravenous injection and monitoring, so he needed a bed for 4 to 6 hours while the arrhythmia was treated, and then he went back home. So he was understandably very anxious. He ought to have been seen regularly in the doctor's surgery for monitoring as he was fit and active otherwise but he wanted home visits.

So these are all patients who wanted to be treated outside hospital, and were, but it is not a cheap option. In every case regular admissions to hospital were essential to keeping the situation going, and respite care, in an NHS facility or more likely in a private care home, was very helpful. Relatives, even when they are healthy themselves and have the ability and the wish to care for the patients, can only do so much. Sometimes the situation becomes impossible and the patients are admitted to hospital and then become 'bed blockers'. The official name for this is 'delayed transfers of care' or DTOCs, an abbreviation which causes some hilarity at first when people think that the discussion is about drug users. In many areas there are places where these patients stay for years, such as 'cottage hospitals' or 'intermediate care' homes, run either privately or by the NHS, but usually these patients have no resources so the state picks up the tab. While it is very expensive to keep these patients in long-term beds, the main disadvantage to the patient is that a hospital bed is not where anyone would want to live their life. People in care homes get a much better environment, and it may well be cheaper to look after them there, so the problem becomes a financial matter for administrators who are of course from various agencies – social services, NHS and the County Council or equivalent. It is a very long-running saga with political implications as each agency tries to protect its own budget, and the fact that the money all comes from taxpayers in the end is forgotten. All such care, and the funding for it, should be integrated, but 'integrated care pilots' where GPs, social services hospital specialists and managers try to work together and pool resources are having a very bumpy ride.

I don't have a solution of course any more than any one else. But I do think that insisting on care at home at all costs can be counterproductive. In one area the social services chief was very much against all kinds of institutional care and so social services would not fund many patients in local care homes, or if they did it was at a low rate. Not surprisingly most of the homes in that area closed or relocated, and the bed-blocking problem in hospitals grew (not his problem of course).

Social services also often did not understand the trajectory the patient was on and would spend large amounts of money adapting a patient's home with showers, lifts, handrails etc only to find that the patient soon became too dependent to stay there and went into hospital anyway. It is very difficult to predict which old person will manage years with suitable adaptation and those who are on a deteriorating slope, which is going to end in hospitalisation and death in the next 6 months, but a GP often has a good idea. And when an old person is on such a path, it requires a lot of planning and thought to make sure that she can stay in her own home. Sometimes too, a really good care home can ease the way, with regular 'respite' admissions where frequent admissions to hospital can be prevented because the patient feels safe and valued.

One very real difficulty with elderly patients, and particularly elderly patients with diabetes, is providing proper joined-up care within hospitals and between primary and secondary care. How often do patients complain that they go to one department after another with different problems – say, one for their feet, another for blood pressure, another for dizziness – and no-one knows anything about them? If they are admitted to hospital the doctors start from scratch again. Sometimes the notes don't arrive or the computer system isn't working. While GPs have good clinical computer systems, they are not integrated with the hospital's own system. Computerised central records will take a long time coming – witness the failure of the large English computer system. The failure was due to many things but one main problem was confidentiality and consequently the fact that many patients refused to give permission to upload their data. Smaller more local systems will have to be improved.

One big advance is that in England patients are to be able to hold their own GP records and be able to check them and use them by 2015. This will be a big change, and GPs who have already tried it say that it will actually reduce patient contact time, not increase it, and reduce overall costs. Knowledge as ever is key. A big advance that has already happened in some areas was a system in which the out-of-hours computer system, which was run as a separate system, was able to use some of the key information on the GP systems so that the on-call doctors could access basic information about the patients, and this then was available if they had to be admitted. But once inside the hospital, especially large ones, there are difficulties in sharing information between departments, which is quite incredible considering how we can share information so easily through global systems. As a result time is wasted, doctors hesitate to make decisions because they are unsure of the facts and sometimes the wrong decisions are made. It is very upsetting for patients to be admitted time after time with no progress being made. Of course it goes without saying that information is not shared with social services or mental health services.

There have been many attempts to improve the integration of services for patients between hospital and home. A recent report on the lessons learnt from a two-year independent study of 16 integrated care pilots[136] that were intended to address these problems and improve the quality of care for people with complex care needs who were leaving hospital, showed surprising results. Staff reported that they were working more productively as teams and were happier in their jobs, and they thought that the quality of care to their patients had improved, but this was not reflected in the experiences of the patients and service users themselves. The report said 'Although patients reported receiving care plans more frequently and most felt that care was being better co-ordinated after a discharge from hospital, people found it significantly more difficult to see a doctor or nurse of their choice, were less involved in decisions about their care, and were listened to less frequently'. The fact is that the process of integrated care did not necessarily involve the patients, who felt less empowered and in control rather than more. Recent research has found that continuity of care and personal relationships are very important to patients' well-being,[137] probably even more than getting the latest specialist treatment. And it affects people's life chances. As a GP I certainly felt that good generalist medical care, and nursing care that made the patient feel safe and valued, are more important than the latest medical advances, and good care both at home and in care homes can prevent admissions and excessive treatment that the patient does not want.

A situation that is commonly faced by a GP is an elderly patient who lives on their own and who has had a fall, may have become confused, or has 'gone off their legs'. This group is often referred to as 'the frail elderly'. All too often these patients are admitted to hospital because the health service does not provide an alternative to admission.

But we also know that any admission to hospital if a patient is on the edge, can result in the 'going, going, gone' syndrome,[138] as a professor in care of the elderly put it. For a frail elderly person in their own home, who is normally managing or perhaps just coping, any sort of incident – an infection, a problem with medication, a fall or an increase in anxiety because a carer is going on holiday – can result in the person having a crisis and 'going off': going off her legs, not eating, calling on neighbours and family frequently. Then everyone thinks this means they have to go to hospital, to be on the safe side. So then the waiting game begins, first an ambulance to A&E, then to an admissions or transition ward, sometimes a surgical ward, sometimes on a trolley in a corridor.

Going, going ... Tests and investigations and then treatment are done over days and weeks, before a review with senior consultants and nurses, and a Discharge Plan is produced. A multidisciplinary team is contacted and risks worked out and discussed with relatives, who will have their own ideas. There is further delay and another review. Eventually a care package is reinstated which improves on the previous one. But while all this is happening the patient gets disorientated because staff come and go and they don't know what is happening, they lose the ability to self care as no-one explains to them what they ought to do, they may not be able to get to the toilet easily so become incontinent, they become immobile because walking is not encouraged. They next get an infection, usually a urinary tract infection, further confusion and then often have a fall. Now they have 'Gone', and become a 'Delayed Discharge' and may stay in institutional care, sometimes until they die.

In order to prevent this spiral, the concept of 'virtual beds' has been mooted – take the hospital to the patient, with specialist nurses able to organise tests at home under the joint direction of GP and community care of the elderly specialist. The funding that otherwise would have gone to the hospital therefore would go to setting up these systems. It is an excellent idea and works well in some areas. It takes a shift of emphasis though, especially for GPs. Most GPs recognise the problems at home and if you ask them, many will say that what is wanted is a quick admission – in to get the immediate problem (bedsores, infection or whatever) sorted out and then a quick discharge. They often do not realise that it is impossible to do this, given the system that has to be gone through in the local acute unit, because those patients who really do need a quick intervention have to be recognised quickly. One can't assume that every frail elderly person just needs to go in to hospital for a quick fix and then out again – some do indeed need complex interventions. So GPs sometimes do not want to support these 'virtual beds' – hospitals at home. When they are mostly run by hospital specialities GPs can resent being sidelined, but when the GPs are actively involved they have been heard to complain that it is too much work. And indeed the demarcation line of accountability is frequently very unclear. The GP always has to take responsibility for medication, as this is never funded by the hospital, so they will be told what to prescribe without necessarily being aware of the thinking behind the medication change. It is only possible to set these systems up with very clear communication between primary and secondary care.

While older people develop many degenerative diseases, most of them are in fact compatible with independent living for many years. It is dementia that is the biggest problem as this always leads to complete dependency in the end, with devastating consequences for the sufferer and the family.

There are at least two forms of dementia in old age. One is caused by damage caused by poor blood supply due to atheroma, which causes frequent mini-strokes, and this is known as multi-infarct dementia. To some extent this can be prevented by treating high blood pressure and high cholesterol, in the same way that we try to prevent heart attacks. The most common form of dementia is of course Alzheimer's Disease (AD), which is thought to be caused by plaques of amyloid, an odd sort of protein that can develop in certain areas of the brain. Both types of dementia, as everyone knows, become very common as people age – as high as 50% in the over 80s – and there are other rarer forms of dementia as well, such as Lewy body disease, a hallmark of which is that the patient sees hallucinations. This was vividly portrayed in the film about Margaret Thatcher, who was supposed to see intrusive visions of Denis at frequent intervals, though of course this must be a representation only and may not mean that this is the sort of problem that she actually suffers from.

The early form of the disease, which used to be called pre-senile dementia, occurs in the under 65s and there is definitely a tendency for this to be inherited. Screening for the inherited abnormality can be done, and in some places especially the USA these tests are promoted direct to the general public. This seems a particularly misplaced activity to me. It seems so wrong to test for a disease which is so debilitating and where there is no treatment. Yet people do it, and so they must have been persuaded to ask for screening because of advertising in one form or another. New guidelines in the USA say 'Genetic testing for AD should only occur in the context of genetic counselling…and support by someone with expertise in this area.'[139] Well, yes.

I had two patients who started to develop dementia in their early fifties. One was a man who did a manual job, and he was brought in by his boss, who had noticed him not doing the job properly. It took some time for us to realise that he had AD. He only survived a year after that so it must have been a very aggressive form. The other was a lady who held a responsible job in the council, and eventually she went to one of the council day centres. She thought she was going there as part of her job to help 'the old people'. It was very sad. None of the children of these patients asked for genetic testing fortunately and I was very glad about that. But it must have been hard for them to live with the knowledge that it might be hereditary.

The current drugs for dementia act by inhibiting the enzyme acetylcholinesterase (AChE). AChE is a substance in the brain that helps in the transmission of electrical impulses and the theory is that this is disturbed in AD. These drugs are only marginally effective, however. The trials on which NICE's recommendations were based showed mixed results, and the best outcomes were seen with higher doses when unfortunately there were often more severe side effects, sometimes causing the patient to stop the tablets. NICE guidance for their use is therefore extremely specific, so that they are not used for example in the very early stages of the condition to prevent it getting worse. They are used only when a sufferer's functioning has already deteriorated to a specific level, to a score of between 10 and 20 points according to a memory test – the Mini Mental State Examination [MMSE] (normal is 26 to 30 points).

Even herbs may have positive effects. One study that looked at the effect of Ginkgo Biloba on cognitive function in normal middle-aged and elderly patients (not those who had been diagnosed with AD) showed that after six weeks people who got the treatment improved significantly on how well they could recall a list of appointments, and how well they performed on a test on the ratio of false to correct items. But Ginkgo had no effect on another everyday memory test which asked for recognition of a driving route. The first type of function is known to be sensitive to normal ageing while the second is less critically affected. So there maybe specific actions of Gingko on the ageing brain, and it would be interesting to see a study comparing ginkgo biloba with cholinesterase inhibitors.

So there is no cure, and dementia is one of the most debilitating diseases that come to us as we get older, and is a big cause of the projected costs of an ageing population. The burden on family members, and therefore in some cases the state, is huge.

Having said a lot in this book about having sufficient drugs now, and how difficult it is to afford the very high price the drug companies charge when they are developed, there is one disease that I, along with every one else I know, would agree to pay an enormous amount for, and that is a preventative drug for Alzheimer's disease. Not a cure, because once damage has been done to the nervous system especially the brain, it is next to impossible to reverse. But a drug which would pin point the abnormality that is going to lead to Alzheimer's and stop it in its tracks – now that really would make a difference. To me, it would make sense to develop an international group of researchers (a bit like what happens when a new pandemic is threatened), funded by all the rich countries together, to direct and fund research. It is such a threat to both the older individuals and their families, and to health care systems throughout the world as we all live longer. Yes, you have to die of something. Cancer is mostly a very unpleasant way to go; give me a quick heart attack (or a stroke so long as I didn't survive!), but Alzheimer's disease, the deterioration of every thing you are over so many years – now that is really cruel. Failing a drug, I would want to be able to end my life. All good luck to Terry Pratchett and his campaign, and I do hope he succeeds.

Chapter 31
Emergency medicine

History of being on call – rotas cooperatives and deputising services – new contract of 2004 – EWTD – GP out-of-hours care now – doctors' pay – when things go wrong – psychiatric cases.

Emergency medicine is the most fascinating and challenging of medical work. Each patient I saw with something that was obviously serious, where diagnosis and treatment needed to be started straight away, was memorable, and every event made a story in itself.

Being on call was always stressful. There were several elements to the stress but the worst was being on call itself. It meant that you couldn't settle down to anything, knowing that you could be called at any moment. Calls mostly came regularly throughout your period on call so if the phone didn't ring for a bit of time you would worry that the calls hadn't been switched through! At night it was difficult to get to sleep because you felt it was hardly worth it as when you were woken from deep sleep it was much worse than not going to sleep at all. But of course sleep you did, as after a whole day of calls you were tired out. Then there was the stress of the many calls you took when you knew perfectly well from the story that there was no need for a visit – the patient really needed only advice, but people often insisted on a visit. There was absolutely no point in arguing or even questioning whether it was necessary – if the patient got annoyed then all you did was to cause bad feeling which would make the inevitable visit to the house all the more stressful.

And finally there was the stress on the rare occasions when there really was something wrong and you worried in case you didn't get there in time or that you had prioritized a call wrongly. If three or more calls came in quick succession you had to decide how soon to visit each of them. If none of them sounded urgent then you would do in them in geographical area to minimize driving time (which could be considerable in a rural area like ours). Once a man called to say he was having trouble breathing, and he didn't sound too bad on the phone so I did another call (to a not very unwell child) on the way. But when I got to him he was very breathless indeed with asthma. I called the ambulance myself as soon as I saw him and then treated him with intravenous steroids and a nebuliser, but he deteriorated and needed ventilation in hospital. The delay had only been 45 minutes but that was too long for him, although I doubt if it made any difference in the end. He survived but people did die of asthma then and still do.

Once early on in my career I was called at 2 am to a man with abdominal pain who had collapsed. The caller said, 'please come quickly – I think he's dying', so I alerted the ambulance and got there myself quite quickly, but he died shortly after I arrived. It was very upsetting for everybody. He actually died of an abdominal aneurysm and almost nothing would have saved him. Another time I was called in the early hours to a farmer. The message I got from the caller was that his wife was dying but I got very little more than that and did not know whether to call the ambulance or not. When I got there the story was quite different. His wife had actually died in hospital an hour or previously – in childbirth. She was in her early forties and had five children already and there had been complications during the birth. The child did not survive and she developed disseminated intravascular thrombosis where the blood didn't clot and they couldn't save her. I was called to calm down the poor man who was beside himself. There was so little I could do but perhaps my visit helped. At any rate he regularly came to see me in the surgery and after a year or two brought his new wife to register with me. They were a great pair and together brought up his teenage children and her five year old.

Organising immediate care in the community is fraught with difficulties and there were severe limitations as to what GP with a small bag and a car could do for real emergencies. I was never quite sure why it took so long for the message to go out that if a patient or caller was desperately worried about a health problem then they should call an ambulance straight away and not wait for the GP. GPs, though they grumbled about it, mostly accepted that they should attend whatever, and many thought that it was the right thing to do. Administrators were happy with the situation because the load on the ambulance service was already great in an underfunded service and waiting times for an ambulance to arrive were very long. It was cheaper for the doctor to visit first, to triage those calls where the patient didn't need to go to hospital. Eventually though it was coronary care which tipped the balance, as it became clear that the delay in calling a GP first was costing lives, and GPs were advised in 2001 not to attend but to call 999 instead. Patients were encouraged to call an ambulance immediately. However it took time for the message to sink in, and I remember a casual conversation with a senior doctor (in dermatology) who told me that he had had to go to hospital four times with chest pains and nothing had been found and why wouldn't his GP visit? He resented having to go to hospital, and wanted his personal physician to visit. A colleague pointed out that this would cost lives if everyone did it, but he was still dissatisfied with us GPs.

Nowadays, therefore, everything is better organised with triage systems set up by NHS Direct and other organisations, and patients being advised to call an ambulance first for certain well-defined conditions. Systems for ensuring that there is a safe and effective way for patients to get into hospital as an emergency are crucial in any developed health system, but it has always been a challenge to achieve. It means that there always has to be a well-trained group of doctors on call at any time of day or night, or 24/7 in modern parlance, to receive those patients who arrive at the hospital, and then to treat them as expeditiously as possible. In A&E and hospitals generally this work is done by junior doctors, (all grades below consultant grade), and emergencies occupy the bulk of their day to day work, necessitating complicated rotas to make sure that every hour is adequately covered.

My first house jobs were typical of the time in the early 1970s, with periods of continuous 30 hours on call, followed by 18 hours off, most of which would be spent sleeping. Weekends would be one in two, so that we might be on call for 56 hours continuously. It was impossible to have any sort of life beyond the hospital; you couldn't go to the bank, have your hair done or attend to any of the necessities of life. The hospital of course recognised this and a room and all your meals were provided, and at first you had someone to clean your room (a 'bedder', usually a motherly sort of lady who would look after 'her' doctors) and you could get a hot meal in the middle of the night if you were up working. It was tough even so, as though nights were quiet by today's standards, a night's uninterrupted sleep was rare, so we were all sleep deprived. Pay was about the same as a young teacher would get, despite the huge differences in hours worked.

I don't think working conditions improved much over the next two decades. Rotas of one week in two became rarer but still existed when there were staff shortages because of sickness or holidays, and rotas of one in three or one in four were more common. But the intensity of work at night increased as more interventions could be done and more lives saved, and quite soon the privileges of junior doctors were taken away. First the bedder went, then the night food (replaced by a vending machine that might or might not work), then the separate area for medics in the dining area, so that you had to join a long queue with all the other staff. Sometimes just as you got to the head of the queue your emergency bleep would go off and that was the end of your lunch. But there was good camaraderie in the doctors' mess, and patients were very grateful, as you attended to them personally throughout their stay. They certainly wondered if we ever got any sleep, and sometimes were more concerned for us than about themselves!

Those who went on to specialise in hospital medicine continued with these rotas throughout their careers, but as they became more senior they of course had their own juniors to do the bulk of the routine work. This consisted of 'clerking' of patients, which meant taking the history of the reason for the illness that had brought them into hospital, finding out what medication they were on (which usually then meant sorting through a plastic bag with assorted bottles of tablets which the patient might or might not have been taking before he came in), and then organising preliminary tests and treatment if it was immediately necessary. There might be twenty or more admissions on a 'take', the 24 hours when the firm you were assigned to was on call for all emergencies, and if many of them were really ill, you didn't stop. Each firm had a consultant at the top, and then either a senior registrar (a doctor who had had about six years' experience in that speciality and would soon be ready to get a consultant job herself), or a registrar, a doctor who had passed the first examination in that speciality and needed lots of ward experience, and there might be a senior house officer (SHO), who was at the beginning of speciality training. In small peripheral hospitals though there might only be a consultant and an SHO and if you were the SHO that could be very scary.

In fact the whole thing was scary at times. Doctors were trained to be 'action men'; quickly acquiring skills and knowledge they would need and had very little support. The rule about any sort of new procedure such as a lumbar puncture, a chest drain or whatever was 'see one, do one, teach one' – and hopefully you would have someone who was experienced enough to do it properly when you 'saw' one, otherwise you might perpetuate all their mistakes! Sometimes you were reduced to doing one using a textbook to guide you.

Because of the constraints of staffing in the NHS – and systems elsewhere, come to that – this level of overwork continued and quite possibly would be the case now if it weren't for the EWTD – the European Working Time Directive. This sought to get rid of excessive hours in all walks of life, but was much more difficult to implement in medicine, (and in veterinary medicine as well), and in many areas the law is broken even now. The idea was that no one should work more than 52 hours a week, and though many managerial hours have been spent on this there is no easy solution to the fact that there has to be 24/7 cover for all hospitals yet there are a finite numbers of souls to supply the staffing. Indeed there is opposition from doctors as well, as surgeons in particular say they need more hours of training than they can get if their hours are restricted, and would like to see exceptions to the rule. But more usually doctors still have to work more hours than they should because otherwise the patients would not get the care they need.

General practice therefore was seen a soft option. Even in my early days GPs were getting together in large rotas to cover the out-of-hours periods and in my first GP job I had an absolutely luxurious one-in-nine rota, so we were on call only one night in nine and a weekend only one in nine weekends. The downside was though that you would be working the whole day, often until 7 pm, after a busy night on call, not a restricted day as was usual in hospital, and you were on call from Friday evening till Monday p.m. Everyone soon realised this was impossible as by the end of the weekend, if it had been busy, you were incapable of doing anything constructive and were probably very unsafe, not to mention bad-tempered. So then the weekends were split and you did one day of a weekend, either a Saturday or a Sunday every 4 weekends. This was manageable and this rota stood for over thirty years.

However in city areas another system was possible, as GPs were independent contractors and could therefore contract out their work to others. Deputising services therefore were set up as private organisations, which would arrange GPs to do out-of-hours sessions, pay them and then doctors would pay in to have their out-of-hours commitment covered. The cost was high; in the late 1990s it would be about a quarter of our net income, although it was tax-deductible, and not many GPs would subcontract all their out-of-hours work. But it could be very flexible, and doctors could choose which sessions they would pay to get covered and also which extra sessions they would work if they needed more pay. Occasionally there would be a complaint that hit the headlines about the service provided in an individual case if a patient was harmed by a poor GP consultation out of hours, and successive governments of the time were unhappy about the arrangements. At one point the Government tried to prevent GPs subcontracting all their out-of-hours work, but it did seem rather vindictive, objecting solely because the system was seen as being as out of their control, and they were losing out on the tax, as GPs could claim the cost of using the service against tax. These deputising services flourished, though they perpetuated the idea that most out-of-hours care should be provided by home visits for far longer than was sensible, remaining enshrined in the NHS rules and regulations, and it was popular with patients. There was in fact a better way to do it – the setting up of GP cooperatives, which were non-commercial and had the best of all worlds. GPs could trade sessions, no money changed hands and there was excellent back up for the doctors. This could work only in fairly urban areas though, and our rural area continued to run on a rota system, though towards the end of its life we sometimes paid locums to do the weekend and overnight slots that were the most onerous.

On the whole, out-of-hours care in general practice provided a good safe service to patients for many years. GPs set great store by continuity of care so that even if they did not themselves do all the out-of-hours care for their patients, they usually could communicate with the doctors who did the emergency work and could continue the care of the patent the next day. It was stressful, but then emergency work is always stressful, but it is also very satisfying when it goes well and is interesting and rewarding.

So what happened to change things with the GP's contract of 2004?

I think what happened was this. By the early 2000s, general practice recruitment was becoming increasingly difficult. More and more young doctors were choosing hospital medicine, and becoming a specialist was again being seen as a route to a more satisfying career. There were many reasons for this, mostly reflecting the huge advances in technology and sophistication in hospitals compared with the work done in general practice, and of course all medical students were and are trained in the hospital setting for most of the time. The out-of-hours system was also seen as a detraction, as there is no doubt the system was often abused by people who had an expectation of a 24/7 service for all minor ailments, and would often call doctors with very trivial complaints, even in the middle of the night where there was no deputising service. The Government listened as the perception – and indeed the evidence – pointed to a healthy primary care service as being central to an efficient health service, and governments in general are keen to see that this is properly resourced. The new contract of 2004 was there-fore negotiated to address some of these problems.

The consensus of the media and the general public was that the resulting contract was very advantageous to doctors, in getting rid of the 24-hour commitment of GPs to their patients completely. Indeed most of us were surprised that even the Saturday morning commitment was removed. But it was inevitable that with the move to more family-friendly working practices generally and the imminent re-quirement of the EWTD, that the 24-hour commitment had to go. It also paved the way to a much more sensible way of organising the service so that patients would usually expect to be seen in a well equipped primary care centre with a doctor who was not overworked, rather than at home under impossible condi-tions for anything remotely medical to be done.

The basic pay rise that GPs got was actually not that great; the great win of the BMA over the government of the time being the introduction of the quality im-provement exercise (QOF), which is quite revolutionary and is described else-where. The Government (and probably the BMA too) greatly underestimated how effectively doctors would work to improve the quality of care for their pa-tients under the scheme, which is basically a bonus for meeting quality targets, and this success (which reflected a lot of extra hard work by practices) accounted for a large part of the increase in GPs pay. Also there was a big variation in the amount GPs actually took home in different practices, with some large practices being extremely profitable while others were still struggling, despite offering good services. Very, very few GPs earned the vast sums talked about in the media at that time. Since then of course GP's pay had been frozen and has now fallen for several years in succession because expenses have risen, as austerity bites.

On the whole the replacement services for out-of-hours GP care have been rea-sonably successful. They are run through contracts from PCTs or Health Boards, sometimes by private companies, and sometimes by hospital trusts. Many doctors regret the passing of the cooperatives, none of which managed to win contracts with the new deal. The opening hours for patients are now less than ideal and there are moves in many places to try to extend GPs' hours in many places. PCTs have offered extra money to persuade surgeries to open on Saturday and sometimes Sunday mornings, but they have not been very successful, and just recently, as payment for these has been cut, GPs are withdrawing from them. The problem is that paying a receptionist, opening the surgery with heating costs, setting up the telephone systems and so on are expensive, and the GP isn't left with very much after the bills have been paid. If the out-of-hours service has enough centres for people to reach easily and the service is good, then opening the surgery at weekends really isn't needed.

There are other problems though, as setting these up has intensified the push for patients to get everything they need on a 24/7 basis, including repeat prescriptions. This year in one area 10–15% of calls to 'Out Of Hours' on a Saturday morning were taken up by repeat prescriptions for current medications, and this reached a peak on the bank holiday for the Royal wedding, with 25% of calls at 9 am being for repeat prescriptions. GPs running the service said the calls were mostly for regular medication such as asthma inhalers and the contraceptive pill, but, before the system changed, patients didn't expect to get these on a Saturday morning. And it isn't simple to arrange such a repeat prescription either, as the out-of-hours doctor does not know the patient and patients sometimes do not bring the current authorisation from their GP that what they are asking for is what they are currently prescribed (although these systems are getting better). The prescribing doctor has to take full medico-legal responsibility for what happens so will often want to see the patient face to face. There is often a problem with patients 'trying it on' to get medication their own doctor would not prescribe, so the whole exercise is very difficult. There have been schemes whereby patients can go to an out-of-hours pharmacist to get a few days' supply (maximum 3 days) of medication that is already on a repeat prescription, and this can work, but there isn't a system by which pharmacists can be reimbursed for the extra work (although if truth be told it usually isn't a lot of work if nothing extra is supplied, and they do get their normal dispensing fee). It is of course partly a reflection of the fact that GPs' surgeries are closed for such long periods, but when GPs worked in rotas they only rarely agreed to supply extra medication to tide people over. It is more a culture that has developed whereby people expect to get a service over these periods when previously they knew they would have to stock up in advance.

Problems also arise when there is difficulty staffing the sessions, and then doctors have been brought in from other countries without proper training or knowledge of primary care in this country, such as in the case of David Gray, a man who died after an overdose of a painkiller given by a doctor from Germany who had no primary care experience in the UK. All doctors staffing these centres should be doctors who are well trained in family medicine and who know the NHS, and they usually have excellent back up and facilities with which to provide a good service.

I hope I have clearly shown in my account of doing the work that on call work is not for the faint-hearted, and it is therefore absolutely imperative that doctors doing sessions for out-of-hours providers should also be properly trained and supported by the organisations employing them. The doctors often do not have their networks of support as in daytime work, and if they do not know the area and the local hospitals or, more seriously, have an inadequate command of colloquial English or what is in the bag of drugs supplied to them by the out-of-hours organisations and how to use them, then there will be very unsafe service. It seems that at bottom the problem in the David Gray case was that there were two sorts of vials for injection for pain relief in the bag supplied, one of them for ordinary acute pain, and another normally used for palliative care for patients with severe cancer pain. The doctor was unfamiliar with one of these drugs, as it was not used on the Continent, where he usually worked, and so he used the stronger one by mistake. The much higher dose, which would have been appropriate for a patient with cancer who had a high tolerance for opiates, killed the patient, who needed the smaller dose for patients with acute pain only. So efforts are now being made to ensure that doctors from Europe and other places outside the UK are not employed on such work at all.

Another solution would be to triage all patients who need strong pain relief to go to hospital and not to visit them at home. As a matter of fact after the Shipman case, patients were often obviously worried when I suggested an injection for pain relief, and I remember several patients who, although in pain, refused to have an injection and we had to use a patch medication. So this procedure would be sensible, though upsetting for some patients, as it would rarely be wrong to ensure that the patients get more investigation as to what the real problem is. At the same time, the system would have to make sure that cancer patients who need regular pain relief could get pain relief at home. Fortunately palliative care is usually well organised, in a system where local pharmacies, GPs (usually their own GPs during the day) and community nurses who are the key people in this scenario, get together to make sure that appropriate strong medication is there ready for use if needed out of hours.

The rate of home visits done by doctors in primary centres has reduced considerably compared with deputising services but still varies very widely. Many calls are now dealt with on the phone, and of the rest where the patient is actually seen face-to-face, the rate of home visits varies from about 10% to 40%. These will include house visits for terminal or palliative care, where this is the only way such patients should be seen, so most cases are probably appropriate, and those to acutely ill elderly people living on their own or where parents with sick children have real difficulty getting to a centre.

The occasional severe psychiatric problem is also best seen at home or sometimes wherever they are. Many is the time I have been told of a case of someone wandering around who seems to be confused or psychotic, but finding them is often difficult. It is the police who are the greatest help here, and they can be rather essential. I do remember one case where I was called out because the caller's son was coming back to the house and had two guns in his possession, and she was worried (quite understandably) and called me. I called the police and we arranged to meet at the patient's house together. However I got there well before they did and the caller met me at the door. 'He's upstairs,' she said. 'He has still got the guns and he is intending to shoot a neighbour who he said was going to harm Prince Charles'. He was of course acutely psychotic, and it had happened before, she said. She did not seem all that anxious and then the son came down the stairs still brandishing a gun. We had no option but to try to talk him down, and indeed apart from being convinced that the neighbour was going to attack Prince Charles he seemed quite calm. So we sat quietly in the front room and between us we persuaded him that he ought to go with the police to 'get the problem sorted out'. The police (six of them in an armoured car) came but fortunately got the measure of the situation and one officer came out, took the gun, and escorted him into the van. I heard later that he responded well to treatment and went back to his job as an office worker.

So, having successfully got yourself to a primary care centre, or having been seen at home, by a health professional, what happens then? In most cases of course you will be treated with medication or a small, procedure or given a prescription, but sometimes the doctor will decide to send you to hospital. And that is the next chapter.

Chapter 32
Hospital admission

Local GP or A&E services – entitlement to NHS services – inappropriate attenders

As stated in the previous chapter, there is always a problem as to whether a patient should go to their own GP or go to an emergency department in a hospital. The interface between the two is complex but most people have a good idea about where to take their minor accidents or illnesses. In rural areas GPs will do more with minor accidents – cuts and bruises – than in cities, but each area has had to develop ways of paying the GPs for this work as it is not in their basic contract. Traditionally it has been with payments through bed funds of cottage hospitals where the GPs also have contracts, but these have been reduced and altered in many areas. For patients, though, to travel many miles to a hospital is a big disincentive. It is an important consideration and can be difficult to solve. A patient going 30 miles for a boil to be lanced on a weekend is not a happy situation.

But in cities the reverse is often true – it is much easier to go to the local A&E department and wait. Inappropriate attendances are frequent and there is no doubt that the patient needs clear guidance on where to go, and carrots and sticks to encourage them to do so would help. GPs are often blamed because it is assumed that it is difficult to get appointments, and this is often what patients say is the reason for their attendance at A&E. Hence the requirement for immediate or same day GP appointments and the many patient surveys to ensure that this is the case, on which some of the doctors pay will be based. Managers want to reduce the load on A&E as much as possible, and obviously want to ensure that GPs play their part. In fact, some people just need to be made aware that their GP is the place to go, but where people go is not often something the GP can influence, even during the day when the surgeries are open and still less out of hours.

There are also those who either have no GP, or aren't entitled to GP services, such as foreign nationals including refugees. Apparently there is a problem in some cities where middlemen extort lots of money out of illegal immigrants, to get them onto a GP's list and hence to free NHS treatment in hospitals. It is completely unclear whether they are entitled to treatment or not. Several times we got directives saying we had to challenge people from abroad about their eligibility, and sometimes we did and sometimes we didn't. Then we would get another directive saying that all patients were to be treated on the NHS unless they were 'health tourists'! How on earth were we to tell? They didn't often say they were health tourists! The usual thing was that a patient, originally from another country such as India or Nigeria, or with family there, would bring the relative in and say either that he had become ill suddenly (then they were entitled to emergency treatment) or that he was now staying permanently. Either way there was really nothing we could do without getting into an involved situation about legal residency and visas. True illegal immigrants in big cities, especially if they are working and contributing to our economy, need medical care the same as anyone else, and there are legal firms who will challenge refusal of care and say they haven't lost a case yet. The NHS was never set up to deal with taking money from patients and NHS hospitals undoubtedly lose millions from fraudulent use of the NHS. But the rules need to be a lot clearer before this will stop.

There are also people with language difficulties or who are unable to manage the process of making an appointment, such as people under the influence of drink or drugs and those with psychiatric problems. Considerable effort has been made to reach these people to encourage them to use GP services but it s an uphill battle. A walk-in service is always going to be more accessible – you know that if you sit and wait some one will attend to you, but it does rather depend on making sure the waits are a bit of a discouragement otherwise they would fill up with lots of people who know that they ought to see a GP or ring the GP service out of hours. However, waiting times in A&E got so bad that the government introduced the four-hour wait target, which meant that every A&E department had to take action on every patient within four hours. While a good idea in theory, this led to many unforeseen effects as it meant that patients who were being assessed but needed a period of observation to see whether admission was necessary found themselves being admitted anyway so as not to breach the 4 hour target.

NHS Direct and other telephone- or web-based information centres have proved very useful. Since the new NHS Direct Wales website was launched in February 2007, the number of web visits grew from 338,000 to 450,000 in 2008–2009.[140] In England in 2009–2010 it was estimated that 2.4 million unnecessary GP appointments and 1.2 unnecessary ambulance journeys or visits to an Accident and Emergency department were avoided. Ask any GP though and you may get a different answer as they think such services actually increase a GP's workload, although they might well save money elsewhere.

However patients get to hospital, it is imperative that they are assessed early and admitted, investigated, or discharged in an effective manner. Since the four-hour target was introduced, there have been many ways of ensuring that patients are seen quickly, the most famous being the 'hello' nurse with a clipboard who goes through a proforma to quickly assess the patient. Often it is obvious from this exercise that the patient should not be at A&E at all. Then what happens? Often a patient will be re-directed to the nearest GP out-of-hours centre and if this is nearby then it will be an excellent solution. If not, and the patient has difficulty in getting to another centre she may still be treated in A&E and may think therefore it is best to go there every time. A patient can then become a 'frequent attendee at accident and emergency' on whom a lot of managerial energy is consumed.

These patients can often be identified by GP surgeries, as when a patient is seen in A&E, a practice will usually receive a written summary of the reason for attendance and the action taken. Theoretically, a practice could discuss attendances with the patient and try to ensure that they are seen in the practice instead if that is more appropriate, and certainly the practice should look at whether there are any barriers to the patient coming to see them first. Another method would be to stop walk-in A&E attendances, and triage all patients over the telephone before coming to A&E, for instance using GP out-of-hours services or NHS Direct. It would be revolutionary but in these days of near-universal access to mobile phones, it may actually improve the system.

For those patients who are properly in the A&E setting, and who need assessment, treatment and possible admission, there is an imperative for the treatment to be as effective as possible to save lives. Emergency services for road traffic accidents and major incidents are nowadays available only in large hospitals that are properly equipped to deal with them, and smaller hospitals have lost their major trauma centres. Every time there is talk of a hospital losing its A&E centre there is a big public outcry, but there are good arguments for centralizing admissions in bigger units, such as increasing the expertise of staff and centralizing the expensive equipment. But patients can lose out – there is evidence that some people have died because they had to travel much further, though other lives have also been saved by having the expertise and equipment for serious injuries concentrated in one place. The costs and benefits will therefore depend on the numbers in each group and the types of injuries most likely to occur in that locality. There are no perfect solutions, but is definitely one for the whole community to consider. It will inevitably get political, but one hopes that the politicians and communities are guided by evidence and not just keep the status quo by default.

The other big problem is getting the admission rate down. The days of patients being admitted to hospital for trivia are long gone, and managers spend a lot of energy on looking at admission rates, discharge rates and length of stay. There are international comparisons and league tables on how well countries do it, as it can make a difference to whether a health service is affordable to a population or not. Hospital admissions are an extremely expensive way of sorting out the patient's problems and should be used only when there is an absolute need. This is especially true of emergency admissions to hospital at night and weekends, which are distressing for patients and disruptive for hospitals. So if you are a health service manager, you will need to look at why and how patients arrive at hospital and what happens to them. Inappropriate admission of people who could have been treated at home or sent home for further treatment without admission is therefore an important topic, as this costs extra money.

The ambulance system now has sophisticated software that is able to identify frequent callers from a specific geographical area and within a specific timescale. Reviewing of people who have made three or more calls during a 6-month period may detect individuals who are already known to have high clinical need, and may also identify those with poor control of their condition or who frankly abuse the system. In Austria they have even more sophisticated equipment which enables the ambulance staff to see which hospital has the shortest waiting times for non-urgent cases to be seen. I availed myself of this when I was in Vienna, as I cut my leg rather badly when I fell off my bike when riding down the path alongside the Danube. I went back to the conference centre where I was a delegate and was seen by one of the 2000 GPs who were attending, and he called an ambulance to take me for stitching. (It did seem a shame that none of them could do it on the spot, but it did need about 30 stitches!) He said, 'The hospital is only five minutes away. You will be back within the hour'. Fifty minutes later we were still in the ambulance heading to the southwest corner of Vienna, in search of the hospital with available slots, and when we got there, there were doctors standing around and I got seen and stitched up straight away. The doctor stitching me was talking about chess all the way through as he was a chess grandmaster. Everything seemed very relaxed and quiet – I don't think that would have been the case in the UK! It was by the way completely free. Don't forget to take your EHIC card to show when you travel to Europe!

GPs are now being asked to look at the case notes of their patients who have repeated admissions through the out-of-hours service, especially those who have 5 or more admissions in a short space of time. GPs are rewarded through the QOF if they do it effectively, and suggest new local pathways of care, which could be implemented by a commissioning group. The practice should then take action to prevent future inappropriate admissions. Obviously this would be a much better outcome for the patients concerned if they could have their care better coordinated at home. This was the focus when employing 'community matrons', specially trained nurses who would visit and look after these patients, but unfortunately this scheme was not always successful. Sometimes whatever managers might want, there are patients who are just unstable and who may need the expertise of a hospital to sort the problems out. But where there are social problems, a link worker of some sort should be able to bring on the appropriate help in time to prevent an unnecessary admission.

A common occurrence is the weekend admission that comes from visiting relatives who haven't seen the patient for an extended period. They may live a long way away, have busy jobs and lives, and put off coming. When they finally arrive, they then realise that the patient is a lot more ill than they thought, and then out of real concern, but also often out of guilt because they haven't been to see them before, call the on-call doctor and insist on admission to hospital. The on-call doctor may not know the patient well, and even though the patient is in fact being well looked after at home by teams of nurses and care staff, bow to the relative's wishes, rather than risk an unpleasant situation. That relieves the relatives anxiety and guilt, and they go back after the weekend thinking they have done well. But they don't understand that this has perhaps caused the patient to be in hospital for a long stay because once in hospital, older people can lose their coping skills very rapidly as explained in Chapter 30.

It can happen to people who are being looked after well in care homes too. At the end of their lives people often have unpleasant symptoms such as bed sores, but these are usually very well managed in care homes and would be less well in hospital, and there might be no need to admit the patient. Sometimes, consultants in hospitals complain that many people who are admitted to hospital on their take are in fact obviously dying. Someone somewhere has panicked, but the patient would almost certainly have been better left in peace at home with carers or in a care home. When people panic like this, though it is an understandable reaction, it does no good at all to their loved one.

It is unlikely that this happens more since GPs stopped routinely working weekends. The fact that out-of-hours rotas and deputising services were so frequently used rather than the patient's own doctor or practice meant that the on-call doctor did not know the patient anyway. For the patients who are sent to A&E after being seen or assessed by GPs, whether within normal hours by their own GP between 8 am and 6:30 pm, or after hours by GPs working for out-of-hours services, there has been no change in referral rates for admission since GPs stopped being on 24/7 call. This is not surprising as in most cases it is still the same GPs doing the work – the difference is only in how they are employed.

The groups of patients that have already been seen by their GP usually go straight to a medical acute assessment unit (MAU, called by various acronyms in different hospitals), which is quite separate from the A&E department, and assessed by the resident medical team there. Hopefully they will be treated there and then sent home. GPs of course will vary as to whether they have judged correctly whether a patient needs to be admitted to hospital. Patient behaviour will also influence what happens; an anxious patient, a young person or an inexperienced parent, or a patient and family with poor coping skills may mean it is more likely that the patient will be admitted to hospital. Some people think that a hospital is the only place where anything gets done, and others are at bottom showing attention-seeking behaviour. This sort of situation demands very good communication between hospital staff, patient, and GP to make sure it is managed properly and the real concerns of the patient, which may not lie in the health domain at all, are addressed.

I found this to be true in our local area. When we looked at the rates of referral to MAU we found that one doctor was sending down three times as many as the other doctors, and they were mostly children. This doctor was very underconfident and apparently had not done a paediatric job before going into general practice (as most do) and so was erring on the side of caution. However these children had a journey of nearly 15 miles to the local hospital and most of them were discharged almost immediately. So the practice had to organise as special training course for the doctor concerned and also give extra support. In fact another doctor reviewed every case before the patient was sent down, and this helped to educate the doctor. So the problem was contained but it does show that proper training of GPs in paediatrics is essential, and certainly the practice should look at whether there are any barriers to the patient coming to see them first.

'Assessing out' or in other words seeing patients effectively and organising their further investigation and destination, is an organisational matter that some hospitals do better than others, but in almost all cases the patient will be happier to go home with a clear plan of what is going to happen next, than to sit in a hospital bed. Lots of things influence whether a patient is admitted or sent home, such as the experience or otherwise of the admitting doctor (newly qualified doctors or nurse practitioners sometimes quite sensibly play safe), whether immediate crucial investigations are available within a four-hour window, inefficiency within the department so that patient is in danger of breaching the four-hour window for non-clinical reasons, the culture of the speciality (some would rather admit than consider outpatient investigation), and the availability of 'hot clinics' (see below). It is hard to get it right. Most GPs have had the experience that when they manage to contact a hospital doctor directly to see whether the patient can be spared admission, the result is a grunted 'Oh, just send them in' from a rather tired and overworked doctor, but usually not the most junior doctor who will then have to receive and 'clerk' the patient!

The reason for ensuring that people go to the right place in an emergency is of course to ensure that the staff are able to concentrate on the true emergencies and not on those who needn't be there. A very important part of this part of the system is to make sure that investigations such as blood tests, X-rays, and scans are done very quickly, and this usually requires a good complement of staff on hand to do these things. Provision of more diagnostic or other interventions that can be done more locally can save the patients having to come back to the hospital. In many hospitals it has been decided to put the most experienced doctors in the forefront of admissions, because experienced doctors will be quicker and more accurate in deciding how to manage patients. This also goes for GPs. Many hospitals have set up dedicated clinics ('hot clinics') where the patient can be referred so that their management and investigation can then proceed in a less pressured environment, but it is essential to make sure that these clinics are not overloaded by patients attending who otherwise would have waited a long time for an outpatient appointment, but would not otherwise be going to a A&E department.

What to do with the four-hour target? Hospitals were required to meet a target of so many (usually over 90%) of patients being seen within four hours, but this is being abolished now, as it provides some perverse incentives to admit those whose investigations aren't complete or who really need more time to be assessed. But I expect something else will be put into its place – it would be difficult to get away from some sort of target.

However it has always been difficult to convince patients, and especially their relatives that admission is not necessary. When I first became a GP, patients, especially lonely old folk, used to beg me to send them into hospital 'for a rest'. And certainly in the cottage hospitals that we used to have then, and some bigger hospitals too, there was a free and easy route to hospitals for not very sick people. That soon stopped though, as medical care and interventions soared in the 1980s and 1990s, and a stay in hospital became anything but a rest. Patients and their relatives, especially when ill and anxious, feel 'safe' in hospitals and this has bedevilled attempts to get more patients treated at home or in community settings.

I remember an elderly man with multiple problems including cancer and Alzheimer's disease, whom I knew very well and saw every week or so in the surgery. He began to get paranoid and was accusing his wife of poisoning him. I visited, and found the man was not any more ill than he had been but was very aggressive at times and his wife was frightened. I contacted the local psychiatric team and they promised to see him urgently, but the following day the wife called for a visit and specifically asked for another GP to call. So another partner went and had to send the man to an acute medical ward. That really wasn't the best place for either him or the other patients, but obviously the wife had reached breaking point. She never really forgave me for not admitting him the day before. He stayed in a few days and was seen by the Psychiatric team and discharged back home again on medication. However over the next few weeks his physical problems deteriorated and he was admitted again to hospital and died shortly after. This was another example of the trajectory – this man was at the end of his life, and probably the best solution for him would have been expert palliative care in a hospice. But that is with hindsight, and it is never that clear at the time. To tackle such problems administrators have to look at the whole pathway of care.

Once the decision to admit the patient is made, it is necessary to have a bed in a ward available for the patient to go to and this may be a big problem. Hospital beds have been cut dramatically in the last ten years and many people think there are now not enough beds available in the system. The result is that patients have to wait on trolleys in corridors, sometimes for hours. The backlog even extends to ambulances, which are not allowed to transfer the patient into the hospital until there is a bed actually available, despite the fact that admission for these patients has usually already been agreed between the GP who has seen the patient and the admitting junior doctor. Sometimes ambulances will queue for hours outside a hospital with their patients still on board, and so then there aren't any ambulances available to attend to new emergencies and the waiting times for ambulances to arrive at an emergency reaches dangerous levels. So organising the throughput of patients efficiently is crucial. And partly the problem is that a bed is generically considered to be a bed with everything available, when a range of beds with various types of backup would be better, such as step up step down beds, beds for palliative care, and 'virtual beds' at home.

Once we tried to close a local 'hospital' which had long since morphed into a very expensive care home – but a care home with none of the 'homely' feeling that could have been provided, as it was still a 'hospital'. All the patients were suitable for discharge, either home or to a private care home, yet it took five years, costing huge amounts of public money to close it. Local people objected strongly, but it seemed this was an emotional reaction to the loss of a 'friend' rather than a reasoned stance. This was a typical example of the difficulties managers have all round the country when facilities are closed or downgraded. Politicians then find themselves supporting facilities right against the evidence.

Many areas now are looking at integrated pathways of care between GPs, social services departments, and consultants in care of the elderly, in order to make sure admissions to hospital are only made when really essential. They concentrate on patients, usually elderly people with lots of chronic diseases, who go into hospital frequently in a 'revolving door' pattern. But there are problems. In one scheme, which was set up to try a new way of working, staff tried hard to break down barriers between clinicians inside and outside hospitals, but found it very difficult to get everyone working together.[141] There had been a lot of distrust between GPs and consultants in the past, and working together was a new experience for many. They also found it very difficult to get the funding to enable work to go on between the various services; such is the monolithic and inflexible payment structure in the NHS. But they eventually succeeded and their admission rate to hospital actually went down, while in other areas around them the rates continued to increase.

Community rapid response teams are another way of trying to reduce unnecessary admissions. They consist of a team of community nurses and therapists who work to prevent the inappropriate admission of complex patients (those who have a combination of healthcare and social care needs or who may have more than one long-term condition) to hospital. The team can be contacted to help in the management of frail elderly patients, and active management of patients who have frequent falls. Community geriatricians – consultant doctors with considerable experience in hospital care, but who work with GPs and nursing teams – can help improve the care and prevent avoidable admissions for those who are at high risk of admissions.

Acute assessment can be an alternative to admission: an outpatient appointment costs between £100 and £300 and an acute admission is in excess of £1000, but all too often the appointment is too far into the future, and the patient requires urgent assessment rather than an acute admission. The development of an assessment unit that can assess, investigate, and potentially discharge patients is a possible alternative to admission.

Of course, people want to know – how many beds are enough? The number of hospital beds has declined in most countries over the last ten years and according to health economists, this is a reflection of efficiency. It is achieved through mergers of hospitals, by closing wards, or by accelerating the move from inpatient hospitalisation towards outpatient care and day surgery. Oddly, the country that has taken this furthest is the US. The number of curative care hospital beds in the US was 2.6 per 1000 people in 2009, the latest year available,[142] lower than the OECD average of 3.4 beds. This decline has coincided with a reduction in average length of stays in hospitals and an increase in day surgery. In the UK in 2005 the number of beds was 4.2 per 1000 people.[143] I can't find any more up-to-date figures but it is unlikely that the numbers are higher now. In France there were 8 beds per 1000 people in 2000 and in 2011 there were 6.6; and in Austria 7.9, reducing very slightly to 7.7 in 2011.[143] Japan has by far the most hospital beds with 14.7 in 2000 reducing to 13.7 in 2009. So how do countries use their beds?

Clearly in Austria they aren't trying to reduce costs, as yet anyway, if my experience in Vienna was anything to go by. The GPs I met from Japan said that their patients knew exactly which hospital they wanted to go to, and there was competition between hospitals for patients. I think that has also been the case in France. So if the general public is prepared to pay the cost of lots of available beds, they have been able to have it up to now.

The result in the UK of hospitals striving to get maximum efficiency by maximising the use of beds, is that bed occupancy rates of well over 87% are usual.[144] If then there is a sudden emergency such as a flu epidemic, pressure on beds is intense and usually all routine admissions are cancelled to allow for these expected emergencies. The Royal College of Surgeons thinks that bed occupancy as high as this can be dangerous, because such high occupancy rates do not allow thorough cleaning of equipment between patients.[145] Most GPs would say there aren't enough beds because they often can't get their patients in to hospital during an epidemic. However the pressures on any health system are too intense for a return to having more expensive beds, and so the focus is always on 'throughput' and shortening the length of stay.

But the main obstacle to 'efficiency' is discharge rates not admission rates. I attended a symposium once where a game was made of it. We sat at five tables, and each table had to decide how to set the various rates, which were admission rates, length of stay, rate of investigation, rate of treatment, and rate of discharge. The organisers entered all our estimates into a computer which calculated the waiting times for admission following each decision. Whether the computer programme was realistic I don't know, but the result was that the only rate that made any difference was the rate of discharge (compared to rate of admission), which is only common sense really. What happened in between had no effect. So once you have made sure that only the people who need to be there get admitted, your next task is to concentrate on discharge. The main recommendation was therefore that consultants during a ward round should start with those who could probably be discharged pretty soon and get all their investigations and treatment arranged before looking at the patients who have just been admitted – a very counter intuitive way of working, but on the evidence essential to quick patient flow. Every ward round should start with those who are not quite ready to go home!

Of course what prevents discharge is as often as not the social circumstances of the patients and this can really be a very hard nut to crack. All hospitals are now ranked according to average length of stay (LOS), which should be between certain parameters depending on the type of hospital, but so-called bed-blockers, delayed transfers of care (DTOCs), are a real problem. Discharge planning needs to start as soon as patients have been admitted, so you need robust nurse-led discharge procedures. They are not always followed though; some hospitals have much better relationships with their community colleagues than others, and some have many more services in the community than others. Alas, old habits die hard and when funds are scarce it is these community systems that tend to be cut because the hospital has to be there for those really ill patients. It is a really difficult problem that won't be solved easily. All countries are grappling with these problems, but the expense of care of the elderly is huge and increasing. It is difficult to get an entirely fair system of payment but my personal view is that it is right that the elderly should contribute to their own care. The present elderly generation has done very well and it is the younger generation that will have to pay for their care, when they themselves are not going to be able to have such big pensions or such expensive houses.

In the future more and more people will be treated in their own homes, and GPs will be the ones caring for them. All I can say is that this whole problem has to be tackled so that people have a choice in the matter, and are offered alternatives to hospital admission that are actually better for them and their families.

Part 10

Management of the NHS

Dilemmas and vested interests

Chapter 33
Rationing of care: musculoskeletal problems – who should be treated?

Rise in orthopaedic referrals – multi-disciplinary teams – podiatrists and operations – hip and knee replacements – problems with weight

Orthopaedic surgery

'"Timebomb" fear as "rationing by stealth" of operations hits NHS' was a head-line in the Telegraph in September 2011.[146]

> Department of Health statistics show the number of referrals made by GPs in the year up to July was 4.7 per cent lower than for the same period in 2010. These referrals had shown a 3.5 per cent increase at the same stage last year, according to the department. The number of patients attending for outpatient appointments has also fallen, by 2.7 per cent.

To Professor Norman Williams, president of the Royal College of Surgeons, these figures were 'extremely disturbing' – rationing by stealth he called it. Such a steep reduction in the number of referrals by GPs suggested to him that patients are being given limited access to specialists' clinical advice and so are missing out on treatments.

Well, he would say that, wouldn't he? He is aware of all the wonderful things that surgeons can do to save lives and improve the quality of people's lives, and so to him more must be better. But even so how can we explain the huge rise in referrals to orthopaedic clinics made over the last 10 years? If we consider people needing surgery, yes there will be older people needing more joint replacements year on year. But 17% more attendances to orthopaedic clinics in one year? Surely not due to that many more operations being needed. Yet this was the rate of increase of referrals to orthopaedic clinics in our local area in 2006-7. There had been a steady increase in referrals, but not the same increase in operations performed. There are other factors at work here, and the answer to better health care is often not more specialist intervention. People need access to a range of different therapies and solutions, but too often the glamorous specialist high-tech approach has grabbed all the money in a cash-strapped environment. This must change if health is to improve without bankrupting the nation.

Joint and bone problems tend to be painful and also stop you doing things. If you sprain your knee or your ankle, getting around can be difficult and a fracture is just an awful nuisance. Diseases such as arthritis and back pain are horrible. So it is understandable that bone and joint pain is a very common reason for people to seek some sort of medical help, and of course there is a lot of help available, from over-the-counter bandages, painkillers, or anti-inflammatory medication, and exercises, to physiotherapy, acupuncture, chiropractice, podiatry, GP services and on up to orthopaedic surgeons. All of these therapies can be helpful for different conditions, but the orthopaedic surgeon is at the top of the tree, with the longest training, the widest scope of treatments available (from expert advice to cutting-edge operations), the most up-to-date investigations available to them and also probably the safest service as they will certainly diagnose serious disease such as cancer or nerve involvement that the other professionals might miss. And they are free! So theoretically everyone should go to orthopaedic surgeons first (through their GP of course), and then if their problem doesn't need their services, then they could see someone with other, more general skills. Shouldn't they?

Well, some orthopaedic surgeons might think so, but of course patients will want to make their own decision whom they want to see. The drawback to seeing an orthopaedic surgeon is that the patient will have to wait. Unless it is an absolute emergency such as a tumour or a cauda equina lesion (lower back problem where the patient might end up paralysed without treatment), the patient will first have to see a GP, then be referred to the specialist and may have to wait up to 18 weeks. If an operation isn't needed and a simpler treatment such as physiotherapy will work, the patient has to wait again to see the physiotherapist, by which time the crucial window for treating this condition early will have been missed.

So there is a balance, a tradeoff, where people will decide for themselves, with advice from family or friends, and influenced by advertisements and media articles, which treatment they are going to go for depending on what sort of a problem it is. This is therefore a marketplace where each professional will jockey for position in the local environment, and it can be competitive at times. Don't think that an experienced orthopaedic surgeon is immune from this need to compete. Hip and knee replacements aside, most of the other bone and joint problems can be treated in many different ways. If an orthopaedic surgeon saw only patients who had to have an operation (there being no other effective treatment), orthopaedic clinics would be empty, their waiting lists would be short and many of them would have to look for other employment. So they do need to make sure that patients keep coming with conditions that are not so clear cut, and that they are seen to offer the best solutions for as many problems as they think they are clinically the best at treating.

This basic need of orthopaedic surgeons to hold their position in the market is at bottom why historically so few other forms of treatment for musculoskeletal conditions have been available free on the NHS. When I started in general practice, NHS physiotherapists were all hospital based and attached to and controlled by orthopaedic specialists, who of course were all surgeons. So my patients could only get NHS physiotherapy by first waiting to see an orthopaedic specialist. In fact I heard one consultant say that physio was something that they needed to control in order to offer the patient something if they didn't need an operation! NHS physiotherapy was in effect marginalised – only getting to see the patients at the end of a very long process to exclude conditions which surgery might help. By this time physio sometimes was not of much use – either the patient had got better on their own (most did), or had got beyond any help and had to live with the problem. I remember that it was not until 1992 that our practice first got direct access to physiotherapists. The NHS did indeed work on the assumption that every person with a musculoskeletal problem should see an Orthopaedic surgeon, if their GP couldn't deal with it.

The reason for this assumption at first was the knowledge that only doctors could ensure patient safety. The medical profession had been properly regulated for a long time and some of the newer disciplines had had very little regulation until recently. Patients have to be protected from rogue non-medical health professionals, and in any case the human body is so complex that possibly only doctors with their long training and greater expertise could be sure that there was not anything more serious (like cancer) going on which needed to be spotted early. It is true that some seemingly mechanical problems like back pain, especially in the elderly, can be due to serious diseases, and it is the GP's job to pick these up early. Now, however, other health professionals have developed their own charters and clinical governance systems, and many are as safe and as well regulated as doctors. So recently, with the emphasis on care in the community, more and more other health professionals have been able to get a say in the planning of services. New multidisciplinary teams, involving physiotherapists, podiatrists, osteopaths, chiropractors, and specialist nurses, have been set up and are proving very useful in providing effective treatment and advice outside hospital, although many are still regulated and trained by orthopaedic specialists.

However the orthopaedic surgeons' strategy of keeping NHS treatment mostly confined to doctors has been very successful, so that year on year orthopaedic clinic attendances have soared, and the number of orthopaedic surgeons has increased enormously at great cost to the public purse. So more and more people have come to the conclusion that really this is the wrong way round. Patients should be encouraged to look at all ways of dealing with their problem. All health professionals should be accredited (even if not all of them may be allowed to give treatment free on the NHS), and only the people who are very likely to need the services of orthopaedic surgeons specifically should be channelled towards them.

How can this be arranged? Of course it will have to rely on patients' wishes and on the ability of GPs to triage patients more effectively than ever before, and that may also mean a change in attitude of GPs. GPs have been trained to think in terms of orthopaedic management first, and many have needed convincing that physiotherapists, chiropractors, and the like can offer an acceptable service. So when new systems have been set up all over the country to allow GPs to use the services of other professionals they have not always been willing to change their referral patterns. There is also no reason why a patient would need to see a GP first – many see their own physiotherapist privately anyway and sometimes this can be arranged on the NHS.

The multidisciplinary service just mentioned was set up with new money and was run jointly by senior physiotherapists and orthopaedic surgeons, but was held away from the big district general hospitals with their overloaded clinics, in community hospitals, in health centres, and in GP surgeries. Patients were referred by their GP and were seen by an experienced physiotherapist who triaged them into those that needed routine physio and those who might need 'extended range' physio, which might include more targeted physio, injections, or further investigation. These physiotherapists were allowed to ask for more investigations than the GPs were, and also could refer on to various specialist services if needed – such as orthopaedic surgeons, pain clinics, rheumatologists, and so on. However, three or four months into the service, GPs were referring very few patients, despite a lot of publicity from the Health Board, and it was necessary to do more to persuade GPs to think of alternatives to hospital referral by looking at their referrals in more detail.

Previously GPs had been reluctant to send patients to an untried service, which wasn't another doctor, often because they thought that the patients wouldn't like it. Patients indeed at the beginning often felt they were being 'fobbed off' with an inferior service, and thought that the NHS just wanted to save money. But after a lot of work communicating the benefits to everybody, satisfaction ratings rose considerably. Patients liked the fact that they didn't have to travel to the local district general hospital with all the attendant parking problems, and felt that the community setting was much more approachable and friendly.

Waiting times were critical to the acceptance of the new system. It had to be arranged so that a patient could see a physio very quickly, within two weeks or a month at most, as physiotherapists found that the earlier they got to the problem the better the outcome and fewer patients needed to go to the hospital. It was crucial that the funding was there to give a quick service to the patient. Enhanced physio had also to be more easily and more quickly available, with a maximum wait of six to eight weeks. Usually the wait to see an orthopaedic specialist was longer.

Most orthopaedic surgeons were happy with the new system, as they were seeing patients that they could best help. Not all were happy of course. We had a particular problem with some orthopaedic surgeons who specialised in foot problems. They were competing directly with podiatrists, and recently podiatrists had been extending their training to do straightforward foot operations such as bunions and removal of lumps and bumps, and the surgeons felt this was a step too far. However there was not a lot they could do to stop it at first, because there was a first-rate podiatry clinic in a nearby authority where our health organisation had a contract. Patients could go there and have their bunion operation done as a day case, and then get their GP to do their dressings in the surgery, whereas it was a two-day stay at least to have it done in hospital (the podiatrists had a slightly different way of operating). The waiting times in this podiatry service were much shorter and frankly it was a much more user-friendly sort of service. The obvious solution was to train our podiatrists up to do this operation but the orthopaedic surgeons opposed it vigorously, and despite the fact that it would have been much cheaper and the patients would have preferred it, it never got done. Eventually GPs were stopped from referring to this service altogether because it was out of the area and therefore had to be paid for separately. My experience of podiatrists who operated (and I was one of the GPs whose patients went there) was extremely positive and I wish them luck in their struggle to get acceptance in the NHS. Podiatrists are very interested in the biomechanics of the foot and at least now they can prescribe the full range of orthoses such as inserts and special shoes. In my opinion all patients with a foot problem should be able to see a NHS podiatrist before being referred to hospital. Bio-mechanical foot pain, dropped arches, calcaneal spur, heel pain and plantar fasciitis, and achilles tendon problems are all treated well by experienced podiatrists, who are able to give a wide range of useful treatments, such as orthotics, taping, and stretching techniques, all of which will work for some patients. Some physiotherapists also work closely with podiatrists and deal with problems with the ankle and knee which are caused by over-pronation and other gait problems. Everything has a downside of course and patients then found that they could not get a NHS podiatrist to do simple tasks like cutting toenails! They have moved beyond it. Patients sometimes still need such things done for them, therefore other workers such as health care assistants have had be trained to fill the role, usually organised by the GP.

Hip and knee replacements

Hip operations are one of the big successes during my career. Treatment for fracture of the head of the femur, a fracture common after falls in the elderly, used to signal the end of life. Even previously healthy people would deteriorate rapidly and most would be dead within six months. Severe arthritis of the hip was a painful crippling condition and I remember patients with completely 'frozen hips' who could barely sit in a wheelchair let alone walk. When hip replacements were first introduced they started very slowly and there was a big backload of patients who needed the operation, so patients waited for very lengthy periods for them. But once such operations really got going it made such a difference. I can hardly think of a case where an operation did not completely transform a patient's life. From the start there were few complications and patients got walking very quickly after the operation. Eventually even young people would get them, even though the artificial prosthesis had a limited life and eventually they would need two or more 'revisions' – i.e. replacements. One young soldier had had both hips replaced after an unusual degenerative disease, and went back to the Army. However we thought his wish to do para-jumping was probably a step too far!

Knee replacements came shortly after, and at first were definitely not so successful. Although people were pain-free afterwards, for many the joints were stiff and there seemed to be a high rate of complications. Now these too are almost as successful as hip operations. Recently though there have been big problems with certain prostheses, metal on metal, which were used for younger patients and which were supposed to be harder wearing. They are made of a chromium-cobalt alloy and it has been found that some of them leak cobalt ions into the body. Cobalt is highly toxic[147] and can cause neurological damage, with patients complaining of confusion and paralysis, and there have been concerns about cancer. As local tissue reactions associated with ions from metal hips were first described in 1975, in 2000 NICE recommended that patients should be warned of the uncertainty about long-term effects, yet these prostheses are still being used, and this amounts to a huge regulatory failure. The BMJ says, 'Commercialism, medical vested interests, and regulatory inertia and overload all seem to have played a part'.[148] Most patients are pleased with the outcomes of their orthopaedic surgery. Though David Cameron said recently that many people with knee prostheses did not have a better outcome, it seems the survey he was quoting referred to patients' general health not their knee health. Surgeons were quick to point out that the January 2012 Patient Reported Outcomes Measures Report showed that 82.2% of patients rate their knee operation as good or excellent,[149] and this certainly agrees with the experiences of my patients.

But there are limits. A recent paper[150] indicated that 30% of new prostheses introduced in the last 5 years have not benefited the patient and that were associated with 'a significantly worse outcome,' some of which needed to be 'revised'. It may mean that companies are trying too hard to improve on something that is already good. Or it may mean that people are having their hips and knees operated on too early. In my practice I observed that when waiting times for operations came down, so did the criteria for operations. Instead of having to be being crippled with pain, some of my patients were getting operations when they had minimal disability, for instance they could walk on the flat for miles but had pain when going down hill. Obviously these joints, having been put in much earlier than in previous times, were going to have to take much more wear and tear and will have to be replaced more often. All good grist to the mill of the prosthesis market of course.

The unfortunate fact about knee problems though is that they are totally bound up with a patient's weight. The knees are the biggest joint in the body and take its whole weight, and as we are all getting heavier so knee problems get worse and more common. Wear and tear of cartilage especially will result in damage to the knee over years. So in primary care the most important advice we can give to our patients with knee problems who are overweight is to lose weight, difficult as that is. Certainly massive weight loss improves pain and function and decreases low-grade inflammation (this was from a study[151] where patients had lost a lot of weight through bariatric surgery – the stomach banding operation). The other thing that is crucial to knee health is to exercise – but not too much. Pounding the pavements can definitely lead to later knee problems, and just passive exercising – moving the knees without weight bearing can significantly reduce knee pain and improve knee function in overweight and obese people with knee pain. The study showed that there were changes in levels of joint biomarkers with weight loss, suggesting a structural effect on cartilage. I always gave advice on weight loss and leaflets giving instructions on simple quadriceps exercises to anybody who came in with knee pain, from almost any cause. There is also evidence that strengthening the muscles around the knee can stabilize the knees and prevent damage this way.

Referral to hospital by GPs can be difficult to get right, as it was easy to overload the orthopaedic department without much benefit to the patient. Consultants were of course even more aware of the importance of exercise and losing weight before an operation. Some years ago patients who saw consultants privately were much more likely to get an arthroscopy, where the surgeon looked inside the joint to see what was going on, and sometimes were able to 'clear out' some of the debris in the knee. That, though, was an uncomfortable investigation and there were many patients who hobbled around for days or even weeks after it. Any benefit also did not last, as it was a diagnostic rather than a truly therapeutic procedure. So after a while we stopped referring patients until they had done exercises and if necessary lost weight, and they seemed to get better just as well. MRI scans are very useful for investigating knee pain of course and these don't cause as much pain as arthroscopies!

Cartilage problems are very common especially in active people and orthopaedic surgeons say that if knee pain is caused by an unstable meniscal (cartilage) tear then to remove the affected part relieves knee pain completely. One surgeon told me that there is little evidence that these patients treated in the early stage by arthroscopic surgery progress to osteoarthritis. However I have failed to find any recent evidence as to whether this is the case or not. Referral guidelines are important here to decide whether a MRI referral or arthroscopy is best.

Back pain

Back pain is one of the commonest causes of absence from work and many patients are disabled with it. Management here has changed a lot – when I first started in practice the advice was to rest for at least 10 days. Some patients were happy to do this, because at first it can be almost too painful to move much. Many a time I would do a house visit to give a morphine injection for someone with a really excruciating painful back. But soon the evidence was clear that in fact this did more harm than good and the best outcome came when patients were encouraged to move about and get back to usual activity as soon as possible. But it was then difficult to explain this to patients after the bed rest theory had been the recommended advice for so long. So public health specialists developed patient advice leaflets and tools on desktop computers to explain symptoms to patients and advice to stay active as far as possible.

While outcomes for patients are better when they do this, there is still a high proportion of patients who suffer from back pain long term even if they do keep active. The trouble is that the human back is just not designed to do some of the things we want or need to do – especially lifting, digging and twisting; another 'Scar of Evolution' as Elaine Morgan put it.[152] So sometimes people do have to accept that they might have to give up these activities and this is hard if it is your job. So it is important to know about local employment contacts and advice on changing career and training.

One of the first things GPs will do apart from giving painkillers (this is very important; in general straightforward paracetamol and ibuprofen are as good as any new wonder drug) is to refer to physiotherapy to supervise the graded exercise needed. Physiotherapists and some GPs can also give injections such as epidurals and manipulation in the same way that chiropractors and osteopaths do, and all these treatments have been shown to work in many cases. So firstly if GP decides that the back pain is due to mechanical problems, the patient can be informed of self-help skills, appropriate exercises and analgesics. If the pain is severe, or not responding to treatment, GPs will refer to physiotherapy (very few need orthopaedic referral) or a back pain clinic for further investigation. That clinic can do injections and manipulation if needed. I found when I referred patients that in general the outcome was good only if the patient himself really worked hard on exercises and activity.

So who does need to be referred to orthopaedic consultants? There are still more back referrals to orthopaedic surgeons than the evidence would justify. Many areas now have a pathway for spinal and neck pain and there are red flag symptoms, which make it mandatory to refer, and all health professionals dealing with back problems will know them.

The first is evidence of cancer on an x-ray, and cancer can indeed be diagnosed in some cases when the GP knows what she is looking for. Then there is the rare surgical emergency when the nerves to the bladder and bowel are damaged by the back problem (cauda equina lesions). The important test here if the symptoms sound suspicious is to test for reduced sensation in the skin around the anus. This is very rare, but, if not referred for a back operation, the patient may suffer paralysis.

Sciatica is caused by one of the discs (basically a cartilaginous shock absorber) between the vertebrae in the back 'slipping' out from the position it should be in, and in doing so pressing on one of the nerves which comes out of the spinal cord which runs along the spine. This pressure on the nerve causes very acute pain. Operations to correct the problem, usually by removing the central part of the disc, have been done since 1971 and there have been considerable advances in technique to allow more precise removal of the fragments causing the most harm, or complete removal of the affected disc 'aggressive discectomy'. More recently surgeons are replacing the worn disc with an artificial prosthesis. A recent review[153] indicated that these operations can help, with most patients having very little pain between 6 months and 2 years after the operation, though 14% still had severe pain, and the results were slightly worse with the more aggressive discectomy (though these may have been the patients with the severest problem). However this study did not look at those patients who had other forms of treatment. A more recent study in the BMJ[154] which compared the two treatments, surgery or rehabilitation, was not conclusive. The authors, from Norway, conclude that though the improvement scores in the operated group were higher, the difference was not clear enough for it to be certain that an operation was better as a sizable group of the rehabilitation group had also improved considerably.

I certainly felt that an operation ought to work. I had a patient, a nurse in her fifties, who had a great deal of pain and the local surgeons were very reluctant to operate. She asked to be referred to a surgeon in a nearby area, and I did so. The surgeon wrote me a letter saying that she really did need this operation and he could not understand why it had not been offered by our local surgeons. He operated on her within three weeks (unheard of then as it was many years ago) and initially she seemed to do well and said the pain was much improved. But when I saw her again four months later the pain was just as bad as it had been before. In any case she had to retire from nursing. Nurses of course have had a high incidence of back problems and this might have stemmed form the fact that years ago we did not really understand how the back came to be injured by lifting patients. Now there is much more advice for nurses and much better occupational management of their work.

So the current advice is to keep active. The evidence for and against an operation such as disc surgery changes all the time, but rarely does it competely solve the problem.

Whiplash

Whiplash injury is a new diagnosis that came in with the eighties. Before that I would see a few patients with a sore neck and headache for a day or so after an injury, but it seemed to clear up very quickly. Now it is a sorry story with insurance companies and lawyers getting in on the act so that now it is one of the commonest reasons for litigation and compensation. Nearly everyone benefits – the patient who has had a sore neck for a while and gets a large pay out, the lawyers, the doctors who write specialist reports for the courts, and even the insurance companies who accept the situation and do not challenge the payouts in the courts. The only loser is the ordinary punter who wants car insurance who has to pay much higher premiums.

What of the doctors who write the reports? In a marketplace the money is in a successful claim and so only reports from doctors whose report is helpful to the claim are used. These doctors may or may not have clinical evidence to back up their opinion – as noted earlier courts are not huge users of evidence based medicine. It is definitely a nice little earner for some. Jack Straw recently claimed that third-rate doctors, in the pay of claims management companies or personal injury lawyers, were the ones giving these whiplash diagnoses and he has tried to change the law to reduce or ban insurance companies taking referral fees from lawyers. Whether that would help isn't entirely clear, but from a medical point of view it is sad that so much is spent on a relatively minor injury.

When it gets to the point that racketeers will deliberately drive in front of a vehicle and brake suddenly so as to try to get a collision in which whiplash injury compensation can be claimed, then the diagnosis is out of control. This happened to a patient I knew a year or two back, and the patient braked so hard that he did not hit the car in front but lost control and his car went off the road and turned over several times. Both he and his wife were injured but fortunately not seriously, as modern cars have lots of safety features which saved their lives in this case. In fact car accidents have been reducing for years and the roads are actually safer than ever, so that the increased incidence of such claims is anomalous. The car that braked sped off into the distance of course.

Shoulder pain

Shoulder pain is another condition where the world has changed out of all recognition. I was taught that acute shoulder pain, whatever its cause (and there were certainly quite a few diagnoses around even then), can get chronic and if so, it would take up to two years to get better. And indeed this seemed to be the case. It can be a very painful condition, and certainly limits activities. As well as giving simple exercises and painkillers we often used to inject the shoulder with corticosteroids ands this clearly seemed to help in the short term at least. But by eighteen months to two years almost everyone seemed to have recovered and very few reported any marked disability. But now with the advent of scans and more use of specialised X-rays people are being referred to orthopaedic clinics much earlier and a high proportion are getting operations. It is a complicated field as there are various possible diagnoses, from neck problems to sub acromial impingement where ligaments are compressed, and tears of the ligament, and sometimes patients get a 'frozen shoulder' where the shoulder is very stiff and movement is severely limited, which lasts a long time. In the USA it seems that people do not want to wait many months for the problem to get better on its own, and more and more are opting for operations at an early stage.

The problem is though that in the initial stages after the operation the shoulder gets much more painful and movements are much more limited than they would have been before, and then improve only slowly while recovery takes place. The average time a patient had off work was 11 weeks, longer for those with manual jobs, so it is no quick fix. Recent evidence indicates that an operation should not be considered until non-operative treatment has been tried for at least six months, and in many cases it should be tried for up to eighteen months. Fortunately in the UK there is now a RCT multi-centre trial (called CSAW!) that aims to find out in which cases shoulder operations really are necessary and this should report in a year or so.

Two studies recently caught my eye. In a recent Swedish study[155] strengthening exercises such as eccentric exercises (resisting a weight as it comes down) for the rotator cuff – muscles and ligaments surrounding the shoulder – and concentric (pushing a weight up) and eccentric exercises for the scapula stabiliser muscles – those muscles behind the shoulder – were used for an experimental group of patients and more general exercises for the control group of similar patients, and after 12 weeks, 69% of those in the specific exercise group reported a large improvement or recovery compared with 24% in the control group. Only 20% of the specific exercise group subsequently chose to have surgery, compared with 63% of the control group. In my experience all exercises were helpful, as if you don't put your shoulder through a full range of movements even if it is painful to do it, you are bound to get a very stiff shoulder. Corticosteroid injections also provide short-term relief while waiting for the problem to get better on its own, and I always offered at least one injection early on, and patients found them very helpful. So I was pleased to see another controlled trial[156] with people receiving steroid injections compared to those receiving a painkilling injection of local anaesthetic, which showed that only three patients in the steroid group still had moderate per severe pain compared with 25 in the control group, and they had a much bigger range of active movement in the shoulder as well. A more recent study[157] showed that exercise was just as good at 14 weeks, however it did not measure the pain suffered in the short term. So it seems that while shoulder operations may well be very helpful for the minority of severe cases, in most cases it is wise to carry on with simpler measures. A friend of mine in the USA had an operation on her shoulder after only eight weeks of symptoms and had an awful time with her arm in a sling for months with a lot of pain. It got better after six months but I think it was likely to have been unnecessary. Because she was only partly insured for this procedure she also had to pay $600 herself. I do hope this trend does not cross the Atlantic!

Specialist injections, usually of corticosteroids, for other conditions can be performed within the practice by GPs who have been trained to give them. These include injections for trigger finger, tennis elbow, plantar fasciitis, and carpal tunnel syndrome, and all of them have at least some evidence that they work and save an operation. If the GP can't do it there are usually other NHS local clinics where GPs can send you that will do them, and these are often run by orthopaedic consultants or consultant physiotherapists, who are otherwise known as extended scope physiotherapists.

Other conditions

There are other conditions that are sent to orthopaedic clinics such as ganglions and other lumps and bumps. Ganglions are the lumps that often occur on the back of the hand. The traditional treatment is to hit the lesion hard with the family bible (or other larger object) in order to try to rupture the capsule, but this has gone out of fashion (and there aren't so many heavy bibles or any heavy books around!). The rule at present is that they should only be removed in an orthopaedic clinic only if significantly interfering with function, not just because they are there.

There are many children's orthopaedic problems such as knock knees, intoeing, and similar gait disorders to that can be seen in podiatry or children's clinic rather than an orthopaedic clinic, as these don't as a rule need surgery. Similarly knee pain in adolescents, a common problem often due to chondromalacia patellae, an irritation of the undersurface of the kneecap, is best seen by specialist physiotherapists, and orthopaedic referral is rarely indicated.

This all means that well-trained and effective professionals in local community settings are treating more and more musculoskeletal conditions. So I do not think Professor Norman Williams should worry at all about the small fall in referrals to orthopaedic clinics last year. It does not mean that patients are not getting the care they need or that rationing by stealth is happening. It means that patients are being referred to and using other services that have a very important place in a modern health service, and that this is to be encouraged, not only in orthopaedics but in other specialities as well. In fact if we do not diversify in this way, the Health Service will certainly grind to a stop, whatever reforms are made to its structure.

Chapter 34
Private health care

History of private care in the UK – conflict of interest – failures of regulation – cost–rent scheme – the Private Finance Initiative – Diagnostic and Treatment Centres – staffing in hospitals.

Private care in the UK

Private care is an integral part of health care in the UK, as in nearly all other countries in the world, with Cuba being a notable exception. It is a fundamental right of people to spend their money as they wish in a democracy, and so all these countries in fact have a two-tier system. The amount the private sector contributes to health spending as a percentage of GDP differs in each country of course, and also whether it is contributed by an insurance company or direct spend. In the UK the private sector spend is the lowest of any of the countries in the OECD and so when most people talk about medical care they usually mean the NHS. There is a tendency to talk about the private sector with disdain as if it is a very minor and slightly disreputable area where profit rules everything.

This is far from the truth of course as the private sector in the UK is absolutely essential to a functioning system. There is a two-tier system in the UK just as there is in Austria, though not so well developed. Historically, private work has always gone on concurrently with the NHS ever since its inception, but it has affected consultants and GPs in different ways. The two groups were treated differently by the NHS act of 1947. GPs were allowed to keep their independence and become contractors for services rather than employees and this continues to the present day. Consultants were forced to become salaried employees, but crucially could continue private practice outside the NHS.

Unfortunately the GPs' contract at the beginning of the NHS was a very disadvantageous one, and it seems they only signed up to it because many GPs were hardly scraping a living at all in a free-market system, where for every full-paying patient they had to treat several for a reduced fee. For the first 15 years of the NHS

GPs had a terrible time, with overcrowded surgeries, dilapidated buildings, on call all hours and very few staff. I have mentioned before how the threat of 80% of GPs leaving the NHS improved the situation for GPs. However, even at the beginning when the service was frankly awful, very few GPs did private practice.

Oddly enough, I worked for one such in my early years as a doctor. The GP I worked for, in a very leafy part of the South of England, had a small list of NHS patients – just enough to qualify for the basic allowance, which was given to every doctor who had 750 patients, and the rest of the work was done privately. But all private patients had to be extremely rich as they not only had to pay the doctor but also had to pay the full price for all medication. One private patient lived in a mansion with a long drive and several gates so it took over three quarters of an hour to get there and the same to get back to the surgery. Local NHS doctors had been very reluctant to take her on. The doctor I was working for visited her every day in the last weeks of her life (she was dying of cancer), and I thought he gave a very good service. I remember he charged £10 per visit (in 1971) but the total bill came to well over £1000 with drugs and extras, and the solicitors for her estate after she died queried the bill and didn't pay it until he threatened to take them to court. I don't think the solicitors realised that spending so much time on one patient was bound to be very expensive, as everyone took a GP's time for granted. I am not at all sure how a NHS doctor of the time would have coped; he probably would have given a pretty good service too, but just not earned so much. Even then with the few drugs available it was expensive, but as time went on it became completely uneconomic. Nowadays the NHS service supplied by GPs in most areas is good, so insurance companies very rarely include GP care in their products. There is something of a market for private GP services in big cities catering for visitors and some who are dissatisfied with their GP, but it is still bound to be very expensive and only for those who don't need regular expensive prescriptions.

Things got better for GPs in the 1970s and 1980s, and things changed for consultants too. At first they could do unlimited private work, and there were many examples of private work being done in NHS time. When I was a houseman in a big teaching hospital, it was part of my contract to look after the patients in the private wing, often getting up in the middle of the night to attend to them. In some cases the patients were far from happy, as I had only been qualified a few months, when I appeared at 2 am to a quite seriously ill private patient. Consultants even then lived far from the hospital and it wasn't easy for them to come in quickly in an emergency if they weren't on call for the NHS, yet that was what was promised to the patient. In time, depending on the government in power, private work for consultants was either encouraged or discouraged but it continues to play a big part in provision of health services in the UK.

I was often happy when a patient asked to go privately, especially when I did not think she needed to be referred anyway! It took the load off the NHS (and me) as all I had to do was ring up the consultant's secretary (in working hours of course – not out of hours in a real emergency) and the problem would be sorted between the patient and the consultant directly. This was something my Australian colleagues really like too; only they are often able to do this with their public patients as well.

In an ideal world the two sectors would be entirely separate, and there would be one group of doctors working for the public sector and another group working separately, as then there would be no conflict of interest. But that is not how it is in most systems. Very few doctors can do all their work privately and make a good living. Irish GPs can't and there is competition to get the public sector jobs – and they are often very critical of the way in which they have to work in private practice. Austrian GPs also compete to get the public work, which is a much more reliable income stream. Consultants in the UK can only make money out of private practice when they have been trained by and worked in the NHS for years. No mainstream specialist in the UK can make a living entirely outside the NHS, so many top up their NHS income with private work. When they are at the top of the tree they can minimise or stop NHS work, and concentrate on private work, but that is rare, as most of them tell me they prefer the NHS work which is more exciting and more rewarding, professionally if not financially.

But where private practice is popular, either because many people buy private medical insurance, or because there are waiting lists, the private clinics can be almost as rushed as NHS clinics, because outside the big cities there may not be many consultants available to do the private work on top of their very busy schedule in the NHS. I suppose a well-trained registrar who is looking for a consultant post could theoretically do private work, but it never happens. The patients would not go to anybody they thought was not fully trained (unless of course it was very cheap but that would indeed be very risky). So there is an inherent conflict of interest here, with specialists always working for both sectors, and when the public medicine is performing badly there are the greatest opportunities for private practice.

This is where GPs can be very aware of situations which are questionable, and this is a thread running through this book, even though in the vast majority of cases senior members of specialist colleges will be entirely ethical in all their dealing with managers and GPs in the NHS. But the refusal of consultant committees to allow GPs access to services such as physiotherapy in the 1970s and 1980s was in part due to the desire of consultants to keep and develop their private work. I knew because they told me so. I worked on developing services locally with a consultant who did no private work, and she said she used to get fed up with her colleagues' insistence that things should not change, and so it was not surprising that GPs did not get access to services that would improve their ability to care for their patients immeasurably. At that time (1991) we had a lecture on management of orthopaedic problems from a visiting Australian orthopaedic surgeon, telling us about the service that he had arranged jointly with GPs there. He was assuming that we had at least some access to physiotherapy but when we said we didn't, he was dumbstruck. It was very embarrassing for our orthopaedic surgeons, as they had invited him and they had to explain why GPs couldn't have it. Actually I think that was a tipping point, and soon afterwards a small pilot scheme was arranged.

Also of course during the dreadful times from about 1991 to 2002 when waiting times became incredibly extended in some specialities – up to 5 years in some areas – a huge rise in private referrals was the result. One audit I did in 2004 showed that private work increased to 25% of all referrals in orthopaedics, and it was not a wealthy area.

Unsurprisingly, we found that private referrals varied by speciality and area. In our study in 2009, the wealthiest of the areas where we were working in had an overall rate of 20% for private referrals to hospital (all specialities) and a much poorer area with a lot of deprivation had a rate of only 2%, and I am sure this is replicated across the UK. In really wealthy areas and in London it will probably be much higher. I think this vast amount of private funding for first consultant appointments may need to be taken into account when designing NHS services.

When waiting times were so long, even people with very little spare cash would spend their savings on private appointments with the consultant. I think we all, GPs and consultants, felt very bad about this, especially when the patient was in real need. It is one thing for a patient to take out private medical insurance because they want the extra convenience and certainty of getting the consultant rather than a trainee registrar, but quite another when patients had to spend money they couldn't spare to get a very basic service. Once seen, of course, at that time they could jump the waiting list to have further treatment on the NHS, sometimes being seen quicker than people already on the waiting list. This encouraged even more people to pay privately. Then there was a move to stop this happening, but no-one was very sure of exactly what went on. Once the waiting times got to more reasonable levels of course the demand for private treatment fell away; in our area it fell by about 3% a year.

The cost–rent scheme and the private finance initiative

The government has always procured some services for patients through the private market, without the patient paying for them themselves, so all the while the private market was continuing grow in other areas. The scheme to develop GP surgeries from 1964 to 2004, the cost–rent scheme, was also a private scheme akin to the current private finance initiative (PFI). A partnership of GPs could design and build a surgery with money borrowed from the bank. The loan was then guaranteed by the Government by granting a rent paid from a central fund to the doctors to fund the mortgage. The GPs owned the building and therefore when they retired they could sell their share and retire with a hefty lump sum, as the property market continued to rise. As the rent nearly always covered the mortgage this was an excellent deal for the doctors. And when fundholding came in in the 1990s the doctor could use fundholding savings to invest in their premises, on which further rent would be paid, thus ensuring a very nice profit when they retired – if they could persuade some young partner to buy them out. This became less likely as property prices later slumped, but the valuation of the surgery building remained high because of the guaranteed rent. In any case the remaining partners could and can always go on collecting rent even when they leave the practice.

Actually the scheme did succeed very well in providing excellent GP premises in most areas of the country. Even in very poor areas GPs could and did develop their own surgeries under the scheme, but of course there was no great increase in property values in some deprived areas and so such GPs might even land up in negative equity. It was a private scheme with some GPs being great winners (those in prosperous areas) and those GPs in poorer areas where the workload was much higher being much worse off in retirement. It was never as expensive to the public purse as the PFI, however.

When you think of the whole range of services the NHS provides, there has always been a mix of publicly and privately procured services, while the service to the patient is still free at the point of delivery. Now that the coalition government's Health and Social Care Bill has been passed, lots of parts of the NHS are being offered to the private sector in order to 'free up the market' and 'get the advantages of competition', so it is crucial to make sure the private sector is properly regulated. Two recent cases have cast doubt on this: the case of the care home for adults with learning disabilities, and the breast implant problem. In the first case the company that ran the home ran into financial trouble after selling off its properties and leasing them back via another company, and then had to cut costs by reducing staff training and pay and conditions. Poor regulation meant that the home went unchecked and it took a BBC investigation to show that the patients were being seriously ill-treated. The second case was the French firm that used breast implants made of industrial-type silicone that would never have passed safety tests, yet the company managed to elude the regulators for many years. Then it went out of business, and some of women who had had the implants done by private firms needed them removed by the NHS, because of leakage. So there was an argument as to whether the NHS should also replace them, which seemed very unfair to the taxpayer.

In both cases it was failure of regulation in an industry that was very competitive that caused the problem, compounded by moral hazard. In both cases it wasn't the companies that had to pay the price, as they either went bankrupt or were able to just close down the business, but the patients and the NHS. There was no requirement that companies had to have insurance to compensate patients and in every case it was the NHS that had to pick up the bill, which of course the companies had known would happen, and so they felt able to avoid the costs of insurance against it. So what place does the private sector have in a modern health system?

The Private Finance Initiative (PFI) scheme in England (Wales never took part and Scotland had only a few) was similar in a way. Here the hospitals were built with finance put up by development companies that then ran the hospitals, while government money paid all costs, including a rental amount year by year. This enabled many old hospital buildings owned by the Government to be sold off and the sites redeveloped, so ensuring an influx of funds in the short term to the Exchequer. The funds always had to be returned centrally – they were never retained by the local hospital organisation. But with a PFI scheme the hospital trusts have to pay rent to the developer for at least 30 years – and often, especially in the early years, these rents are crippling. These costs are some of the reasons why the NHS is now costing more and more to run. In fact some trusts are now going bankrupt as a direct result of the costs of the scheme. The private firms had to have the cake sweetened before they would bite, and undoubtedly the contracts were too generous, as people like Allyson Pollock, professor of public health research and policy at Queen Mary, University of London, argued from the outset.[158]

Diagnostic and Treatment Centres

Diagnostic and Treatment Centres (DTCs) are privately-run, freestanding healthcare facilities with no emergency beds. They support the rest of the NHS by providing essential diagnostic services that are under pressure, such as MRI scanning, endoscopies and others. They also perform much-needed routine surgical operations for which people used to wait for years – hips, cataracts and hernias, as many as possible as day cases. They were set up in the UK from 2004, and their main purpose was to increase capacity, and so to reduce waiting lists, and they succeeded in doing this very well. They get their surgeons from the UK or abroad; people who become specialized in these operations but cannot do the whole range of work that a consultant surgeon can do in this country. However, because they do them continually they may get better results than general surgeons who do a wide mix of cases. There is no waiting list: beds are always available because the centres don't accept emergencies (they have to go to the local hospital), and for the same reasons MRSA and other infections are less of a problem, because it is always possible to screen patients thoroughly in advance and to treat those with MRSA before they come in, thus preventing its spread within the centre. For mainstream hospitals this is much more difficult when patients come in as an emergency and have to be treated straight away.

There are some problems however. If a complication does arise from an operation done by a DTC after the first 48 hours, or if an operation goes badly wrong, then of course the patient goes straight back to the local hospital, with the cost picked up by the NHS. So you would think that the price paid by the NHS for these operations in the centres should be a lot less than the amount the hospital would be paid by the NHS. This however is not necessarily so because the private companies that run them had to be persuaded to take them on and invest in the separate facilities.

In some cases there has been a problem with their management. In NHS hospitals consultant surgeons have the final say in what prosthesis, for example for an artificial knee, is used. Cost is taken into account but is never the only consideration. They then gain familiarity with this particular product and are used to working with it. However in DTCs, at least at first, the choice of prosthesis was made by the managers of the centre – they would procure these using excellent advice from experienced surgeons and with the latest evidence (we presume). They also hired the surgeons, who might come from the NHS but also might come from abroad. They did not necessarily have any experience at all with the particular prosthesis that the managers had chosen. So a drawback was that some operations were in fact experiments with the surgeons finding out what were the strengths and weaknesses of the prostheses by trial and error and without help from a surgeon used to dealing with this prosthesis. This was a big problem in one area in 2007, where at least three operations went wrong. The Health Authority I worked for then had to arrange for the operations to be re-done on the NHS and the patients compensated.

There is another problem that senior consultant surgeons were keen to highlight, and that was that training young surgeons is made harder when many of these operations are outside the NHS district hospitals, as these cases are the bread and butter on which young surgeons practice their skills in the NHS. Training young surgeons is a job the NHS does very well; British training is considered one of the best in the world and that is why young doctors come here from everywhere. Doctors in training perform many of these operations under careful supervision in the health service. Of course if patients knew this, they might well say that they would prefer to go to a DTC for treatment by experienced doctors, not trainees! However these centres are privately run for profit, so they are using the services of surgeons who have been expensively trained elsewhere, (usually within the NHS) without in turn training the next generation of surgeons.

In the NHS, once the junior doctors been trained in these operations and have their quota, the operations still need to be done. So who performs the operations that the juniors don't need to do? They should go back to the experienced surgeons, but the latter are needed for more complex operations and to train juniors in them. So simple or straightforward operations then go to the end of the queue, adding to waiting lists. Of course theoretically some of the training needs could be done by short-term attachments to these centres, although I don't know of this being done up to now. In fact there is an army of non-consultant grade doctors called staff grade doctors in hospitals who will often do straightforward operations. They earn much less than consultants, but the scheme works well in most cases. However when doctors, often from abroad, are appointed to this grade they do not realise that they will not get any further training, and this can cause problems. The mix of senior and junior doctors in hospitals is crucial to the good functioning of a hospital and in rural areas it is very difficult to get it right. The Royal Colleges try, but sometimes you end up with doctors having reached the end of a long and arduous training schedule and finding that there are no consultant jobs for them. Yet it is not possible for them to provide a private service, and some then emigrate, taking all that experience with them.

The DTCs have to be completely stand-alone centres, to protect them from acute service pressures. The NHS has the sole responsibility for dealing with the huge volume of extra emergency work. There are always pressures on NHS beds in the wintertime because people get ill during this period with medical problems such as chest infections. These patients then fill beds in surgical wards, as there are a fixed number of beds in a hospital. So operations are cancelled and the waiting list for routine surgery lengthens. This is a big reason why waiting lists increase and why the extra capacity is needed.

So with a DTC in the area, theoretically the surgical teams in NHS hospitals can offload some of these operations and can then concentrate on training the next generation of doctors, and allow other well qualified doctors specializing only in a limited area of expertise to mop up the vast amount of routine work, thereby slashing waiting lists. However, some senior surgeons in the NHS were not happy with this and opposed the centres at first. They realised well enough that the reason they had come into being was to increase capacity in the NHS, and this actually was not in their interests. There are a limited number of surgeons in the NHS at the top of the tree, with tremendous power, not so much within NHS bureaucracy itself but emanating from their professional colleges – the Royal Colleges. The Royal Colleges have a big say in the appointment of surgeons and how many are allowed in each region; this is to ensure the quality of the service. Also of course appointing an extra surgeon is always expensive as the NHS also has to ensure that there is enough theatre space, anaesthetists and so on. All this means that capacity is limited, but this actually was in the interests of the surgeons who can take up the slack with their private work. These diagnostic and treatment centres were originally to be staffed by people from outside the NHS, as at first there was a ban on surgeons moonlighting from NHS hospitals, as this would defeat the object of increasing capacity. So the Royal Colleges began to shroud wave, saying that the centres would be bad for the NHS and would destabilize it.

It was also necessary to persuade GPs to refer to the centres rather than their local hospitals, or rather persuade patients to choose them with the 'Choose and Book' system, which came in at the same time. In some cases GPs did not refer enough patients (many patients really just want to go to the local hospital for convenience rather than to some hospital some where else which was said to be 'better') and so sometimes the private companies treated far fewer cases than the NHS had contracted but still were paid for the contractual number.

Eventually some successful centres have continued to provide services, while others have failed and the work has reverted to the NHS, which has no option but to ask its NHS surgeons to take up the extra work. Now there may be regular 'red' bulletins to local GPs telling them to refer to these centres, so they do that, and eventually the centres may be close to capacity. However the patient has to be seen, and if the private hospital contract is 'over-performed' by a small margin the NHS might have to pay for a single operation as well. We don't know how much extra has to be paid because such information is closely guarded by the Department of Health as 'commercially sensitive'.

Of course another objection to this is that a firm is taking a profit out of the money available for the NHS. Why couldn't the NHS set up these centres and recruit personnel itself?

So the place of the private sector in a publically funded health system must clearly be thought out. There has to be regulation that is even more effective than in a public system, as there is more (financial) incentive to 'cook the books' or provide substandard care as it costs less. At present the private sector is regulated much less well than the public sector. It must have at least some integration with the NHS, as surgeons and other doctors working in the private sector must be aware of what is the norm in the NHS, and there should be a level playing field so that if the private sector does not provide follow-up or emergency services the payment should be less. The contract would have to be carefully worked out so that the private company gets paid for what it does and is not paid for work it does not do, and when it does extra this again should be at a reasonable rate. Most of all, the private sector should not automatically assume that the NHS will pick up the pieces if things go wrong, and should pay to insure itself in the usual commercial way. The problem is that if this all happens, if profits are not assured the private sector will walk away.

Chapter 35
Saving money: looking at GP referrals

Electronic referrals – outcomes of out-patient appointments – improving GP's referrals – devolving services to local communities – patients' views – importance of interpersonal skills of doctors – second opinions – urgency.

Referrals to hospital cost money. GPs have always held the reins here – a patient cannot get treatment in an NHS hospital without a referral from a GP, but GPs have also had freedom to refer to whomever they wished. With the drive to using every penny wisely, the quality and quantity of GP referrals has been of great interest in the last six years or so.

During my time as a medical manager, we looked at many GP referrals to hospital in detail. We found that the old saw – a GP would scribble a note to the hospital consultant saying, 'Please see, query chest' and the consultant could write back, 'Dear Doctor, chest present' had not been accurate for a very long time. I do remember some very poor letters from GPs of course when I was on the receiving end, and probably wrote some myself, but that was many years ago. Nowadays GPs' referrals usually contain all the information the hospital is likely to need and we found over 90% were of high quality as judged by their peers.

Electronic referrals

In most countries now electronic referrals are the rule, and the letter can be sent to the correct department of a hospital in hours rather than weeks, the GP typing on the computer keyboard. This must be saving a lot of money as well improving the efficiency of the service. A big problem had been that there was no way of checking where the letter had got to in the system and there were many delays in seeing urgent cases. A rule of thumb was that you waited four to five days for the letter to be dictated, written, signed, and sent off by the doctor; a day for the letter to arrive at the hospital (if there was an efficient collection system); and at least eight days for the letter to arrive in the right department and seen by the consultant, or whoever was prioritizing the letters.

These delays were accepted as part of a very long wait to see the specialist, and the problem was always how to send the urgent ones quickly – usually by a telephone call that may or may not have been quick to make. Electronic templates have been developed to remind GPs of the information that needs to be put in, although both GPs and consultants sometimes prefer a straightforward letter. Managers worked at electronic templates for GPs to make referrals to specialists for several years, and spent a huge amount of senior clinicians' time on large meetings, but some templates are still gathering dust. I asked a colleague, still working as a GP, whether he had heard of any, and he said no. If someone had asked the GPs before this work started whether they wanted such templates they would have said no. But no one did; the work got started but was a complete waste.

Ordinary letters are certainly better than electronic summaries, which GPs send off at a push of a button including practically the whole patient record. Patients may think this is good, but the consultant cannot possibly sift through it to find out what is wanted quickly. So the modern method is very much better, and saves much secretarial time, and it is remarkable how long it took to implement it, since all the letters for some time now have been in MS Word at both ends. In one area I know of they had a system in late 2007; in another they had to wait until 2010. There just did not seem to be a way of getting it past intrinsic resistance to change in management, and it was incredibly frustrating. Security was obviously a very important issue, but if money transfers can be made securely, surely it could be done with patient records. Ironically, many GPs from other countries where there is a strong private sector still find this very difficult, as specialists working from private offices do not develop consistent computerised record systems, making the delay longer in the private than in the public system.

Refining referrals

The big question that interested managers was 'Are GPs referring the right patient to the right place for effective treatment?', so that data on actual outcomes for patients were interesting. These were systematically coded when the consultants' letters came back and we could see what had actually happened following the referral.

We found that of 422 consecutive referrals to orthopaedics:

- In 32% there was no documented action at all. Some of the patients concerned may have been given advice, but they were almost certainly discharged back to their GP straightaway, with no change in diagnosis.

- In 26% of the cases there was some sort of further investigation, usually further X-rays or scans. Of these, some undoubtedly would have had another procedure at some time. We weren't able to follow up the patients to discharge so we did not know whether any of these patients eventually got an operation or not.

- In only 10% of those referred was there an offer of an immediate operation. This is a low percentage as in a surgical speciality managers would hope that at least 30% of referrals would be of a sort that led to an operation, for maximum efficiency.

- In 12% of cases it was documented that there was an 'other action'. This might have been that the patient was referred to another speciality such as to the pain clinic, rheumatology, or other related speciality.

- For 6.2% there was an offer of review in clinic without any other action in the meantime, and 3.6% were referred directly to physiotherapy.

- Some 2.4% were advised to change their medication and 6% were not seen (the patient did not attend or another reason was given).

We also looked at medical specialities such as neurology, and here:

- 74% of the patients had been referred for diagnosis or further investigation, 19% for advice on further management, and 5% were classified as Patient Demand.

- The results showed that 72% were seen again in the clinic and most of those were investigated by the hospital, 20% were discharged after the visit, and 8% were referred to another speciality.

So the proportion of patients only seen once was much lower, which indicates that most patients needed an investigation that the GPs were not able to organise, (although a fifth of patients still only got seen once).

So less than half of the patients had any immediate action that the GP could not have arranged, and there was a very low percentage of patients who were immediately listed for an operation when the GPs thought they might need one. The majority of patients going to an outpatient appointment seemed to be there for reassurance, possible advice, and review, which might indicate that some of the patients might have been spared a journey to the hospital and managed in primary care.

I am never sure what patients think of this. We know that in general a patient is very unlikely to complain if they have been offered an appointment, and very few patients will say their consultation was unnecessary. Yet we also know that a sizable proportion (up to about 10%) never actually turn up for their appointment, even when given several appointments. Some doctors now routinely give a copy of the referral letter to patients, and I found several times that the patient then had a better understanding of why I thought the patient should be referred. But on one occasion a patient came back and said that the letter to the consultant reassured him and now he didn't really want to go! So I think it is very good practice to do this. Sometimes in a short consultation it is difficult to communicate everything correctly and the copy of the letter will then concentrate everyone's mind about what exactly it is hoped will be achieved.

In some cases of course we know that the doctor did not think the patient needed an appointment with the consultant, but because the patient really wanted one, or the doctor was afraid of a complaint being made, the referral was made. In other cases the GP might have thought further investigation was required but had got it wrong. There is nothing incorrect in any of this of course but if you are looking at using every penny of public money as efficiently as possible you have to send only the patient who clearly needs to be seen to the hospital. It is different when the patient is paying privately – in these cases it is the consumer who is getting the value that he puts on his own money.

Just recently, and especially because commissioning groups (established with the re-organisation of 2012) are trying to make the process of referral more efficient and save money, GPs are incentivised through the QOF to discuss their referrals with each other and collaborate with the authorities on which would be the best pathways to develop. This might work, as a study we did showed that they then alter their referral activity.[159] The highest-referring doctors will tend to reduce their referrals quite considerably, but also the lowest-referring doctors are likely to increase theirs, thus reducing the variation. This should be a good thing. In the past GPs used to get very little feedback about their referrals apart from the consultant's letter. Consultants would never actively criticize a referral even if they privately thought that the referral should have been made earlier or that it wasn't necessary. We asked consultants if they would give feedback to GPs and the GPs told them that they really wanted to know if their referrals were not appropriate, but it never happened. The only feedback a GP would get was from the patients, and sometimes that could be very helpful, but a patient's satisfaction was more likely to come from the way they were treated rather than the outcome. Sometimes when things went wrong the patient would be supportive of the consultant because he had 'tried', and even when they weren't actually given much in the way of treatment because it wasn't necessary, they were satisfied because 'now we know'.

So GPs are more able to give each other feedback. GPs who are at the lower end of the referring range realise that other GPs are referring cases that they did not usually refer, and they can be shown the benefits of this for the patient. Other GPs will realise that their referral rates were hugely higher than everyone else's. When this happens some are very taken aback, and hopefully realise the value of alternative services and start to use them. The aim is to reduce the variation in referral rates so that patients are more likely to get a referral if most GPs would agree that they should.

There were some groups of GPs whose referral patterns differed from the norm. The most obvious of these were the doctors in training – GP registrars. Registrars are the most inexperienced referrers. We did not have very much data on their referrals as there were not many training practices at the time of the study and we do not know how many patients they actually saw. Certainly in the early part of their training they can have a very light load. However one practice with three registrars noted that in July when the registrars were seeing more patients, because partners were on holiday, the referral rate for orthopaedics jumped from an average of 40 per month to 76 per month. A proportion of that increase was due to increased numbers of registrar referrals, and the practice looked at these referrals in detail. As a result they found that some referrals were inappropriate or wrongly directed and the practice then made a policy of checking all registrar referrals before sending them off. The partners took steps to increase the supervision of registrar referrals and to provide more teaching, and they did this for all specialities, not only the ones the practice was discussing at the time.

Locums also tended to have a higher rate. In one practice where a partner was on maternity leave during the study the locums who came in to cover had a referral rate double the remaining partners. This is likely to be a pattern repeated everywhere, as locums have to refer more as they cannot follow up patients within the surgery. So it is important to ensure that locums are given as much information on where and whom, to refer according to local patterns. It does indicate that there will be a cost to the NHS in increased referrals if more and more locums are used to cover for GPs away doing commissioning or other management work.

A problem with commissioning and the new reforms is that with the emphasis on competition GPs and consultants won't easily be able to get together to make sure that the patients get the best treatment. Consensual working is much more likely to get good results, and I think in the past that GPs and consultants have not discussed referral patterns nearly often enough. When this does happen it can be very useful, particularly when consultants 'give permission' for GPs to refer to alternative pathways outside hospital (physio, optometry, nurses). In the past GPs had expected to refer only to other doctors and not to other health professionals. But this was what ultimately had resulted in waiting lists of two or more years, and this had caused bad feeling between primary and secondary care doctors. Some GPs felt that they had been excluded from decisions in the past and would be very keen to work with consultants, and to influence future developments. So I hope that the new commissioning groups will be able to get GPs and consultants together wherever it would be useful.

Patients' views

All health systems in the world are grappling with the problem of making sure that all work that can be devolved to primary care is transferred there. Theoretically there should be an orderly transition of work downwards in any health system, so that specialists can develop and refine new technologies which make such a difference to patient care at the cutting edge, and eventually those technologies that have been standardised and well honed in the hospital setting can then be usefully transferred to less specialised environments. The economies that would be released would enable money to be released which can partly pay for the new treatments. But of course there will be some consultants and some GPs who will resist this. I certainly knew of consultants who were actively against any attempt to refer to non-medical personnel instead of their department, and there were GPs who were very unwilling to stop referring patients to the consultants of their choice.

But patients also need to be convinced of this. We did a survey of patients[160] who had been through the traditional route to a hospital specialist compared with patients who had been to an alternative more local service. We wanted to find out from patients what their experiences were of being referred to alternative community services. So we distributed a questionnaire to a total of 52 patients, which focused on whether patients felt they were given enough information about the referral from their GP, on waiting times to be seen and whether they thought this was reasonable, and their level of satisfaction overall with regard to their referral. The key aim of these interviews was to find out from patients what they valued about the care or services they received and how their care and treatment could have been improved.

We were pleased to find that most patients said they were happy with whatever service they used, and though there were a few who would have preferred to see a specialist in hospital, most were very happy with the alternative. There were some who were very dissatisfied with the hospital specialist too, especially when the patient disagreed with the diagnosis, or they felt they had been waiting too long so that the problem had got worse.

We interviewed five patients in detail to give their 'patient stories' and these are detailed here. (Pseudonyms have been used throughout.) A number of themes emerged: organisation of services, inter-personal skills and 'alternative' services.

Overall patients were very positive about their experiences and commented on the excellent care and treatment they had received. They also reflected on aspects of their care and treatment and aspects of the health service in general that they thought could have been improved.

Several patients highlighted how impressed they were with the way the health services were organised. For example, Dick was given an appointment to see the hospital consultant in the evening:

> It was great – it suited us down to the ground... we were only out [of the house] an hour... I wasn't sat there 2 minutes before I went in to see the consultant. I had my scans very quickly afterwards – it was really slick.

Dick was also impressed with the care he had received in the past from other services within the NHS:

> I have found the NHS fantastic – brilliant! Particularly the local people in occupational therapy –there were handrails everywhere, bed raisers, and stair lifts –unbelievable – it totally changed our life because [my wife] was having to lift me up the stairs.

But he also had some thoughts on how things could be improved:

> You don't ever see the same person twice... that's important because as the patient you imagine they know what's wrong with you – they remember you. its all about human relationships.

Andy also highlighted the importance of consistency and talked of his frustration with the way services were sometimes run. When he first went to the GP, he felt his complaint was not taken sufficiently seriously and subsequent visits to the surgery to see different GPs highlighted what he saw as an inconsistency in approach and treatment.

He spoke of having to 'push a little to get what I wanted', and how, as a patient, 'you have to work the system to your favour'. Unhappy with his initial care, Andy was subsequently referred to the local physiotherapy-led service for an assessment, and it was at this point that he felt his complaint was taken more seriously, and things began to improve.

> I was lucky in that I saw someone after 12 months who wanted to get to the bottom of it and was interested in what I'd done and where I wanted to go.

In addition to service organisation, one of the other key themes to emerge from the patient stories relates to the interpersonal and communication skills of health care professionals. This area was one which appeared to be a 'make or break factor' in-patient experiences and illustrates the importance of compassion, empathy and patient centred care.

Dick in particular was disappointed with his initial appointment to see the hospital consultant. Despite being impressed with the organisation of his care, the experience was marred by the attitude of the consultant he first saw.

> I didn't think much of the consultant – so laid back and un-caring. There was no eye contact – he was yawning all the time. I was relying on him to sort out my pain – it was a major thing for me, but he had nothing to offer.

Dick compared this encounter with his subsequent visit to the hospital – on this occasion he saw a different consultant:

> The second guy was a lot better – he had a lot more empathy with people. He explained what was wrong with me – there was a world of difference between the two.

Sally also highlighted the importance of good interpersonal skills and a caring attitude when she underwent a procedure which she had found very difficult:

> It was the worst thing I've had done in my whole life. I thought I was going to die – it was vile… horrid…. The staff were kind and very lovely. They were fantastic – calm and caring.

The attitude of staff had been the most positive aspect of her experiences.

Andy also identified the importance of good communication skills. He found it frustrating not knowing where he was in the 'system' whilst waiting for an out-patient appointment:

> I was always having to chase where I was in the system – how long I might have to wait. If people tell you, you feel better'

Andy recommended (written) guidance for patients to help them understand how the outpatient system works and what they could expect in terms of waiting times.

The final theme relates to patient's experiences of 'alternative services'. Those patients who had been referred to alternative services were asked about their experiences and how they felt such services compared to the more traditional, hospital based services.

Mary had been seen by the physiotherapy-led service whilst waiting for a hospital appointment and was pleased with the care she received – in particular she commented on the homely environment and the convenience of the local 'cottage' hospital where she was seen.

> It was so much easier, its local and smaller and more homely, the [main District General Hospitals] are more impersonal – so many people milling around. The parking was easier and it was easy for me to get to – virtually on my doorstep. It's a heck of a long way to walk from the car park at [the District General Hospital] to orthopaedics.

Others shared this view. For example, although Sally had initially been seen at the District General Hospital for treatment, she subsequently went to the local hospital for follow-up treatment and was very impressed with the care she received. Sally highlighted the advantages of being seen more locally in terms of the convenience, ease of travel (Sally didn't drive) and its more homely feel.

> Going to [the District General Hospital] was logistically a bit of a pain. Going to the community hospital for my follow-on appointment was much easier. Not everybody has a car – like me – and I have to get a bus or get someone to take me.

> Going to [the local hospital] is like how the old cottage hospitals used to be – it's like a little community – get to know people – they are local people who work there. It's just as effective – there is less waiting around in big impersonal waiting rooms in hospitals.

Reflecting on why some people may prefer to be seen at the District General Hospital by a consultant, Sally commented:

> Some people just want to see a consultant don't they – maybe older people; 'that's the person I need to see'.

This was not Sally's view however, and she highlighted what she saw as another benefit of being seen in the local setting:

Sometimes you get referred to the consultant [in secondary care], who then refers you back to see a physio and it's a waste of time.

This sentiment was echoed by Dick who commented of his first hospital appointment with the consultant: 'it was a waste of time – he just re-iterated what the GP had said.'

From their previous experiences, the time spent waiting to be seen once they had arrived at the District General Hospital was also a cause of irritation for patients, as Frank commented:

The biggest problem is how long you have to wait once you are there…you are just one in a crowd of a 100.

Frank compared this with his experiences of attending the local services:

It's smaller – more personal – it's more a family run thing, everyone knows everyone and what everyone is doing… I felt much more at ease because they were very, very friendly – they seemed to be enjoying what they were doing – they cared.

The personal, friendly atmosphere of where the local services were provided seems to have been significant for patients. When asked how the experience of going to there (to the local services) compared to his previous experiences of going to the District General Hospital, Frank commented 'It doesn't – it's far superior.'

Frank was also impressed with how quickly his appointment with the local service had come through (2-3 weeks). 'I didn't think I'd be seen that quickly!' Reflecting on the most positive aspect of his experiences, Frank added: 'I suppose the person who saw me – they knew what they were doing and helped me a lot.'

Andy was similarly pleased with the services and care offered by the physio service.

I saw the Physio and they got to the bottom of it … it was a bit of a relief – people seemed to know what they were doing. I would have appreciated being referred to them from the start – this happened a year into the process – if it had happened initially I could have been sorted out much sooner.

Andy also commented on how quickly and smoothly things had progressed after his initial visit with rapid referral for further scans and consultant appointment. He was also impressed with the fact that staff had access to his previous scans: 'It was refreshing – it really helped the consultation.'

None of the patients who were interviewed and who had been referred to the physiotherapy-led service had any reservations about the appropriateness of their referral. Indeed, the patient stories suggest that community-based services run by other health professionals can offer a timely and effective alternative to the more traditional, hospital-based consultant-led care – which is just as well, as this is a big thrust of 'improvement' in services from health managers in just about every country you look at. But the main thing that came out of it is the usual thing – it proves once again that what the patients value most is to talk to some one who really takes an interest and tries to help, rather irrespective of the actual outcome.

At bottom it does all depend on the skill of the GP in steering the patient towards a good outcome and communicating with them well throughout the process. From a patient's perspective there is a variety of choices between doing something active about the problem, or not. There have always been patients who are quite reluctant to undergo further investigation or treatment, but most people do see a medical solution as being a main plank in their search for a solution. It is the GP's job to fit the patient's life beliefs and aspirations into a recommendation for referral and most GPs are extremely skilled at this. The GP is usually the one with more accurate knowledge of what is available and may need to correct some beliefs that the patient has gleaned from the many sources in the public domain. It may sometimes take more time and skill than the GP has at her disposal to persuade a patient that the course of action the patient wants is not the best course amongst those the GP thinks are on offer, and so some investigations or referrals are done without good reason. The GP knows that that there are other ways of dealing with the problem that she feels would be more appropriate, but she is unable to persuade a patient of this. The action, an investigation or referral, is therefore done.

It is assumed in every case that the patient will not come to any harm in doing this – the worst that happens usually is that the patient has an unnecessary journey to see a specialist who reassures him that all is well. But there are some cases in this category where a patient has an unnecessary intervention, and it is known that in some cases a patient is worse off.[161] It is absolutely essential that GPs, as well as the surgeon who offers an intervention, give the patient as much information as possible about possible harms, and patients may not then choose to be referred.

From many other surveys of patient outcome that have been done, most people are satisfied, certainly for well proven operations such as hip or knee replacements – over 80% in 2010 – but the satisfaction rate for other operations some of which have a less secure evidence base is lower, down to 60% who are completely satisfied with the results of an intervention. The most important thing is that the process at every stage involves explaining the options and likely results to the patient. The GP will know that to refuse a referral against patient's wishes after full explanation is unwise, both for medico-legal reasons and to protect the doctor patient relationship. GPs however will differ in their ability to go through the whole process of full explanation in the time available and it is sometimes easier to just do what the patient wants.

When patients are unhappy with a consultation in hospital they have a right to a second opinion. This was enshrined in the original NHS Act of 1947, and we found that some of the referrals which were made despite the doctor thinking they weren't strictly necessary were because of patient dissatisfaction with the first opinion that they had. We did not have the data to find out whether the patients actually did get a different opinion from the second doctor, but there is no doubt that doctors should try to communicate better the second time round. As many complaints against doctors in the NHS are fundamentally about poor communication rather than faulty treatment, it is important to get this right first time. If a patient requests a second consultant opinion because of dissatisfaction with the first consultant, it may be appropriate to write to the first consultant and ask them to arrange the second opinion if necessary. This way at least the first consultant will know there has been a problem and perhaps will reassess wither the way he handled the problem or the treatment offered. If a patient insists on getting a certain treatment against the evidence, though, it can be difficult not to give in.

Routine and urgent referrals

As part of looking at referrals we looked at whether they were classified as 'Routine' or 'Urgent' as this should give an indication of how long a patient would have to wait for their appointment. It varied quite a lot from doctor to doctor but not from practice to practice as it averaged out. It bore very little relation to the waits patients have, as the percentage seen within two months was the same for both groups. So GPs who put the classification on the letter and consultants who prioritize whom to see don't usually agree, and it is almost impossible to be sure that people who ultimately turn out to need urgent treatment are seen first. It depends on the speciality and on whether it is the consultants who decide who should be seen first, or whether it is a nurse or a manager, and GPs can sometimes disagree with the classification of urgency put on it by the hospital. This would give credence to the idea that it is most important to have shorter waits for everyone rather than very short waits for some and longer ones for others.

In primary care GPs often refer to each other within the practice. Not every GP's training is identical, and many GPs have 'specializations' because of particular hospital jobs they have done in the past, lectures they have attended, or special qualifications they have obtained in different branches of practice. The common ones are in musculoskeletal medicine, child health and women's health and reproduction, but there are lots of others. Sometimes the doctor with special expertise does not advertise his strengths within the practice, and then his colleagues may not know exactly what he can treat so it is important to advertise this! Practice leaflets have helped here.

Other countries report problems with the referral process too. In Norway, GPs told me that the referral process is getting very difficult for them.[162] They feel the process is too one-sided, and the consultant will sometimes refuse to see a patient that the GP has referred. This is particularly true in psychiatry, because GPs are expected to see the majority of psychiatric patients themselves. A recent article from Norway[163] looked at referrals to psychiatric services, and found that there was very little agreement between the doctors who referred and the doctors who received a referral on what constituted a routine or an urgent referral. This may be because psychiatry consultations can be very subjective and there are few objective reasons for urgency, but this is likely to be true in other specialities as well.

So GPs in Norway too wanted a dialogue with consultants about their patients. GPs there seem to feel more disempowered about referrals in general, with GPs seeing the referral process as asymmetric and sometimes humiliating, which is something that never cropped up in our discussions about referrals. I think this is likely to be because GPs in the UK do in fact have more 'clout' because of the past history of fundholding and now the emphasis on GP commissioning, so that although in some managerial systems it is easy to keep GPs out of the loop, they can often soon get back in again.

Politicians frequently say that clinicians should be in charge and that they should all work together. The NHS would benefit from more communication, not less and it will be a challenge to keep this at the front of commissioning in the future, especially when the gap between what GPs, managers and consultants all want may get wider.

Part 11

Changes over the years and in the future

Chapter 36
Reorganisation and commissioning

Cost of reorganisations – saving money – looking at the bureaucracy of the NHS –
Social Services – inverse care law – reducing health inequality – fundholding

Cost of reorganisations

Most people are both unaware and uninterested in exactly how the NHS is run in their area. As well they might be, because as soon as a system has become familiar, it will be reorganised. Most people are aware that the template for employment of GPs is a contract for services, not direct employment. That contract, which is negotiated by the BMA and the Government, has been administered successively in my time in the NHS by the Executive Council, the Family Practitioner Committee, the Family Health Service Authority, the Primary Care Group and recently the Primary Care Organisations (Primary Care Trust in England, Health Boards in Wales and Scotland, and Health and Social Care Trusts in Northern Ireland). The various 'New Contracts' for GPs have been detailed already, and these were sometimes negotiated and often imposed. Now in England in the new reorganisation, primary care trusts have been abolished and Commissioning Groups established. It is enough to make anyone weep.

In each case the local body has been answerable to different local agencies such as Strategic Health Authorities, in order to put a distance between decisions on the ground and the mandarins in London. When devolution came along, the Trusts or Boards answered directly to the devolved government in Scotland, Wales and Northern Ireland. Total root and branch reorganisations have happened roughly every seven years. As one might imagine, the reason for this is that none of them has delivered the goods, and politicians, who have unfettered control over the structure of the system, always think that somewhere round the corner is a better structure which will best fit their particular brand of localism and accountability.

It is well known that each reorganisation costs billions. The Kings Fund has said,[164] 'It is well established that organisations entering periods of restructuring

413

become less effective. Reorganisations are a clumsy reform tool and seldom deliver the promised goals they were set out to achieve'. Usually it is found that more people are employed rather than fewer, and there are also costs to do with redundancy pay of those who are not found jobs in the new environment. The main cost however is in the effect on the people working in the service, who find that they have to reapply for their jobs every few years, and even if they get new jobs they may be working at different tasks and not using the expertise that they have built up previously. Projects get suddenly dumped, and work plans are derailed. Politics runs all and morale sinks very low.

I have witnessed two such reorganisations recently: the abolition of local health groups in Wales in 2004, and the abolition of their successors, Local Health Boards in 2009. In both cases talented people were ejected from the system and promotion seemed not to follow ability in the job but was related to your ability in networking around making yourself conspicuous. Nevertheless, some people who were never any good at their jobs seemed to manage to hold on by their fingertips. In the other direction one excellent senior manager spent several years working very hard at establishing active commissioning groups, only to be told after a change of (Welsh) government that commissioning was a dirty word, and the changes she had worked so hard on would not happen. She was completely demoralized and left the NHS early. If she had been working in England of course she would have done well! Politics trumps everything in the NHS.

During a reorganisation, very little work is done as all people can talk about is what jobs are likely to come up and who is on line to get them. I can't emphasise enough how disrupting this is. The raison d'être of management, in a system where the price paid by the consumer is not the driver of change, is to decommission ineffective services and introduce new ones. In fact that does not happen for a while before reorganisation nor for two years after it, as the expertise in the various areas is lost and people take time to work out what is going on.

In any case in my time in management, the only period in which there were new developments was when new money came along. Often managers would get very little warning that the money was coming and then were left scrabbling to cobble up a new service to 'bid' for the new money. There was never any time for detailed planning, and so new services then sprung up without adequate research into whether they were needed or not. To be fair, organisations did try to work up likely projects in anticipation of money coming along, but there were always restrictions on what you could do with the money so you could never put a bid up for something you had really researched thoroughly. When money was available in hospitals, specialist teams would develop new services, automatically assuming that the new service would be used and the service would 'grow', but it did not always do that. Old out of date services are never dropped, as that is the difficult part. The old service might be creaking and inefficient, but people are used to it and unaware of how much things could be made more efficient, and the benefit to patients of 'efficiency' is usually unclear as it actually means spending less money, and so people campaign against the changes. Also the providers of the old service have to be moved and, if efficiency is to be improved, need to lose their jobs and the staff certainly don't like that. Then, by the time austerity comes along (as it always does), the people who understand the system have moved on and cuts are then usually made entirely on cost and convenience, i.e. the least resistance from staff and consumer groups, not on efficiency and evidence.

Saving money – looking at the bureaucracy of the NHS

From the point of view of most GPs and many hospital doctors, managers are employed to do very little constructive work. This is because the front line of clinical care goes on regardless of any management changes and reorganisation. What most managers do rarely impacts on a doctor's working life. The adminis-trators who run GP contracts and pay the hospital bills are essential of course, but that is 'pay and rations', not changes in working practice. However to think that managers are useless is a damaging misconception. When change is managed successfully it can improve patient care immeasurably. However it is not easy to do. Managers can work on making changes for years but very little happens. Very few of the advances that people were planning when I was working have come to fruition since I left and new people continue to work away at the same problems, and come up against the same barriers – and then are reorganised out of sight. That of course is particularly true of Wales as few of the latest innovations have come that way, and in England there has been too much change.

Politicians know that it can be a very popular strategy to mock the increasing bureaucracy and escalation of administrators, managers and non-clinical staff in the NHS. Indeed one of the aims of each successive health reform is always to reduce the number of managers. But according to the Kings Fund report of 2011,[165] this is unlikely to come true. Historically, because there has been no need to bill patients, get the money, chase debts, or reimburse patients after they had paid, and the procurement process was kept lean, the proportion of managers and administrative staff in the NHS was a fraction of that in other countries. Until 2002, that is, when payment by results came in in England. This was, and still is, a system whereby hospitals are paid by activity, particularly for the 'elective' procedures: those, usually surgical, activities for which there had been long waiting times – hip operations, cataracts and so on – and the point of it is that hospitals are encouraged to increase throughput of such operations. The more operations a hospital does, the more money it gets. Despite the costs of billing and itemising this process it is said to be very successful and hospitals do indeed do far more work, certainly when money was being poured into the system. It is also very good at reducing lengths of stay in hospital and encouraging more day cases – all things that benefit both the patient and the system as a whole. However now that saving money and making sure that every operation is absolutely cost effective are established priorities, the system may well need a bit of tweaking. Money should follow quality of care and the success of the outcome for the patient. The new Commissioning Boards will find it a challenge to do this, when the system up to now has just been to reward the activity only.

Despite the recent rise in management costs due to this system of payment by results, the Kings Fund said that if anything the NHS was under-managed, and better management would increase efficiency.[166] Most of the increasing costs in the organisations I worked in were directly due to demands from above: the need to supervise and manage improvements in quality and implement targets. Each new initiative from above required new work but it was hardly ever possible to reorganise the work so that somebody could stop doing the work they were previously doing to take it on. The rules and directives from above were always too rigid. New staff were always employed, especially when the overall pot was getting bigger.

But there was often a problem with people spending their time on useless work, time-consuming meetings where nothing was decided, people going off at a tangent to do work that had already been done before without success. Another problem was it was almost impossible to sack anybody, for whatever reason, whether because their skills were not needed or because they were not up to the job. In Wales jobs were totally protected and redundancies forbidden, even during a reorganisation. This meant that when budgets were static or cut, very few new people could be employed, thus depriving the organisations of new talent. However, it was in England that the rise in administrators and managers was greatest, due to the system being micromanaged with so many targets, and the health reforms are likely to make things worse. Experienced people have already left the NHS, but overall the cost of managers is likely to rise not fall.

The terms and conditions of all workers in the NHS, medical, nursing, and all others, are good. Pensions in the past have been very generous and of course reducing them is a prime way of saving money. There is not much the unions can do about it in these times of austerity, but the effect on morale is likely to be large. Sick pay is still very generous – it is not unheard of for someone to have eighteen months off work after a family tragedy, and then to come back managing to do only three days work a week, for full-time pay, for two years. This would be unheard of in the private sector. Undoubtedly therefore there are inefficiencies in the system, but it is unlikely that huge savings are ever going to be made because management of change in any organisation is difficult and needs excellent leadership and motivated people. It is very important to keep talented people in the NHS.

There was a big push to get Social Services and Health to consult with one another to develop joint services, as we knew that, for instance, poor planning and lack of appropriate services in the community often delay discharge from hospital. This is a problem that really must be tackled and most Health Economists recommend doing it, and our organisations tackled it enthusiastically. But we did not get very far. The difference between cultures in the two organisations is just too wide. The public elect their representatives in local government and don't in healthcare. Social care is means tested, health care is not, the budgets are quite separate and the temptation for each to push services on to the other, rather than work together, is irresistible when budgets are tight. As I have mentioned before, the social service chief in one area did not support care homes, which therefore were not developed. Yes, he had an ideology that everyone had to have a front door – in other words had to have privacy and be in their own home – and this is a perfectly reasonable argument. But it may also have been because care homes are a direct cost to Social Services budgets but not to the Health budget, and the effect of this was higher costs for the health service in unplanned hospitalization. Joining these services up is all very difficult to do, and if we were to do it we wouldn't start from here (as they say).

When I started as a medical manager the main focus of managerial effort was in designing and building a spanking new hospital with state-of-the-art facilities. One of the main considerations was first to decide whether it was actually needed (an alternative would have been to further develop the facilities we already had), but this stage was quickly bypassed in favour of detailed planning of exactly the number and types of real and virtual beds that would be available. They had not even agreed on a site, due to competing political interests, by the time the inevitable plug was pulled due to lack of money. But the amount of time wasted by senior doctors and managers, and money spent on advisory firms, was phenomenal.

About that time I happened to meet a long retired consultant in general medicine, whom I knew very well, and I enthused to her about what wonders were in store for us. She looks at me quizzically and said 'do you know, when I first came for interview to this area, they said, "you are coming at a very exciting time. We are just about to start to build a new and very up to date hospital and we will be in the leading edge of work in your speciality." That was 40 years ago!' Things don't change quickly! Of course, the way that new hospital could have been built was by a PFI scheme, but Wales had turned its back on PFI. The result would have been a brand new state-of-the-art hospital and a huge unsustainable debt for the next thirty years, which could have bankrupted the hospital and the local community, as has happened in England recently. One wonders why new hospitals could not have been built using money borrowed by the Government, which was the way it used to be done. The Government could borrow more cheaply than anyone else. I think it was because the debt would be added to the Public Sector Borrowing Requirement. Now we are in austerity, this way is not going to be open to us, but in the years when NHS money was increasing it would to me have been a lot more sensible.

Nearly all the managers I worked with were committed people, who really cared about the Health Service. The debate about whether the NHS is under- or over-managed goes on year after year, but my perspective was that leadership was rare, and a lot of very useless work went on. It is certainly true that, as business leaders are keen to point out, that if you ran a business like that it would go bust. But health care is not a business in the usual sense, and business skills are not always as useful. The need is to develop services to a model that promotes effectiveness at ground level and then to work up to the more complicated secondary and tertiary services. This need is recognised time and time again, but it conflicts with the power of those in top positions in medicine and medical management who have a world view that specialised treatments and exciting new developments should be their priority. There is also a problem with the political class having ever-changing views on what would be best.

Market forces and patient choice

So each successive group of politicians has its own idea of what constitutes an effective health service. The main differentiating views are between, on the one hand, those who believe a health service should actively strive to reduce health inequalities, and develop new services and treatments everywhere as fairly as possible, and on the other hand those who believe that market forces are the only ones likely to bring about cutting-edge treatments, and that allowing free rein will ultimately benefit every one, including the disadvantaged, by a trickle-down mechanism. Other fault lines underlie the tensions between localism and centralism, with the issue of accountability to the tax-paying public, and also the argument between those who would keep health separate and those who would want to join it with social care, as the two issues can be very closely intertwined.

Most GPs I talk to agree that reducing health inequality is a very important aim. Once a patient, a man in his early thirties, accused me of not giving him enough attention, and said he thought he would have got more treatment if he had been wealthy. 'You doctors always favour the middle classes', he said. I had not given him a prescription for a drug he thought he needed, and it had never crossed my mind that anyone would have thought I had one rule for the well off and another for ordinary folk. When I thought about it, it seemed to me that it usually went the other way, as experience had taught me that the poorer people were, the more likely they were to have unmet health needs, and so they tended to get more in terms of prescriptions and other treatments. If there was any doubt about whether antibiotics were to be given for a chest infection, I had two rules, that if

419

a patient smoked or if they lived in poor social conditions they were more likely to get antibiotics. And in many other situations GPs are often more inclined to be proactive with people with fewer advantages. The man was too angry to argue with although I would have liked to assure him that it wasn't the case.

On a population level though the inverse health care law still applies. It was first described by Julian Tudor Hart, a GP in South Wales in 1971, and says 'The availability of good medical care tends to vary inversely with the needs of the population served'.[167] You can see how this will definitely be the case where market forces are involved, as in the USA and private medicine within the UK – better health care is what you pay for. With universal health coverage though as in the UK, the expectation was that everyone would get the same level of care regardless of income level and it was a surprise when paper after paper since 2000 showed that it is not so.[168] Reasons include NHS GPs and hospitals giving a poorer level of service to deprived groups, usually because such areas are not as attractive to the most ambitious and innovative clinicians, and also reasons rooted in the population they serve, such as unwillingness to visit doctors or take up offers of vaccinations, and similar issues, which usually derive from ignorance or lack of understanding of the benefits. This is now called 'low health literacy' and we are recognising how important it is. Conversely the well-educated may actively seek out treatment for less serious ailments when they are available, and may indeed be fooled into getting treatments they may not need or that may even harm them.

So how can any health system get it right? To me a health system should try to get the best evidence-based treatment, and only that treatment, to as many people as possible who would benefit from it. And that may mean restricting market forces within a publicly funded service wherever they tend to work towards experimental high cost treatments for the few at the expense of more routine care for the many. Where market forces can be harnessed in an equitable way of course they should be used, as it is getting the balance right that is the problem. It is exactly like privatisation of the railways and post office. There are gains and losses with both systems.

But this is still only a part of what medicine is. The other factor in the equation is 'patient choice' and we have been trying to go down this path for some time now, with mixed results. There is no doubt that medicine is much more than evidence-based medicine, and a patient's views about her care are crucial to deciding on the best course of action. The patient should be at least an equal party to decisions about her care. Compassion and empathy are integral to medicine, however evidence-based it may be. Choice must be informed choice but if it is that, it has to be respected and built into the system.

However I was told recently in a lecture that patient satisfaction is positively correlated with mortality. I think that means that satisfied patients have a higher death rate, so patient satisfaction with treatment does not necessarily mean they are getting effective treatment! I really don't know if that can be true, but we do know that patients may be very satisfied with unnecessary or even frankly bad care, which actually harms them and may even kill them, provided it is delivered in an empathetic and caring manner. (Think about Dr Shipman again!). Conversely they might be very dissatisfied when they don't get what they want even if the chances are that it would harm them.

So the patient needs to be aware of the evidence base behind the decision to go for treatment, and also know how good the person giving the treatment is at his job. In many countries and certainly the UK and US, governments are passing legislation to allow patients to see league tables of how well hospitals surgeons and GPs perform and this is very much to be welcomed provided the data is presented in a fair manner, taking into account case mix for instance so the doctors and hospital dealing with the iller patients aren't disadvantaged.

Rather than 'pure' patient choice or 'pure' evidence, there has to be a balance and that balance can be mediated by a drive towards patient-centred care – 'no decision about me without me'. Harnessing the power of the patient to contribute to her own care will also immeasurably improve both the health experience and its outcome.

Care commissioning

Back to the organisation of services then, the philosophy of the commissioners tends to influence which services to 'commission'. Originally at the beginning of the NHS, the decisions on what service to develop and which to discard were in the hands of clinicians – usually senior doctors in the hospitals. There were so called 'cogwheel' divisions within each hospital where doctors would discuss where the money should be spent. Not surprisingly, most of the money went to operating theatres and surgeons and the big medical specialities, and very little to mental health and other 'lowly' specialities. Community care, along with the GP service, did not get very much at all out of the pie until after the contract of 1964. Commissioning care for populations remained much the same for many years after that, with very few people in the NHS having much expertise in deciding where the money should be spent. Anyway there was never very much of it, and the UK rapidly fell behind other countries in spending per GDP, and that was a political decision by successive governments. It was not until 1994 that a new idea was first tried out – to give more power to commission, not to the expensive end, the hospitals, but to the cheaper and to some people the more productive area – to primary care which accounted for over 90% of the actual care given. So GP fundholding was born, with hospital specialists and their departments being financed in part according to GP fundholders' specifications.

Fundholding by groups of GPs, which was around in the early nineties, did indeed commission care, and some fundholding practices and groups were very successful, improving care for patients by wrenching some services from local hospitals and providing new models of care. It was however very unfair, with the patients of those practices which could not commission adequately (because they were too small or did not have the skills or interest required) lost out, but that wasn't why it was stopped. It was stopped fundamentally because it could be too successful and local hospitals could be destabilized in a very destructive way. It was also quite expensive and many GPs did very well out of it personally by using some of the money to build large surgeries which they then owned, and were able to rent to the NHS at a much bigger cost to the public purse. Usually these premises were needed, but sometimes they were white elephants. I saw a surgery recently where a whole suite of rooms, almost a third of the total area of the surgery (which had been built with fundholding savings) were left stripped and unused because the ancillary services that had been expected to relocate there never came. Yet the NHS can be left paying rent for these unused rooms in perpetuity.

But fundholding succeeded only where there was new money to spend, and there was no doubt that that was where the small amount available at the time went. An example of a much better service introduced via fundholding was a day case cataract service locally in 1995. At that time everyone who had cataracts removed stayed in hospital at least one night, even though for some years the anaesthetics

side of eye surgery had progressed to the extent that most people were operated on when awake and recovery was pretty quick. But attempts at changing the
system had got nowhere, so GPs and consultants set up a new day case service
with fundholding money. It was an instant success: patients preferred it, the long
waiting list was bypassed, and of course it was a lot cheaper. However it was only
available to patients of fundholding practices and there was a dreadful situation
locally where a person whose practice was not a fundholder had to wait a year
and have a night in a hospital a long way away to have his cataracts done, and his
neighbour in the same street, whose practice was fundholding, had hers done
within two weeks at the local hospital as a day case. When we tried to get access
to this service for patients of non-fundholding practices, we came up against the
problem that it would cost extra money (£17,000 as I remember!) and this was
just not available to the rest of the NHS in that area which was already overspent,
as it was every year.

The good side of this was that when fundholding died the service was reorganised so that day case cataract operations could happen in local hospitals. When
you think about it, cataracts have been operated on for decades in the third world
in field hospitals by charities, so it really shouldn't have been so difficult to do in
the UK, but this case highlighted the inertia built into the system and the lack of
power of GPs.

Fundholding showed that some GPs are very good at seeing what services their
patients need, and can negotiate very well. The scheme which followed fundholding was called practice-based commissioning (PBC) and again some GPs
grouped together to make improvements. Practice-based commissioning has
been defined as

> A continual process of analysing the needs of a community, designing
> pathways of care, then specifying and procuring services that will deliver
> and improve agreed health and social outcomes, within the resources
> available.[169]

It was introduced to try and achieve greater clinical engagement and ownership of commissioning, but all too often the work was neither practice-based
nor related to commissioning. Excellent results were achieved in some parts of
the country, but in many others, it has so far had little or no impact. Most health

economists want to see clinicians being involved in developing services as they appreciate their directness and knowledge of the working of service configuration, but it is hard to do. Many clinicians have no time for the circumlocution of management systems and everybody, managers included (with the possible exception of some Directors of Finance), get completely tied up in knots with the cumbersome rules of how things are paid for and accounted for in the NHS. Doctors usually go into medicine to do 'doctoring' rather than management, and there are only a few with the interest to get involved. I could certainly see why they don't want to. We had clinical meeting after clinical meeting which were supposed to develop pathways of care and hardly any GPs would come, and those that did often found themselves out on a limb. Consultants came a bit more often because they now have periods timetabled into their job plans to do such things (GPs have to find and pay a locum and the money is reimbursed afterwards) but it was hard going to keep clinicians interested.

The amount of money GPs control by being able to refer to hospital is huge. Keeping a brake on the number of referrals to hospital is something that many countries are looking at, not only in the UK. In Norway it is a big issue, and in the Netherlands some Dutch GPs told me that they have just had an agreement with the Government that they will voluntarily accept a cap on referrals with the possibility that they will be fined if they go over the limit. They were quite worried about what they would do when their quota ran out. In the UK commissioning groups are 'managing referrals' and re-directing them elsewhere. In at least one area, GPs are having to make savings (of £155,000) by reducing their referrals by 10% under management plans to redirect referrals through referral management centres.

While GPs get quite angry about this at times, one can see the problem. If referrals to hospital remained steady until there is a new treatment or operation that has just come on stream, then the system could cope. But that is not the case. In some specialities referrals seem to keep on rising. This is understandable where there are really new treatments available, such as for macular degeneration of the eye, which I discussed in Chapter 25, and innovative uses of monoclonal antibody drugs, originally developed for arthritis. But in other cases where there haven't been such new developments, there must have been an increase in patient perception of need, such as the availability of earlier treatment for joint replacements, and we have no way of measuring this. And yes, the population is getting older and this will drive more referrals as they get more long-term illnesses. But from our figures noted earlier this may well be offset by a reduction in the demography of people in their 40s and 50s, who were the major group being referred in several specialities.

We collected data on those patients who were only referred because the doctor felt the patient would not be satisfied unless they did get referred, and the doctor did not see a need to refer the patient. Over the short time we looked at our data, this stayed constant throughout the year, although it varied slightly from practice to practice. So it is unlikely, in our area at least, that patients are demanding more unnecessary referrals.

What has increased demand from patients is the legitimate wish of a more educated public to access treatment which is advertised and for which they perceive a need. This is probably the source of much of the increase seen in the last few years. While some of this demand is good, I believe there is a lot of media hype which can only be counteracted by more knowledge of the evidence base behind the treatments – for both patients and GPs. The more access the patient has to good quality evidence the better. Also to get consultants and GPs talking together, and working towards developing more local services would be really helpful. GPs and consultants do not always agree but the dialogue is always useful. For GPs there is now a slightly better way of encouraging them to spend time out of the practice in that they can be rewarded by the Quality and Outcomes Framework (QOF) for attending such meetings to discuss referrals and other activities. Meetings dealing with incentive schemes in prescribing to use the most cost-effective, usually generic, drug instead of the most expensive branded drug have worked quite well. In the USA at the moment there is a big push to do this as their prescribing costs are the highest in the world, and it is amazing that they have never done it before. Such schemes include switching from expensive to more cost-effective medications or reviewing how patients obtain blood-glucose testing strips, which cost a huge amount if overused.

But again the problems for GPs attending the meetings are that locums don't do all the work that they themselves do, and patients may find the practice very short-handed, with long waits in surgery, if too many doctors are away doing such things at the same time.

So now we enter a new era, with GPs commissioning care, however unwillingly, and many services offered up to private contractors in England. How will this work? The process of reorganisation will take many more months and it is unclear whether every group of GPs will be able to commission care. Such commissioning will take even more GPs out of their practices. We need to look at exactly what difference it is likely to make.

Chapter 37
The Health and Social Care Bill 2012

Possible effects of the health and social care bill – costs of private provision and market forces – moral hazard – managing change – conflict of interest – universality of treatment – rationing – funding by age rather than deprivation – public health – democratic mandate

In the most recent attempt to change everything, the Health and Social Care Bill 2012, commissioning by GPs became centre stage and a recent book has outlined the power struggles behind the scenes between the political parties that has made it into such a hugely complex and sometimes self-contradictory piece of legislation.[170] One can argue at length as to whether it will free up the system as GP fundholding did in the nineties, albeit rather expensively and patchily, but this time produce a much more cost-effective system away from existing vested interests; or whether it will achieve what most medical staff fear it will achieve – a patchwork of private, possibly more malign, vested interests, and produce so many contradictions that it is no longer able to act as a coherent whole. The example of the NHS equipment report which I wrote about in Chapter 21, which refers to a future lack of any planning in the provision of high-cost radiology equipment,[171] is an example of this fear. Only time will tell.

It has to be said that if handing power to GPs was the aim, there was no need for a new bill. The framework was already there to build on practice-based commissioning as detailed in Chapter 36. The tearing down of PCTs and the building of Commissioning Groups was a stage further, and now we have an NHS Commissioning Board whose task is to oversee them. They have legal responsibilities, which at least should prevent politicians getting involved in day-to-day operations, and no-one would think this is a bad thing.

The main head of discontent was the decisions that everything should be under scrutiny in order to bring in market forces – new private companies to replace hospitals, GP practices and community care services like health visiting. Now of course there is some self-interest at work here, as GP practices and GP livelihoods may be threatened by new companies coming in and winning tenders for patient services, which GPs obviously aren't going to vote for. Similarly consultants are now threatened on two fronts, by the emerging threat from GPs on these new commissioning groups and also by some of their work being offloaded to private companies. So not all the opposition was entirely impartial.

But, as we saw in Chapter 34, there were two recent scares that showed the real dangers of private companies operating within the current NHS system. The case of the PPI implants problem, where when the company concerned went bankrupt, the NHS was left picking up the tab for removing implants in patients who had had them fitted privately, highlighted the fact that the costs of anything going wrong in the private sector will probably have to be picked up by the NHS. It was clear from the coverage of this case that many private companies do not buy insurance precisely because they think that NHS will do that. The second case was of the psychiatric hospital that had to be closed because bad financial decisions by the company had led directly to cost-cutting and extremely poor care for patients. These cases made it clear to everybody that, up to then, private companies weren't being nearly well regulated enough and that this would have to change with more bodies being set up and more bureaucracy to safeguard patients interests, at a further cost to the public purse.

A main concern is the timing of this bill; right in the middle of the biggest austerity problem we have had in the last 50 years. Almost any reform can be made to work if you can spend enough money. The main problem with Health Service management in the past has been managing change so that new services are brought in but without destabilsing the old ones. Purely hypothetically, under the old system if you wanted to transfer podiatry services, including operations like bunions, to other professionals such as podiatric surgeons, managers first needed to pump-prime the service; that is, spend extra money on setting the service up outside hospital, training more podiatrists to a higher level, getting new ancillary staff and so on. Only then when it is running successfully and the patients have been transferred can you either disinvest in your orthopaedic department by reducing operating capacity, or transferring the capacity to other orthopaedic work (of which there is plenty), and redeploying hospital podiatrists to work in the new centres. Even just writing this down now leads one to see the difficulties. Orthopaedic surgeons would need to oversee this process to ensure patient safety and some of them are not going to want to. The savings can be considerable when the process is complete but that could take years. That is why it tends not to happen, but with full cooperation between all health professionals the new scheme would have the benefit of all the infrastructure of the NHS.

Under the new system theoretically you could ask a private company or other group which is bidding for the service to set up a competing service outside hospital, and they would give you a price. But it would cost a lot of money that the private sector would have to bear, including the risk that it would fail and the owners would lose their money. They would need to cover themselves to ensure patient safety, employing orthopaedic specialists to oversee it. Therefore they would want a high price to do it, and historically companies like this such as those running DTCs have had to have highly advantageous contracts in order to 'bite'. So in a situation which every penny counts and huge savings have to be made right now, GPs and managers on commissioning groups may reason that they cannot afford the short-term higher costs to save money later on. A much more likely scenario is that any existing local services will be cut instead. The objective of making a health service more local and more cost-effective will be lost. Spending money now to save money later is something that should be done well with a planning structure, but often isn't because of the byzantine nature of the NHS financial system. But either way if changes like this were to be made they should be done in times of plenty not austerity.

Other problems involve conflicts of interest. False Economy, a TUC research group, found that 22 Commissioning Groups have GPs with an external financial interest in a private company such as Virgin Health,[172] and these individuals could profit from commissioning services in companies running operations such as nursing services and other community services. One provider informed the TUC that there were robust methods to prevent this being a problem, but it is essential that such GPs, and all members of Commissioning Groups, have to declare all relevant interests. At the very least it means that GPs on these groups are hardly your typical GP. Politicians themselves can hardly be said to be disinterested either. A research group has noted that there are 62 Conservative Lords out of a total of 217 peers who have interests in the private healthcare industry.[173] Yet they have voted on the Bill in its passage through the Lords.

There are numerous other concerns that have been raised, and some addressed as the bill was going through Parliament, having the effect of making the Bill almost unbelievably complicated. It has been said that there will have to be yet another reorganisation in the next five years to undo all the mistakes that have been made.

So what are the main risks and consequences of the new bill? Unfortunately the Government refused to publish the risk analysis they themselves commissioned, and this certainly raises suspicion that they were hiding something. One has to conclude that a major result will be to diminish the universality of treatment to allow costs to be reduced. One might say that this is essential as a big problem for the NHS at the moment is that if a patient demands a treatment that has some validity it is difficult legally to deny it. Rationing has always been not only frowned upon in the NHS but also extremely difficult to enforce. The difficulty with enforcement of the 'Not Normally Treated' list is a case in point. I think with the new system the waters will be so muddied, with some people in one area getting a treatment that has been commissioned and people in another area not getting it, that rationing will happen automatically. Commissioners strapped for cash will see other areas quietly dropping treatments and drugs and do the same. Rationing will come upon us *de facto*. One might say that this is essential. For at least the foreseeable future, even in the developed world there is not going to be enough money to allow every treatment to be available in a timely manner for everyone. It also can be pointed out that at the moment the quality of care and outcomes for patients vary considerably from area to area. But previously there was a rationale behind healthcare in the UK which emphasises preventative care and health of populations rather than individual care, and this is at risk, especially with the changes to the public health service in England under the Act, which mean that it is aligned with local authorities instead of the NHS.[174] The Bill definitely seems to allow charging for some services which formerly were free.[175] For instance, some vaccinations will now be excluded from the list of things the Health Service is contracted to procure.

It also throws up many difficulties with temporary residents between England and the devolved nations being excluded. For instance, if you live in Scotland but are staying in England, it may be that the practice near you is part of a commissioning group that refuses to treat you except in an emergency.

These fears seem to be justified when you read that the funding mechanism which in the past has been skewed so that poorer areas are compensated with a bigger share of resources may be changed so that by some calculations, the North East will lose a considerable amount of funding so that there will be more spent on the rich South East. This hasn't happened yet but the very fact that it can be a proposal means that it is clear where we are heading. In addition it seems clear that Commissioning Groups don't necessarily start off on a level playing field, as practices can be, and are being, excluded from a group if they serve a needy population for which it would be disproportionately expensive to commission care. Commissioning Care Groups with practices in very deprived areas will have less money to buy services. The winners will be rich areas where new services can quickly be set up, and these will further disadvantage the others in relative terms.

Yet in another way the Government is planning changes to the GP contract that would have the opposite effect. As mentioned earlier, the GP contract is a contract for services, not for employment, and it is re-negotiated every year by the Department of Health, represented by civil servants, and the BMA, the biggest of the doctors' trades unions. It gets very little publicity because quite frankly it is usually incomprehensible, and this year's discussions are worse than usual in this regard. However what is going on in these discussions shows the way in which services are going to change.

Firstly the government has doctors in their sights in their quest to save a lot of money. There seems to be a feeling that the BMA and the doctors 'won' in 2004, and public sympathy is no longer on the side of the doctors, so they can ignore special pleading by doctors especially on pensions. The government now wants to make big changes to the GP contract that would change the way deprivation and other factors are taken into account, which the doctors are resisting because it will allow private companies to more easily take over GP practices. The government has some arguments on its side and theoretically at least it should take deprivation in the areas GPs work in into account.

The GP contract was originally a capitation-based system whereby a GP received a certain amount of money per patient, thus making sure that GPs have to attract patients to stay in business. All well and good, but in 2004 many other changes were made to the system, to try to make it fairer, using a formula, the 'Car–Hill' formula to reflect practice workload, such as the number of elderly, and number of patients with long-term illnesses. For some reason this would have meant that some practices would have lost out to such an extent that they would have gone out of business. Therefore the government added an extra sum of money called the 'MPIG', (Minimum Practice Income Guarantee) to the 'global sum', the total amount GP's receive in order to provide services to patients. Now the government wants to get rid of this extra money by adding money to the total pool and taking away the MPIG. (I am sure I have lost you already.)

The point is that the GPs who make the most money are those in large practices, and smaller practices often struggle to make a living, even though these are usually the ones patients prefer. In the past the government would have tried hard not to let these practices go out of business, but now with the ethos of market principles coming in, there seems to be a feeling that this would be a good way of ensuring that private providers can more easily enter primary care. So the government seems to be banking on being able to destabilize local practices by altering the terms of the GPs contract from 2013. At the time of writing negotiations have broken down, and the government is saying it will impose a contract as it did in 1990, and the result may be not a fairer way of remunerating GPs, but a wholesale change of ownership of practices.

So is this a good way to go? Are GPs the best people to run local practices or would it be done more efficiently by big corporations? There have certainly been lots of complaints from patients at surgeries which no longer have regular GPs who are totally committed to the practice because they have a financial stake in them (which was the case under the old system), that they can no longer see a GP but see other members of the primary care team instead, because the company is saving money. Is this a good thing? Nurse Practitioners are in my experience extremely effective in many ways and can certainly see many of the sorts of problems that GPs used to deal with. However if they do not have good backing from GPs then they are very likely to refer more patients to the hospital which would the defeat the object of making services more effective.

Most doctors are still opposed to the changes and it has to be said there is pessimism and fear for the future. Those that are actively and enthusiastically embracing the changes are few and far between. One estimate recently was that there are only 25 GPs really totally committed to commissioning in the whole country, though there are many who are going to try their best to work the new system to patients' advantage if they possibly can. The difficulties of mandating GPs to run these changes have been spelled out throughout this book. Hospital doctors too have not supported the changes.

I predict that the sorts of treatments that will not be commissioned will be the treatments within the Cinderella specialities. For instance, now that there is evidence that 'talking treatments' (cognitive behaviour therapy, and psychotherapy) for depression and anxiety actually work and NICE has approved them, one would think that they would become more available, but I think this is unlikely to happen. The market principle will make sure that the power bases behind expensive technologies will ensure that they will still get funded, but the more local services will dry up. So no change there then. We will soon be in a similar situation to the USA where preventative medicine and community care are down graded, with an increase in inequality.

One does wonder about the democratic mandate for all these changes. The election promise was to 'keep the NHS safe' and 'no more re-organisation' and this is what people voted for. It was really a remarkable feat to get the changes through Parliament despite the objections. I personally believe the only reason they did manage to pass the Bill was because at bottom no one understands it, and the many risks have not been clearly spelled out.

It is clear that this is an ideologically driven reform, with the belief that introducing private companies into the NHS will reduce inefficiencies and increase innovation, along market principles. As with other privatized industries such as the railways, and energy and water companies the devil is in the detailed regulation of these industries. One thing is certain though and that is that healthcare will still be in the news and the problems that emerge will be well publicised.

Chapter 38
Health spending

Comparison of health spending between countries – effect of austerity – importance of GPs.

The latest reform in England is now complete. But money is likely to be very scarce for years to come, and we are living longer, with all the associated degenerative diseases that come with old age. Some of us also have very unhealthy lifestyles. So how will the NHS cope?

All countries are now facing a crisis in health care delivery. In most developed countries there has been a year on year increase in spending overall, including the UK, of nearly 5% per year in real terms. In the UK over the period 2000-2009, expenditure on health services increased by a third (32 per cent) from £82.9 billion in 2004–05 to £110.0 billion in 2008–09. In 2010, health spending as a share of GDP remained by far the highest in the United States (17.9% of GDP), followed by the Netherlands (12%), France and Germany (11.9%). and Austria 11.2%.[176] The UK spent 9.8%, a larger percentage than Australia, (9.74) and Spain (9.51), Norway (9.5) and Greece, (9.06). This means that UK spending is now just above the average of OECD countries. In many ways the UK has always had an efficient service with low administrative costs, because historically at least the costs of billing for services were very low, and so if this level of spending is maintained we should be able to keep standards up, and quality high. The lowest shares of national income devoted to health are in Mexico (6.2%) and Turkey (6.1%). In Japan, the share of spending allocated to health has increased substantially in recent years to 9.5%, up from 7.6% in 2000, and is now equal to the OECD average. Japanese have the highest life expectancy of all OECD countries, although the extent to which the figures are influenced by the widespread practice of not registering deaths in country areas – to continue drawing benefits – is questionable!

In 2010 when the financial crisis started to bite in the Americas and Europe, growth in health spending slowed, and then, in those countries hardest hit by the crisis, fell quite dramatically.[177] Overall there has been a fall of 0.5% in public spending for health, but in Ireland, Iceland and Greece it has fallen by 6% or more, in 2011. This may be an underestimate. Many of the family doctors I met at the conference in 2012 were noticing the effects, and as usual it was the waiting time to see a specialist that most GPs complained of. Doctors from Spain and Portugal particularly were talking about a marked deterioration, with patients just not getting the care they needed. Doctors from Greece told us that there was a marked increase in doctors charging patients and getting 'kickbacks' for care that the patients previously would, and should, have got for free. We all thought this was a very unacceptable practice, especially as it appears that doctors in Greece have never paid anything like what they should have paid in tax. Many people are now uninsured in these countries and many are not getting even basic essential medical care.

None of the doctors I met said that their pay had been cut, (although of course, as most delegates there had to pay at least part of their conference costs themselves, this was not very surprising), but, from OECD figures, in Ireland for example most of the reductions have been achieved through cuts in wages or the fees paid to professionals and pharmaceutical companies, and through actual reductions in the number of health workers. This is probably why a GP from Ireland told me that doctors there are trying desperately to hang on to their private patients by giving them exactly what they ask for regardless of evidence or even efficiency. (This is a warning for those doctors in the UK who respond to threats of lowering their pay by saying that they will leave the system and go to work in the private system). Ireland also increased the share of direct payments by households for prescribed medicines and appliances and efficiencies have also been made through mergers of hospitals or ministries, or accelerating the move from inpatient hospitalisation towards out-patient care and day surgery, as is happening in many other countries.

Even in the USA where increases in health spending seem to be set in stone, there has been an increase of only 3% last year. It is well known that the USA spends an inordinate amount of money on healthcare and yet is still amongst the lowest in such overall indices of health such as infant mortality. The U.S. rate, at 6.5 deaths per 1000 live births, is well above the OECD average of 4. There money counts; if you have it you can access the very best of modern healthcare (including a lot you may not really need) and if you don't have money your health will suffer. There is therefore a crisis of both overtreatment and undertreatment. For people without insurance, the system will tend towards denying them treatment that would definitely improve their health; for people with good health insurance, the tendency is to give them treatment they may not need. The money saved from not doing the latter could undoubtedly help fund the treatment of those without the means to pay for it, and would also help to counteract the feeling that treatment is being denied solely on cost grounds.

Oddly enough there are fewer physicians in the USA per capita than in most other OECD countries (although word has it that they work much harder). In 2010, the US had 2.4 practising physicians per 1000 population, below the OECD average of 3.1. On the other hand, there were 11 nurses per 1000 population, a higher number than the average of 8.7 across OECD countries. The higher costs are partly due to the extra cost of all spending, possibly due to inadequate control of costs, for instance the 50 high-selling pharmaceuticals cost 60% more in the United States than in Europe. Medical workers do far more procedures and interventions than in most other countries. The average also hides huge difference in cost, efficiency, and quality in different health care organisations.

So one would think the USA in times of austerity would reduce its health care costs. However their new health act is likely to increase costs, not reduce them, and its obesity epidemic is one of the worst in the world. But it is possible that people in the United States think that publicly owned and operated health care is necessarily unresponsive to people's wishes and the staff are under-motivated. While this can indeed happen, it is far from being the general rule. Many OECD countries have efficient, well-financed, publicly-funded responsive health care systems, at much lower cost than in the United States. But because of this entrenched idea of many people in the USA, I have long since stopped trying to discuss health care with friends and family in the USA. Although many people complain about whatever health plan they have, and they are aware that they are paying more than people anywhere else in the world, they still support the system of self-funding. The political debate is so polarized and so heated that it seems many have been brainwashed by the persistent and sometimes exploitative market in health care. They deride so-called 'socialized medicine' without even trying to understand what, for instance, evidence-based medicine means.

Few other countries want to go even near their system of health care, although the English Health and Social Care Bill in 2012 seemed to want to emulate some of the most problematic aspects of the American system. But precisely because they have so many problems, they have a very well developed knowledge of health economics and the sorts of things that are essential to concentrate on. So this is what authorities in the USA recommended:[178] an emphasis on primary care, to ensure that most care takes place outside of (expensive) hospitals

- a system which encourages use of (cheaper) generic drugs, when there are alternatives to expensive brands
- tight regulations of prices and fees, for at least those services that are paid for by public programs
- adherence to clinical guidelines, so that excessive use of expensive diagnostics or unnecessary health care is prevented

– exactly what most European systems, including the UK, already do. So instead of the UK government trying to emulate the market-oriented system in the USA, it should be the other way around.

In many countries gains in efficiency have been pursued through mergers of hospitals or ministries, or accelerating the move from in-patient hospitalisation towards outpatient care and day surgery. The use of generic drugs has also been expanded in a number of countries.

We in the UK already have good systems in place to implement these essential pre-requisites of a fair and cost-effective health care system. We are in danger however of inadvertently copying some of the American attitudes with a misplaced belief in what the market can provide. There is also an increasing tendency for the media to sensationalise and promote questionable procedures and treatments. One thing the USA does do well though relates to patient-centredness and improving the patient experience, however, and we could take a leaf out of their book here. Private medicine does not necessarily guarantee a good experience for the patient, but I think there is probably a floor of rudeness and lack of due care beneath which a private physician or surgeon is just not going to have any patients coming to her. We can all improve on this aspect and often it doesn't even cost anything.

Changes over the years and in the future

So in conclusion I believe this is an excellent time to extend and improve upon primary care, using doctors, nurses, optometrists, physiotherapists and other professionals allied to medicine to increase the availability of simple procedures near to home, and to stick to the evidence base wherever possible. Any system that can make these changes will work, irrespective of the exact mechanism and structure of delivery, but it will need good leadership. Most of all though people will need more unbiased knowledge of what is really in their best interest, to keep themselves healthy and prevent disease wherever possible. I hope I have contributed to this in some small way.

Chapter 39
Round-up and the way forward

Problems of medicalisation and marketisation – importance of health literacy – consensual working versus competition – loss of universality of NHS – comparison of healthcare in devolved nations

For all its faults, the NHS remains a wonderful institution and I have been very happy and proud to work in it for so many years. It provided a very varied way of life. I mostly worked as a GP of course, but at different times also in child psychiatry, and as an anaesthetist for ECT. I trained GPs, started a female GPs' group, sat on medical service committees and hospital job recognition committees, and promoted the early stages of computer use in general practice. I introduced Clinical Governance, worked for the BMA locally, and after retirement I became a Medical Advisor to a Health Board.

It was all very stimulating even though I never had much influence in any of the jobs I did, and certainly never became a leader myself. I was always a foot soldier, and sometimes a bit of a nuisance. Not that that worried me unduly. As a GP you are protected by the fact that at bottom you are supported by your patients who will always be there, coming back to see you about their problems which were always more interesting than any in Health Service management. And my job was safe – I didn't have to worry about a career as so many in health management had to do, constantly. But it did enable me to see a wide variety of ways of working, the problems, the personalities, the waste, and the funding difficulties at first hand.

My view is therefore the snail's eye view, but with a big geographical coverage. None of the conclusions I have reached about the workings of a Health service are new and most are widespread, if not always accepted. The vision of people who really think and care about the Health Service is remarkably similar, and it is always the implementation that is difficult in a large and creaky organisation subject to meddling by politicians, constrained by a five-year term of office and the need to be re-elected.

So.

The latest reorganisation started from the premise that the Health Service in England had to be fixed because it could not go on as it was, due to funding difficulties, pace of developments and demographic change. No-one can disagree that there are difficulties ahead. The question is what change would make it work better? Would any organisational change make it better?

Well, fairly obviously I don't think so. The drivers of most of our problems in healthcare lie altogether outside the Health Service and in our society. The very success of modern society, in allowing us all to live longer, is to do with wealth and freedom from infection and malnutrition, and has raised expectations that good health is a right, not something that most of us need to do much to preserve, and when one gets a disease it can be fixed by someone else and if it isn't, it is probably someone else's fault.

I have tried to reiterate (as so many influential bodies do nowadays) the point that many of our problems lie in the realm of marketisation of our lifestyles, so that our food is governed by a food industry which has no remit to care about healthy living, only to make profits from selling foodstuffs which are attractive to as many people as possible. Therefore we are now eating foods high in sugar, in fat and in calories, and therein lies the cause of the epidemic of obesity and diabetes. Our physiology is not designed to cope with this. We have to take responsibility ourselves to keep ourselves healthy.

Marketisation also drives many of us to be medicalised towards taking drugs which may indeed help a very few of us live longer but at great cost, and which will definitely harm a few people as well. Procedures and operations are done routinely when there may have been simpler alternatives. The market runs our health system now – and always did to some latent extent; we don't have to wait for the latest reforms to allow it to act. Researchers are often not pure-driven seekers after the general good, but tools of companies needing to make a profit at any cost, and who work in a very competitive environment that can lead to research fraud. Any new initiative is going to come at a very high price and may not do any good. We already have good-enough tools with which to fix most of the health problems we have, and though new developments may be very exciting, they are only likely to benefit the few, or the very wealthy. Gene therapy, cloning, and everlasting life through stem cell technology and replacing body parts can't possibly be for all seven billion of us.

The British health service has always prided itself on its emphasis on equality in healthcare, so that the poorest in society can have at least a chance of the benefits that flow automatically to the better off. Most clinicians in the NHS believe in equality in a way that those in the US do not. Recently I was talking to an eminent professor in preventive medicine in Los Angeles (we were in the same group while walking in the Canaries), and we were talking about the dire situation there of California's inability to balance its budget. I asked, deferentially enough, about how the health service there was coping with so many people uninsured. And he said – 'Well, California wouldn't have a problem if it wasn't for all those illegal immigrants with health problems that the state has to look after [in the public hospitals].' I couldn't believe the gap in our thinking. Presumably these illegal immigrants were working (no benefits for them in the US) and presumably the economy needed them. But for him, their health needs were not the concern of his State. We are worlds apart in our aspirations for health care.

But that is the tenor of the system that is driving our health care system forward under the new reforms in England. Politicians from Margaret Thatcher to Tony Blair and now David Cameron have been eyeing the USA for years and trying to import some of the ideas coming from there. And of course some of the ideas on efficiency and effectiveness are very good indeed – the USA is home to the very best thinking in Health Economics, as well as to some very obvious blind spots like their outright opposition to universal coverage as being 'unconstitutional'.

Our society runs on the market principle, and we aren't going to alter that. But most clinicians do not see the market and a health service as being natural bedfellows. Apart from purely private health care, where the patient pays for each service out of his own pocket rather than through an insurance company, which is quite rare, there never is a real market, because the consumer is not choosing a good or a service by being able to compare one producer with another. The consumer generally does not have the knowledge or the perspective with which to make a reliable choice. Healthcare is or should be integrated so that each intervention ties in with others to make up a cost-effective whole, and while this is done directly by the NHS in the UK, in other European companies this is done by insurance companies. In the US there is an increasing tendency for insurance companies and health maintenance organisations to manage the system, even though it is run on private lines, as true freedom is just too costly, so that the consumer is always completely constrained by intermediaries. In this situation, consumers, many doctors, and of course politicians are also at the mercy of advertising, both directly by the lobbying and claims made by health business interests and indirectly by the media in the ways described throughout this book.

So the way forward in my view has to be a drive to improve the consumer's understanding of what works and what does not. I would look to improving health journalism first and foremost, but also to get a better focus from the scientific knowledge community. It would be good if people were to be inoculated against the claims and temptations of health industries, and to be reminded that most things get better on their own, that those that don't often can often be fixed with low-tech solutions and that doctors don't have the answer to everything. In doing that of course it is also necessary to press home the red flag symptoms that people really should worry about so that serious disease is treated early – in other words improving health literacy at every opportunity, and I have tried to do that in this book. This is where the gap between rich and poor gets so important, as it is likely that many more deaths can be prevented by educating the population and increasing health literacy than by future medical advances.

Medical education should be unbiased and avoid scaremongering. It really should avoid the sort of mindless statement that comes at the end of every bit of information that says 'consult a doctor if you are worried' even when the whole of the previous page has been devoted to telling you what to worry about and what not to worry about. This is done to cover their backs no doubt but it does tend to increase use of health professionals when such information should really enable people to get their own knowledge. Only with true understanding of the natural history of diseases can people be confident of their own health care needs. People with chronic diseases especially are being encouraged to be full partners in treating their illnesses and being experts in prevention of complications and side effects. And it needs to be recognised that turning a healthy 65 year old into a worried wreck by giving him the news that he is 'at risk' for so many diseases that he does not have, that he may never get, and that in only one in a hundred instances would he be saved from the disease if he took the recommended treatment, is not very helpful.

There should be much more active promotion of what evidence-based medicine is all about, more magazine articles which are not promoted by business interests, and an understanding of how special interest groups such as those raising awareness of specific diseases and treatments can distort priorities. Education in fact must try to loosen people's fascination with health, which after all for most of us is just fine and owes nothing to medical science and everything to good nutrition, cleanliness, and wealth. All these are messages that definitely don't come out in the press and online.

Looking over the years at how the system has been, it seems to the observer that far-sighted and evidence based planning is needed, keeping politics out of it as far as possible. Planning should include involving the public, giving people the right to make representations for the types of care they want, and also to integrate the whole system of health and social care, using scientific evidence as far as possible.

But there is a conflict here because the public on the whole isn't interested in evidence and can be unduly influenced by media promotions and anecdotal arguments. However there are lots of subjects where the evidence can be presented to the general public in a way that enables the people in making decisions. For example, if the evidence on whether emergencies should be treated locally by less specialised staff or in more distant hospitals by super specialists is presented objectively, together with the costs of each, then the decision should be made by the local people alone, and the planners should then implement it. But 'planning' evokes thoughts of socialist central planning in Russia, with its evident failures – and is of course completely discredited at the moment. The market is the favoured approach in health care despite being shown to be riddled with self-interest and corruption in the financial sector.

Similarly clinicians need to work consensually across different disciplines to make integrated care a reality, so that one part of the public pool does not undermine another. Consultants and GPs need to cooperate, other health and social professionals should be included whenever possible and a culture of silo working (working on isolation from everyone else) in hospitals and general practice discouraged. The funding of the health service needs to be far more flexible to encourage innovation, not stifling it as it usually does.

From my reading of the future, there is the risk that the universality of the NHS in England will be lost, that instead of a national commitment to improve everyone's health with a clear remit to reduce health inequalities, the new reforms are setting out to promote competition so that there will be areas of good or excellent care, but those losing out in the competition will fail and may have to be replaced. No longer will we worry about the 'post code lottery' as of old, where people in one area have treatment denied to those in other areas, as this will be institutionalised – the postcode will entirely determine what you get. The bug will become the feature.

This is a big adjustment for medical staff to make. Public Health doctors, GPs, and managers have been used to seeing reducing health inequalities as one of the driving forces in their quest for improvements in care. But now there is less emphasis on deprivation as such and more on age. This is because age is the biggest determinant of health need and so resources are going to be channelled to those Clinical Commissioning Groups with the highest proportion of older people. It hasn't happened yet, but the very fact that it can be a proposal means that it is clear where we are heading. We know that age is a major determination of health needs, but we also know that incapacity and being on benefits is also very bad for your health, with people on benefits becoming ill at a greater rate than those in work even if they were well to start with. So many doctors would prefer to see the previous emphasis on reducing deprivation and compensating where possible continued.

The changes to the NHS undoubtedly are going to increase inequality in the population and we know that the UK has some of the greatest structural inequalities of wealth and everyday living in Europe now. We also know that 'happiness' is not clearly related to wealth as such but to relative wealth so that those countries where health inequalities are least come out as 'happier' on survey after survey.[179] Social unrest is also well correlated with inequalities.[180] So it does seem surprising that our political masters wish to take this path.

However, financially we in the UK are in a reasonably good position. Though our spending is still less than other developed countries we are quite efficient at providing good services. So long as we keep our spending proportionate with the level of the other developed countries (a big if) we should be able to provide good care. Our population is also already a lot more accustomed to using services sensibly, as many people and patients are already very circumspect about new claims for huge health benefits. In France the bill for drugs is much higher and many more people expect to get expensive prescriptions. In Spain people visit the doctor almost twice as often as in the UK. All countries are in the same boat financially as the money for increasing health spending dries up. All will have to reduce public expectations, but hopefully in a way that gets rid of over-hyped excessive expectations, and reminds people what real health care is all about.

The changes to the NHS detailed above of course only apply to England. Scotland, Wales and Northern Ireland are remaining true to the original centralized version of the NHS and no immediate changes are planned in any of these countries. Of course commissioning by GPs and modernisation in hospitals can go ahead without any new Acts of Parliament and we hope that incremental changes can be made in the devolved nations in order to improve the patient experience, even in a time of austerity. Looking ahead five or more years therefore we will be able to see in an almost perfect example of a controlled trial (though not of course randomised or double blind!) how the various countries perform on many fronts. It will undoubtedly be an interesting time.

Appendix: Evidence for the effectiveness of Herbs

Depression and Anxiety

St John's Wort is the most researched herbal medicine, with a solid body of evidence behind it, including a Cochrane meta-analysis, which included 29 RCTs with 5,489 patients altogether, 18 comparisons with placebo and 17 comparisons with antidepressants. These confirmed its usefulness for mild to moderate depression, proving that it is as effective as standard antidepressant treatment and associated with fewer adverse effects. These studies were well advertised in early 2002 and I certainly recommended it quite a lot at the time, and on the whole patients were very happy with it. However, NICE guidelines in 2009 recommended against its use, not because it didn't work but because of uncertainty about dosage. This seemed to me a shame, because conventional antidepressants have quite severe side effects, which mostly appear before the beneficial effect so that many patients stop them without giving them a fair trial, and it would be good to have something that does not have so many side effects.

St John's Wort appears to work on transmitter substance in the brain, as of course do antidepressants. One active ingredient appears to be hypericin, and some manufacturers have tried to standardise the amounts of this substance in the tablet, but there may be other constituents in St John's Wort which work in a synergistic way (synergism is when two or more substances work together so that the total effect is greater than the sum of the constituents used separately), so that doing this might reduce the overall efficacy of the medication. Other possible 'active constituents' include hyperforin and various flavonoids.

Which now brings us to the other problem. Herbs that are effective do so because they have definite effects on the physiology or biochemistry of the body, and therefore, just as with conventional medications, there can be side effects or interactions. St John's Wort has been proven to be involved in two distinct mechanisms of enzyme induction causing drug interactions. There is a biochemical pathway – i.e. a series of biochemical reactions, which go on in all the cells of the body as part of how the body works – called the cytochrome p450 3A4 pathway.

This is well known to biochemists, pharmaceutical workers and medical students as an awful nuisance as there are many many well known drugs which are metabolised (got rid of) by this pathway, for instance warfarin (the main anti clotting agent used in medicine), oral contraceptives (the pill), anticonvulsant (for epilepsy), protease inhibitors which are used to treat HIV, and some anticancer drugs such as cyclosporine. The result is that if anyone takes more than one of these drugs there will be an interaction leading to the effects of each being enhanced or reduced. In substances like warfarin, where the therapeutic concentration has to be within certain limits, it can be dangerous to take two such substances together. St John's Wort does indeed interact with this pathway, so that these effects of these other drugs may be reduced if taken concurrently. The substance that causes the interaction is not however hypericin but another substance in St John's Wort, called hyperforin. In some formulations hyperforin may not be present in therapeutic amounts and do not interact, but these also may not work as well. This means that people really should not take St John's Wort, and indeed some other herbal formulations, at the same time as taking some conventional medications without checking with their doctor first that it is safe. But as we have seen many people do not check, and some doctors are unaware of the interactions. It is certainly a difficulty that might have serious consequences.

Hyperforin can also affect absorption of some drugs, most importantly digoxin (used for heart problems, although not so much these days) and vinblastine (an anti cancer drug). St John's Wort certainly reacts with antidepressants themselves and should never be taken at the same time. St John's Wort has also been reported as causing photosensitivity in the skin, but this is not thought to be a real problem – the only clinical study to investigate the subject found no increase in photosensitivity in volunteers with up to three times the usual clinical dose so the risk of such reactions with everyday sun exposure in the UK is extremely low.

There is some evidence that St John's Wort also is useful to reduce hot flushes in menopausal women. It doesn't do so as effectively as HRT, but then HRT as we have seen has severe drawbacks, and I for one would definitely recommend St John's Wort at least to try first.

So taking herbal medicines that actually work can be as fraught with difficulty as taking conventional medicines, although it seems to me that in general their actions are gentler and have fewer side effects than similar conventional medicines.

Ginseng indigenous to Siberia *Rhodiola rosea* (rose root) is what herbalists call an 'adaptogen', which means that it is thought to beneficially affect general resistance to physical and mental stressors, whilst being non-toxic and non-stimulating. I personally do not think this amounts to anything. It can interact with warfarin, causing bleeding.

Chamomile may help to reduce anxiety: one small but adequately powered (n=57) placebo-controlled RCT in mild to moderate generalised anxiety disorder over 8 weeks showed that chamomile extract was clinically effective in reducing Hamilton Anxiety Rating scores,[181] which are a method of measuring the intensity of anxiety. This test isn't used much today in general practice as it has been superseded by better ones, for instance the Beck Anxiety Inventory. There was no excess of adverse events. Regularly drinking tea has not been evaluated for anxiety but there was no effect on vigilance next day. Again more studies are needed.

Valerian Has not been found to work for anything in any study to date.

Herbs where there have been concerns over safety

Kava *(Piper methysticum)* is a member of the pepper family, from whose root a beverage is made which is very important in traditional South Pacific culture. Standardised extracts of kava root have been shown to be effective for anxiety in a Cochrane systematic review of 12 RCTs including 700 participants.[182] A meta-analysis performed on seven of these studies demonstrated a statistically significant effect over placebo in modestly reducing the Hamilton Anxiety score.[183] However it was banned in some countries in 2003 because of reports of liver toxicity.

Black cohosh has been implicated in causing liver problems.[184]

Aristolochia plants might be responsible for the high incidence of urinary tract cancer in Taiwan.[185]

For arthritis and to relieve pain

Arnica Montana has been used medicinally for centuries, and nowadays is used in liniments and ointments for strains and bruises, but there are no scientific studies that indicate any medical effectiveness. It is not entirely inactive however. The roots contain derivatives of thymol, which are used as fungicides and preservatives, and are effective capillary vasodilators. There has been a German study of wound healing after varicose vein surgery, which found a trend towards less bruising.[186] However homeopathic arnica was no more effective than a placebo.[187]

Cat's Claw vine has been used to treat inflammation and arthritis. However there are only small trials so far to indicate that it actually works in patients.[188]

Devil's claw root (*Harpagophytum procumbens*, native to the Namibian desert) has anti-inflammatory, antispasmodic and antioxidant properties, which make it useful to treat arthritis. A high-quality RCT in 88 participants over 6 weeks demonstrated similar benefits for Devil's claw and rofecoxib,[189] one of the recently developed and heavily promoted anti-inflammatory drugs, but rofecoxib was withdrawn due to cardiovascular adverse effects such as heart attacks. But Devil's Claw is highly bitter and may cause gastric upset, as indeed do most of the conventional drugs used to treat arthritis.

Boswellia resin (containing boswellian acids) from the *Boswellia serrata* tree (a species of frankincense) long used in Ayurvedic medicine, works in arthritis of the knee. It possesses anti-inflammatory, anti-arthritic and analgesic activity and has been shown to reduce pain and stiffness more effectively than placebo,[190] but caused some gastro intestinal upset.

This again shows that herbs which are truly effective may suffer from exactly the same sorts of side effects as the conventional drugs. .

Other herbs

Many herbs sometimes taken medicinally are really foods and are regulated as such rather than as MHRA-approved herbal products.

Turmeric, a member of the ginger family native to South Asia, has long been used for both culinary and medicinal purposes in Ayurvedic medicine. Recent research has confirmed multiple anti-inflammatory and antioxidant properties attributed to curcumin, a major constituent.[191] These include effects on prosta-glandin and leukotriene metabolism (very important pathways that I learned about in medical school), and inhibition of NF-kappa B, one of the most impor-tant signal transduction mechanisms in cells. An RCT of 107 patients with knee osteoarthritis compared turmeric extract (2 g per day) with ibuprofen 800 mg per day for 6 weeks. The turmeric extract was similarly effective to ibuprofen, with no difference in adverse events.[192] However, the study was not powered to confirm statistical equivalence. The only adverse effect reported is gastrointesti-nal upset.

Ginger root Ginger root is a commonly used spice, and used as a medicine it can help arthritis of the knee,[193] although other studies have not been so posi-tive. It has been used for nausea and vomiting postoperatively, and according to the American College of Obstetricians and Gynecologists it can be useful for treating hyperemesis gravidum,[194] better known as severe nausea and vomiting in early pregnancy, a condition with a high profile recently! There were no re-ports of adverse effects which is an extremely important consideration in early pregnancy.

Garlic seems to help to reduce low-density lipoprotein (LDL) 'bad' cholesterol and triglyceride levels, in the short term anyway (three to six months)[195] and may help blood pressure and diabetes.[196] The levels of high-density lipoprotein (HDL) 'good' cholesterol were unaffected. Allium compounds from garlic have been shown to inhibit cholesterol synthesis, which would explain how it works. Interestingly garlic supplements with the distinctive odour of garlic removed still retain efficacy. The evidence was inconclusive about garlic's role in protecting against cancer. Dietary garlic may possibly be associated with decreased likeli-hood of some types of cancer such as stomach and colorectal cancer, but the number of available studies was not sufficient to draw firm conclusions.

Omega-3 fatty acids are naturally found in fish, plant, and nut oils, and have also been made into dietary supplements. Fish oil contains both docosahexae-noic acid (DHA) and eicosapentaenoic acid (EPA), which have been proven to lower triglycerides, slow the buildup of atherosclerotic plaques (hardening of the artery walls), lower blood pressure, and reduce risk of death, heart attack, and dangerous abnormal heart beats due to cardiovascular disease.[197]

More specifically, an analysis of 17 clinical studies of the use of fish oil supplements showed that taking three or more grams of fish oil daily significantly reduces blood pressure for people with untreated hypertension.[198]

One clinical study found that overweight, mildly hyperlipidemic men who took four grams of purified DHA per day had lower blood pressure (BP) than did those who took the placebo, olive oil capsules. The study concluded: 'Relative to the placebo group, 24-hour BP fell 5.8/3.3 (systolic/diastolic) mm Hg and daytime BP fell 3.5/2.0 mm Hg with DHA.'[199]

Furthermore, fish oil is effective in reducing high triglyceride levels by 20 to 50%. One fish oil supplement, Lovaza, is now FDA-approved for use to lower triglycerides.[200]

Notes and references

Chapter 1

1   Managing high value capital equipment in the NHS in England. HC 822, National Audit Office, 2011. http://www.nao.org.uk/publications/1011/nhs_high_value_equipment.aspx

2   Health at a Glance 2011: OECD Indicators. OECD, 2011. http://dx.doi.org/10.1787/health_glance-2011-en

Chapter 2

3   Health at a Glance 2011: OECD Indicators. OECD, 2011. http://dx.doi.org/10.1787/health_glance-2011-en

4   Ingleby D, McKee M, Mladovsky P, Rechel B. How the NHS measures up to other health systems. BMJ 2012; 344:e1079. http://dx.doi.org/10.1136/bmj.e1079

Chapter 3

5   Jerant A, Franks P. Body mass index, diabetes, hypertension, and short-term mortality: a population-based observational study, 2000–2006. The Journal of the American Board of Family Medicine 2012; 25:422–431. http://dx.doi.org/10.3122/jabfm.2012.04.110289

6   Bruinsma, J. The Resource Outlook to 2050: By How Much do Land, Water and Crop Yields Need to Increase by 2050? Prepared for the FAO Expert Meeting on 'How to Feed the World in 2050', 24–26 June 2009, Rome. FAO, 2009.

7   Aiking, H. Future protein supply. Trends in Food Science & Technology 2011; 22:112–120. http://dx.doi.org/10.1016/j.tifs.2010.04.005

8   Adams, TD. Health benefits of gastric bypass surgery after 6 years. JAMA: The Journal of the American Medical Association 2012; 308:1122. http://dx.doi.org/10.1001/2012.jama.11164

9   Neovius M. Health care use during 20 years following bariatric surgery. JAMA: The Journal of the American Medical Association 2012; 308:1132. http://dx.doi.org/10.1001/2012.jama.11792

10 Heath, I. The Art of Doing Nothing. Keynote address at the Wonca Conference 2012, Vienna.

11 Goedde HW, Agarwal DP, Fritze G, et al. Distribution of ADH2 and ALDH2 genotypes in different populations. Human Genetics 1992; 88. http://dx.doi.org/10.1007/BF00197271

12 Brooks PJ, Enoch M-A, Goldman D, Li T-K, Yokoyama A. The alcohol flushing response: an unrecognized risk factor for esophageal cancer from alcohol consumption. PLoS Medicine 2009; 6:e50. http://dx.doi.org/10.1371/journal.pmed.1000050.sd001

13 Ørn S, Dickstein K. How do heart failure patients die? European Heart Journal Supplements 2002; 4(suppl D): D59.

14 Castelnuovo A., Costanzo S., Bagnardi V., Donati MB, Iacoviello L, de Gaetano G. Alcohol dosing and total mortality in men and women. Archives of Internal Medicine 2006;166:2437. http://dx.doi.org/10.1001/archinte.166.22.2437

Chapter 5

15 Wagner M, Oehlmann J. Endocrine disruptors in bottled mineral water: total estrogenic burden and migration from plastic bottles. Environmental Science and Pollution Research 2009;16:278–286. http://dx.doi.org/10.1007/s11356-009-0107-7

16 Armstrong LE, Costill DL, Fink WJ. Influence of diuretic-induced dehydration on competitive running performance. Medicine & Science in Sports & Exercise 1985;17(4):456–461. http://dx.doi.org/10.1249/00005768-198508000-00009

17 Heneghan C, Perera R, Nunan D, Mahtani K, Gill P. Forty years of sports performance research and little insight gained. BMJ 2012; 345:e4797. http://dx.doi.org/10.1136/bmj.e4797

18 McCartney M. Waterlogged? BMJ 2011; 343:d4280. http://dx.doi.org/10.1136/bmj.d4280

19 Noakes TD. Commentary: role of hydration in health and exercise. BMJ 2012;345:e4171. http://dx.doi.org/10.1136/bmj.e4171

20 Haldane, JBS. Minerals in food. In Science and Everyday Life. Vigyan Prasar Publication, 1939.

21 Organ donation give the gift of life. Kidney Wales Foundation, 2007. http://www.kidneywales.com/index.php?p=1889

22 Longest organ donor chain links 60 people in US. BBC News, 2012. http://www.bbc.co.uk/news/health-17112314

Chapter 6

23   Grady D, Rubin SM, Petitti DB, Fox CS, Black D, Ettinger B, Ernster VL,
     Cummings SR. Hormone therapy to prevent disease and prolong life in
     postmenopausal women. Annals of Internal Medicine 1992;117:1016–37. http://
     annals.org/article.aspx?articleid=706003

24   Writing Group for the Women's Health Initiative Investigators. Risks and Benefits
     of Estrogen Plus Progestin in Healthy Postmenopausal Women: Principal Results
     From the Women's Health Initiative Randomized Controlled Trial. JAMA: The
     Journal of the American Medical Association 2002;288:321–333. http://dx.doi.
     org/10.1001/jama.288.3.321

25   The million women study. University of Oxford, 2001. http://www.
     millionwomenstudy.org/

26   Barbour, V. Successful intervention by PLoS Medicine and New York Times in
     Federal court grants public access to evidence that drug company 'ghostwrote'
     medical articles about hormone therapy drug, Prempro. PLoS Blogs, 2009. http://v.
     gd/drug_companies_ghostwrite

27   Shapiro S, Farmer RDT, Mueck AO, Seaman H, Stevenson JC. Does hormone
     replacement therapy cause breast cancer? An application of causal principles to
     three studies: Part 2. The Women's Health Initiative: estrogen plus progestogen.
     Journal of Family Planning and Reproductive Health Care 2011;37:165–172. http://
     dx.doi.org/10.1136/jfprhc-2011-0090

28   Schierbeck LL, Rejnmark L, Tofteng CL, et al. Effect of hormone replacement
     therapy on cardiovascular events in recently postmenopausal women: randomised
     trial. BMJ 2012;345:e6409. http://dx.doi.org/10.1136/bmj.e6409

29   Duffy O, Iversen L, Hannaford P. The impact and management of symptoms
     experienced at midlife: a community-based study of women in northeast Scotland.
     BJOG: An International Journal of Obstetrics & Gynaecology 2012;119:554–564.
     http://dx.doi.org/10.1111/j.1471-0528.2012.03276.x

Chapter 7

30   Cochrane A. Effectiveness and efficiency: random reflections on health services.
     Nuffield Provincial Hospitals Trust, 1972.

31   Effects of intensive blood-pressure control in type 2 diabetes mellitus. New
     England Journal of Medicine 2010;362:1575–1585. http://dx.doi.org/10.1056/
     NEJMoa1001286

32   Shaw HL. The Opren scandal. British Medical Journal (Clin Res Ed) 1983;286: 721.

33   Goldacre, B. Bad Science. Harper Perennial, 2010.

34   Tanne JH. Alzheimer's researchers face trial for scientific fraud and defrauding US government. BMJ 2012;344:e3608. http://dx.doi.org/10.1136/bmj.e3608

Chapter 8

35   Evans E, Aiking H, Edwards A. Reducing variation in general practitioner referral rates through clinical engagement. Quality in Primary Care 2011;19(4):263–72.

36   Gabbay J., le May A. Practice-based Evidence for Healthcare: Clinical Mindlines. Routledge, 2010.

37   Two breast cancer drugs not cost effective, says final NICE guidance. NICE, 2012. http://www.nice.org.uk/newsroom/pressreleases/ TwoBreastCancerDrugsNotCostEffective.jsp

38   Rosoff AJ. Evidence-based medicine and the law: the courts confront clinical practice guidelines. Journal of Health Politics, Policy and Law 2001;26(2):327–368. http://dx.doi.org/10.1215/03616878-26-2-327

39   Coleman M, Forman D, Bryant H, et al. Cancer survival in Australia, Canada, Denmark, Norway, Sweden, and the UK, 1995–2007 (the International Cancer Benchmarking Partnership): an analysis of population-based cancer registry data. The Lancet 2011;377(9760):127–138. http://dx.doi.org/10.1016/ S0140-6736(10)62231-3

40   Vedsted P, Olesen F. Are the serious problems in cancer survival partly rooted in gatekeeper principles? An ecologic study. British Journal of General Practice 2011;61(589):508–512. http://dx.doi.org/10.3399/bjgp11X588484

41   Health at a Glance 2011: OECD Indicators. OECD, 2011. http://dx.doi.org/10.1787/ health_glance-2011-en

42   Health at a Glance 2011: OECD Indicators. OECD, 2011. http://dx.doi.org/10.1787/ health_glance-2011-en

43   WHO Global Health Expenditure Database. http://apps.who.int/nha/database/ DataExplorerRegime.aspx

44   Coleman M, Forman D, Bryant H, et al. Cancer survival in Australia, Canada, Denmark, Norway, Sweden, and the UK, 1995–2007 (the International Cancer Benchmarking Partnership): an analysis of population-based cancer registry data. The Lancet 2011;377(9760):127–138. http://dx.doi.org/10.1016/ S0140-6736(10)62231-3

45   Humphrey, LL. Lung cancer screening: an update for the U.S. Preventive Services Task Force. Systematic Evidence Reviews, No. 31. Agency for Healthcare Research and Quality (US), 2004. http://www.ncbi.nlm.nih.gov/books/NBK42872/

Oken MM. Screening by chest radiograph and lung cancer mortality. JAMA: The Journal of the American Medical Association 2011;306(17):1865. http://dx.doi.org/10.1001/jama.2011.1591

46   Fontana RS, Sanderson DR, Woolner LB, et al. Screening for lung cancer. A critique of the Mayo Lung Project. Cancer 1991;67(Suppl):1155–1164.

47   Veronesi G, Maisonneuve P, Bellomi M, Rampinelli C, Durli I, Bertolotti R, Spaggiari L. Estimating overdiagnosis in low-dose computed tomography screening for lung cancer: a cohort study. Annals of Internal Medicine 2012;157(11):776–84.

48   IWelch HG, Black WC. Overdiagnosis in cancer. JNCI Journal of the National Cancer Institute. 2010;102(9):605-613. http://dx.doi.org/10.1093/jnci/djq099

49   Chlebowski RT, Schwartz AG, Wakelee H, et al. Oestrogen plus progestin and lung cancer in postmenopausal women (Women's Health Initiative trial): a post-hoc analysis of a randomised controlled trial. The Lancet 2009;374(9697):1243–1251. http://dx.doi.org/10.1016/S0140-6736(09)61526-9

50   Explaining variations in lung cancer in England. Roy Castle Foundation, 2011. http://v.gd/cancervariation

51   Bowel cancer survival statistics. Cancer Research UK, 2012. http://www.cancerresearchuk.org/cancer-info/cancerstats/types/bowel/survival/bowel-cancer-survival-statistics

52   Morris EJA, Taylor EF, Thomas JD, et al. Thirty-day postoperative mortality after colorectal cancer surgery in England. Gut 2011;60(6):806–813. http://dx.doi.org/10.1136/gut.2010.232181

53   Mayor S. Mammography screening has little or no effect on breast cancer deaths, Swedish data indicate. BMJ 2012;345:e4847. http://dx.doi.org/10.1136/bmj.e4847

54   Esserman L. Rethinking screening for breast cancer and prostate cancer. JAMA: The Journal of the American Medical Association 2009;302(15):1685. http://dx.doi.org/10.1001/jama.2009.1498

55   Mulcahy, N. Most screen-detected breast cancers are low risk. Medscape Today, 2012. http://www.medscape.com/viewarticle/756859

56   Autier P, Koechlin A, Smans M, Vatten L, Boniol M. Mammography screening and breast cancer mortality in sweden. JNCI Journal of the National Cancer Institute 2012;104(14):1080–1093. http://dx.doi.org/10.1093/jnci/djs272

57   Breast cancer: facts and figures 2011–2012. American Cancer Society, 2012. http://v.gd/breastcancerfactsfigures

58   Jacobsen GD, Jacobsen KH. Health awareness campaigns and diagnosis rates: Evidence from National Breast Cancer Awareness Month. Journal of Health Economics 2011;30(1):55–61. http://dx.doi.org/10.1016/j.jhealeco.2010.11.005

59   Cancer advances in focus: prostate cancer. National Institutes of Health, 2010.
      http://www.cancer.gov/cancertopics/factsheet/cancer-advances-in-focus/prostate

Chapter 10

60   Venn-Watson S, Carlin K, Ridgway S. Dolphins as animal models for type 2
      diabetes: Sustained, post-prandial hyperglycemia and hyperinsulinemia. General
      and Comparative Endocrinology 2011;170(1):193–199. http://dx.doi.org/10.1016/j.
      ygcen.2010.10.005

61   Gooßen K, Gräber S. Longer term safety of dipeptidyl peptidase-4 inhibitors
      in patients with type 2 diabetes mellitus: systematic review and meta-
      analysis. Diabetes, Obesity and Metabolism. 2012:no-no. http://dx.doi.
      org/10.1111/j.1463-1326.2012.01610.x

62   Simmons RK, Echouffo-Tcheugui JB, Sharp SJ, et al. Screening for type 2 diabetes
      and population mortality over 10 years (ADDITION-Cambridge): a cluster-
      randomised controlled trial. The Lancet 2012;380(9855):1741–1748. http://dx.doi.
      org/10.1016/S0140-6736(12)61422-6

63   Diabetes Prevention programme (DPP). NIH, 2012. http://diabetes.niddk.nih.gov/
      dm/pubs/preventionprogram/

64   Farmer AJ, Perera R, Ward A, et al. Meta-analysis of individual patient data in
      randomised trials of self monitoring of blood glucose in people with non-insulin
      treated type 2 diabetes. BMJ. 2012;344(1):e486–e486. http://dx.doi.org/10.1136/bmj.
      e486

Chapter 11

65   Thom TJ, Kannel WB. Downward trend in cardiovascular mortality. Annual
      Review of Medicine 1981;32(1):427–434. http://dx.doi.org/10.1146/annurev.
      me.32.020181.00223510.1146/annurev.me.32.020181.002235

66   Myocardial Ischaemia National Audit Project (MINAP).
      Healthcare Quality Improvement Project. http://www.hqip.org.uk/
      myocardial-ischaemia-national-audit-project-minap/

67   Stott D, Dewar R, Garratt C, et al. RCPE UK Consensus Conference on
      'Approaching the comprehensive management of atrial fibrillation: evolution
      or revolution?'. The Journal of the Royal College of Physicians of Edinburgh
      2012;42(1):34–35. http://dx.doi.org/10.4997/JRCPE.2012.S01

      Hobbs FD, Fitzmaurice DA, Mant J, Murray E, Jowett S, Bryan S, Raftery J, Davies
      M, Lip G.A randomised controlled trial and cost-effectiveness study of systematic
      screening (targeted and total population screening) versus routine practice for the
      detection of atrial fibrillation in people aged 65 and over. The SAFE study. Health
      Technology Assessment 2005; 9:40. http://dx.doi.org/10.3310/hta9400

68   Stephanie Seneff. http://people.csail.mit.edu/seneff/

69   Ray KK. Statins and All-Cause Mortality in High-Risk Primary Prevention: A meta-analysis of 11 randomized controlled trials involving 65 229 participants. Archives of Internal Medicine 2010;170(12):1024. http://dx.doi.org/10.1001/archinternmed.2010.182

70   Cholesterol Treatment Trialists' (CTT) Collaborators, Mihaylova B, Emberson J, Blackwell L, Keech A, Simes J, Barnes EH, Voysey M, Gray A, Collins R, Baigent C. The effects of lowering LDL cholesterol with statin therapy in people at low risk of vascular disease: meta-analysis of individual data from 27 randomised trials. Lancet 2012;380(9841):581–90. http://dx.doi.org/10.1016/S0140-6736(12)60367-5

Chapter 12

71   Little P. Importance of patient pressure and perceived pressure and perceived medical need for investigations, referral, and prescribing in primary care: nested observational study. BMJ 2004;328(7437):444–0. http://dx.doi.org/10.1136/bmj.38013.644086.7C

72   Evans E. The Torfaen referral evaluation project. Quality in Primary Care 2009;17(6):423–9.

Chapter 13

73   Iezzoni LI, Rao SR, DesRoches CM, Vogeli C, Campbell EG. Survey shows that at least some physicians are not always open or honest with patients. Health Affairs 2012;31(2):383–391. http://dx.doi.org/10.1377/hlthaff.2010.1137

74   White P, Goldsmith K, Johnson A, et al. Comparison of adaptive pacing therapy, cognitive behaviour therapy, graded exercise therapy, and specialist medical care for chronic fatigue syndrome (PACE): a randomised trial. The Lancet 2011;377(9768):823–836. http://dx.doi.org/10.1016/S0140-6736(11)60096-2

75   A practical guide to the provision of Chronic Pain Services for adults in Primary Care. British Pain Society and RCGP, 2004. http://v.gd/chronicpainservices

Chapter 14

76   Parkes GC, Brostoff J, Whelan K, Sanderson JD. Gastrointestinal microbiota in irritable bowel syndrome: their role in its pathogenesis and treatment. The American Journal of Gastroenterology 2008;103(6):1557–1567. http://dx.doi.org/10.1111/j.1572-0241.2008.01869.x

77   Marshall JK, Thabane M, Garg AX, Clark WF, Salvadori M, Collins SM. Incidence and epidemiology of irritable bowel syndrome after a large waterborne outbreak of bacterial dysentery. Gastroenterology 2006;131(2):445–450. http://dx.doi. org/10.1053/j.gastro.2006.05.053

78   Pumphrey RSH. An epidemiological approach to reducing the risk of fatal anaphylaxis. In Anaphylaxis and Hypersensitivity Reactions, Castells MC, ed. Springer-Verlag, 2011:13–31. http://dx.doi.org/10.1007/978-1-60327-951-2_2

Chapter 15

79   Chalder M, Wiles NJ, Campbell J, et al. Facilitated physical activity as a treatment for depressed adults: randomised controlled trial. BMJ 2012;344:e2758. http:// dx.doi.org/10.1136/bmj.e2758

80   Maunder L, Cameron L, Moss M, et al. Effectiveness of self-help materials for anxiety adapted for use in prison – a pilot study. Journal of Mental Health 2009;18(3):262–271. http://dx.doi.org/10.1080/09638230802522478

81   Website available at http://www.criticalpsychiatry.co.uk/

82   Paid to Prescribe? Exploring the relationship between doctors and the drug industry. Hearing before the Special Committee on Aging, United States Senate, 27 June 2007, no. 110–10. US Government Printing Office, 2008. http://aging.senate. gov/publications/6272007.pdf

83   Ranibizumab and Bevacizumab for Neovascular Age-Related Macular Degeneration. New England Journal of Medicine 2011;364(20):1897–1908. http:// dx.doi.org/10.1056/NEJMoa1102673

84   Avastin and Lucentis are equivalent in treating age-related macular degeneration. National Eye Institute, NIH, 2012. http://www.nei.nih.gov/news/ pressreleases/043012.asp

85   Ghostwriting: The Dirty Little Secret of Medical Publishing That Just Got Bigger. PLoS Medicine 2009;6(9):e1000156. http://dx.doi.org/10.1371/journal. pmed.1000156

86   Gale EAM. Conflicts of interest in guideline panel members. BMJ 2011;343:d5728. http://dx.doi.org/10.1136/bmj.d5728

87   Loewenstein G. The Unintended Consequences of Conflict of Interest Disclosure. JAMA: The Journal of the American Medical Association 2012;307(7):669. http:// dx.doi.org/10.1001/jama.2012.154

Chapter 18

88   Copenhagen Consensus. http://www.copenhagenconsensus.com/

89   Haider BA, Bhutta ZA. The effect of therapeutic zinc supplementation among young children with selected infections: a review of the evidence. Food and Nutrition Bulletin 2009;30(Suppl):S41-59.

90   Maret W, Sandstead HH. Zinc requirements and the risks and benefits of zinc supplementation. Journal of Trace Elements in Medicine and Biology 2006;20(1):3–18. http://dx.doi.org/10.1016/j.jtemb.2006.01.006

91   Schmidt B. Survival without disability to age 5 years after neonatal caffeine therapy for apnea of prematurity. JAMA: The Journal of the American Medical Association 2012;307(3):275. http://dx.doi.org/10.1001/jama.2011.2024

92   Reichenbach S, Sterchi R, Scherer M, Trelle S, Bürgi E, Bürgi U, Dieppe PA, Jüni P. Meta-analysis: chondroitin for osteoarthritis of the knee or hip. Annals of Internal Medicine 2007;146(8):580–90.

93   Wilkens P. Effect of glucosamine on pain-related disability in patients with chronic low back pain and degenerative lumbar osteoarthritis: a randomized controlled trial. JAMA: The Journal of the American Medical Association 2010;304(1):45. http://dx.doi.org/10.1001/jama.2010.893

94   Devitt, M. Complementary Care in the U.K.: Study finds high use of herbal medicine and acupuncture. Acupuncture Today 2000; 1. http://www.acupuncturetoday.com/archives2000/sep/09camuk.html

95   Tsai H-H, Lin H-W, Simon Pickard A, Tsai H-Y, Mahady GB. Evaluation of documented drug interactions and contraindications associated with herbs and dietary supplements: a systematic literature review. International Journal of Clinical Practice 2012;66(11):1056–1078. http://dx.doi.org/10.1111/j.1742-1241.2012.03008.x

96   Ramsay NA, Kenny MW, Davies G, Patel JP. Complimentary and alternative medicine use among patients starting warfarin. British Journal of Haematology 2005;130(5):777-780. http://dx.doi.org/10.1111/j.1365-2141.2005.05689.x.

97   Complementary Medicines – UK – December 2009. Mintel Oxygen, 2009. http://store.mintel.com/complementary-medicines-uk-december-2009

98   Devitt, M. Complementary care in the U.K.: Study finds high use of herbal medicine and acupuncture. Acupuncture Today 2000; 1. http://www.acupuncturetoday.com/archives2000/sep/09camuk.html

99   Barnes MP, Bloom B, Nahin RL. Complementary and alternative medicine use among adults and children: United States, 2007. National Health Statistics Reports 2008; 12. http://www.cdc.gov/nchs/data/nhsr/nhsr012.pdf

100   Ernst E, White A. The BBC survey of complementary medicine use in the UK. Complementary Therapies in Medicine 2000;8(1):32-36. http://dx.doi.org/10.1016/S0965-2299(00)90833-1

101 Shaw A, Noble A, Salisbury C, Sharp D, Thompson E, Peters TJ. Predictors of complementary therapy use among asthma patients: results of a primary care survey. Health & Social Care in the Community 2008;16(2):155–164. http://dx.doi. org/10.1111/j.1365-2524.2007.00738.x

102 Matthews A, Dowswell T, Haas DM, Doyle M, O'Mathúna DP. Cochrane Database of Systematic Reviews 2010; 8:CD007575. http://dx.doi.org/10.1002/14651858. CD007575.pub2

Chapter 19

103 Rabbani N, Alam SS, Riaz S, et al. High-dose thiamine therapy for patients with type 2 diabetes and microalbuminuria: a randomised, double-blind placebo-controlled pilot study. Diabetologia 2009;52(2):208–212. http://dx.doi.org/10.1007/ s00125-008-1224-4

104 Pogge E. Vitamin D and Alzheimer's Disease: is there a link? The Consultant Pharmacist 2010;25(7):440–450. http://dx.doi.org/10.4140/TCP.n.2010.440

105 Ramagopalan SV, Dyment DA, Cader MZ, et al. Rare variants in the CYP27B1 gene are associated with multiple sclerosis. Annals of Neurology 2011;70(6):881–886. http://dx.doi.org/10.1002/ana.22678

106 Bischoff-Ferrari HA, Dawson-Hughes B, Staehelin HB, et al. Fall prevention with supplemental and active forms of vitamin D: a meta-analysis of randomised controlled trials. BMJ 2009;339:b3692. http://dx.doi.org/10.1136/bmj.b3692

107 Binkley N. Is Vitamin D the fountain of youth? Endocrine Practice 2009;15(6):590–596. http://dx.doi.org/10.4158/EP09115.RA

108 Li K, Kaaks R, Linseisen J, Rohrmann S. Associations of dietary calcium intake and calcium supplementation with myocardial infarction and stroke risk and overall cardiovascular mortality in the Heidelberg cohort of the European Prospective Investigation into Cancer and Nutrition study (EPIC-Heidelberg). Heart 2012;98(12):920–925. http://dx.doi.org/10.1136/heartjnl-2011-301345

109 Reid D, Toole BJ, Knox S, et al. The relation between acute changes in the systemic inflammatory response and plasma 25-hydroxyvitamin D concentrations after elective knee arthroplasty. American Journal of Clinical Nutrition 2011;93(5):1006–1011. http://dx.doi.org/10.3945/ajcn.110.008490

110 Williams, S. On the defensive. Casebook 2011;19:8. http://www.medicalprotection. org/uk/casebook-january-2011/On-the-defensive

111 Salisbury AC. Diagnostic blood loss from phlebotomy and hospital-acquired anemia during acute myocardial infarction. Archives of Internal Medicine 2011;171(18):1646. http://dx.doi.org/10.1001/archinternmed.2011.361

Chapter 20

112 Williams R. 'Hospital hopper' given criminal ASBO. Guardian 2 June 2010. http://www.guardian.co.uk/society/2010/jun/02/hospital-hopper-criminal-asbo

113 Wasteful diagnostic testing situations listed by ACP. Journal Watch 17 January 2012. http://firstwatch.jwatch.org/cgi/content/full/2012/117/1

Chapter 21

114 Cherington M, Smith R, Nielsen PJ. The life, legacy, and premature death of Felix Mendelssohn. Semin Neurol. 1999;19(Suppl 1):47–52.

115 Bederson JB, Awad IA, Wiebers DO, et al. Recommendations for the management of patients with unruptured intracranial aneurysms: a statement for healthcare professionals from the Stroke Council of the American Heart Association. Circulation 2000;102(18):2300–2308. http://dx.doi.org/10.1161/01.CIR.102.18.2300

116 Magnetic resonance imaging units, total per million population. In Health: Key Tables from OECD. OECD, 2012. http://dx.doi.org/10.1787/magresimaging-table-2012-2-en

117 Managing high value capital equipment in the NHS in England. HC 822, National Audit Office, 2011. http://www.nao.org.uk/publications/1011/nhs_high_value_equipment.aspx

Chapter 22

118 2006/07 UK General Practice workload survey. NHS Information Centre, 2007. http://www.dhsspsni.gov.uk/gp_workload_survey_2006_07.pdf

119 2006/07 UK General Practice workload survey. NHS Information Centre, 2007. http://www.dhsspsni.gov.uk/gp_workload_survey_2006_07.pdf

120 O'Mahony S, Blank AE, Zallman L, Selwyn PA. The benefits of a hospital-based inpatient palliative care consultation service: preliminary outcome data. Journal of Palliative Medicine 2005;8(5):1033–1039. http://dx.doi.org/10.1089/jpm.2005.8.1033

121 Boccuti C, Moon M. Comparing medicare and private insurers: growth rates in spending over three decades. Health Affairs 2003;22(2):230–237. http://dx.doi.org/10.1377/hlthaff.22.2.230

Chapter 23

122 Whittle B, Ritchie J. Prescription for Murder: The True Story of Harold Shipman. Sphere, 2000.

123 Patients and GPs – Partners in care? Patients' Association, 2012. http://v.gd/partnersincare

124 Williams, S. On the defensive. Casebook 2011;19:8. http://www.medicalprotection.org/uk/casebook-january-2011/On-the-defensive

125 Kessler DP, McClellan M. Do doctors practice defensive medicine? NBER Working Paper No. 5466. National Bureau of Economic Research, 1996. http://www.nber.org/papers/w5466

Chapter 24

126 Morgan, E. The Scars of Evolution. Oxford University Press, 1994.

Chapter 26

127 Andrews PA. Don't use urine microscopy to confirm microscopic haematuria. BMJ 2009;338:b2629. http://dx.doi.org/10.1136/bmj.b2629

128 Wilt TJ, Brawer MK, Jones KM, et al. Radical prostatectomy versus observation for localized prostate cancer. New England Journal of Medicine 2012;367(3):203–213. http://dx.doi.org/10.1056/NEJMoa1113162

Chapter 29

129 Allen-Hall L, Arnason JT, Cano P, Lafrenie RM. Uncaria tomentosa acts as a potent TNF-α inhibitor through NF-κB. Journal of Ethnopharmacology 2010;127(3):685–693. http://dx.doi.org/10.1016/j.jep.2009.12.004

130 Trends in asthma mortality in Great Britain. Factsheet 97/3. Lung & Asthma information agency, 1997. http://www.laia.ac.uk/97_3/97_3.htm

131 Asthma in the US: Growing every year. Centers for Disease Control and Prevention, 2011. http://www.cdc.gov/vitalsigns/Asthma/index.html

132 Health Effects of exposure to secondhand smoke. United States Environmental Protection Agency, 2011. http://www.epa.gov/smokefree/healtheffects.html

133 Arie S. What can we learn from asthma in elite athletes? BMJ 2012;344:e2556. http://dx.doi.org/10.1136/bmj.e2556

134 Aaron SD, Vandemheen KL, Boulet L-P, et al. Overdiagnosis of asthma in obese and nonobese adults. Canadian Medical Association Journal 2008;179(11):1121–1131. http://dx.doi.org/10.1503/cmaj.081332

135 Calderòn-Larrañaga A, Carney L, Soljak M, et al. Association of population and primary healthcare factors with hospital admission rates for chronic obstructive pulmonary disease in England: national cross-sectional study. Thorax 2011;66(3):191–196. http://dx.doi.org/10.1136/thx.2010.147058

Chapter 30

136 Ernst & Young, RAND Europe, University of Cambridge. National evaluation of Department of Health's integrated care pilots. Department of Health, 2012. http://v.gd/integratedcarepilot

137 For example,

Freeman G, Hughes J. Continuity of care and the patient experience. The King's Fund, 2010. http://v.gd/kingsfund_continuity

Saultz JW. Interpersonal continuity of care and patient satisfaction: a critical review. The Annals of Family Medicine 2004;2(5):445–451. http://dx.doi.org/10.1370/afm.91

Cabana MD, Jee SH. Does continuity of care improve patient outcomes? J Fam Pract. 2004 Dec;53(12):974–80. http://www.jfponline.net/Pages.asp?AID=1830

138 Bhowmick B. A steady state: what should intermediate care in Wales look like? National Leadership and Innovation Agency for Healthcare, 2009. http://www.wales.nhs.uk/sitesplus/829/opendoc/144695/

Chapter 32

139 Goldman JS, Hahn SE, Catania JW, et al. Genetic counseling and testing for Alzheimer disease: Joint practice guidelines of the American College of Medical Genetics and the National Society of Genetic Counselors. Genetics in Medicine 2011;13(6):597–605. http://dx.doi.org/10.1097/GIM.0b013e31821d69b8

140 Colman, J. NHS Direct Wales. Wales Audit Office, 2009. http://www.wao.gov.uk/assets/englishdocuments/NHS_Direct_Wales_eng.pdf

141 Vize R. Integrated care: a story of hard won success. BMJ 2012;344:e3529. http://dx.doi.org/10.1136/bmj.e3529

142 Health at a Glance 2009: OECD Indicators. OECD, 2009. http://dx.doi.org/10.1787/health_glance-2009-en

143 Health at a Glance 2012: OECD Indicators. OECD, 2012. http://dx.doi.org/10.1787/health_glance-2012-en

144 Fit for the future? Dr Foster hospital guide 2012. Dr Foster Intelligence, 2012. http://download.drfosterintelligence.co.uk/Hospital_Guide_2012.pdf

145 High NHS hospital bed occupancy remains a big infection risk, says RCS. The Royal College of Surgeons, 2010. http://v.gd/rcsbedoccupancy

Chapter 33

146 Adams, S. 'Timebomb' fear as 'rationing by stealth' of operations hits NHS. The Telegraph, 9 September 2010. http://v.gd/telegraph_timebomb

147 Mao X, Wong AA, Crawford RW. Cobalt toxicity – an emerging clinical problem in patients with metal-on-metal hip prostheses? Medical Journal of Australia 2011 Jun 20;194(12):649–51.

148 Godlee F. Serious risks from metal-on-metal hip implants. BMJ 2012;344:e1539. http://dx.doi.org/10.1136/bmj.e1539

149 Kmietowicz Z. Surgeons condemn Lansley for misinformation on outcomes of knee operations. BMJ 2012;344:e1326–e1326. http://dx.doi.org/10.1136/bmj.e1326.

150 Anand R. What Is the Benefit of Introducing New Hip and Knee Prostheses? The Journal of Bone and Joint Surgery (American) 2011;93(Supplement_3):51. http://dx.doi.org/10.2106/JBJS.K.00867

151 Richette P, Poitou C, Garnero P, et al. Benefits of massive weight loss on symptoms, systemic inflammation and cartilage turnover in obese patients with knee osteoarthritis. Annals of the Rheumatic Diseases 2010;70(1):139–144. http://dx.doi.org/10.1136/ard.2010.134015

152 Morgan, E. The Scars of Evolution. Oxford University Press, 1994.

153 McGirt MJ, Ambrossi GLG, Datoo G, et al. Recurrent disc herniation and long-term back pain after primary lumbar discectomy. Neurosurgery 2009;64(2):338–345. http://dx.doi.org/10.1227/01.NEU.0000337574.58662.E2

154 Hellum C, Johnsen LG, Storheim K, et al. Surgery with disc prosthesis versus rehabilitation in patients with low back pain and degenerative disc: two year follow-up of randomised study. BMJ 2011;342:d2786. http://dx.doi.org/10.1136/bmj.d2786

155 Holmgren T, Bjornsson Hallgren H, Oberg B, Adolfsson L, Johansson K. Effect of specific exercise strategy on need for surgery in patients with subacromial impingement syndrome: randomised controlled study. BMJ 2012;344:e787. http://dx.doi.org/10.1136/bmj.e787

156 Buchbinder R. Short course prednisolone for adhesive capsulitis (frozen shoulder or stiff painful shoulder): a randomised, double blind, placebo controlled trial. Annals of the Rheumatic Diseases 2004;63(11):1460–1469. http://dx.doi.org/10.1136/ard.2003.018218

157 Crawshaw DP, Helliwell PS, Hensor EMA, Hay EM, Aldous SJ, Conaghan PG. Exercise therapy after corticosteroid injection for moderate to severe shoulder pain: large pragmatic randomised trial. BMJ 2010;340:c3037. http://dx.doi.org/10.1136/bmj.c3037

Chapter 34

158 Written evidence submitted by Professor Allyson Pollock, Queen Mary, University of London http://www.publications.parliament.uk/pa/cm201012/cmselect/cmtreasy/1146/1146vw45.htm

Chapter 35

159 Evans E, Aiking H, Edwards A. Reducing variation in general practitioner referral rates through clinical engagement. Quality in Primary Care; 2011;19(4):263–72

160 Hughes A, private communication.

161 Adams, S. Doctors 'not telling patients the pitfalls of surgery'. The Telegraph, 8 November 2012. http://v.gd/telegraph_pitfalls

162 Thorsen O, Hartveit M, Baerheim A. General practitioners' reflections on referring: An asymmetric or non-dialogical process? Scandinavian Journal of Primary Health Care 2012;30(4):241–246. http://dx.doi.org/10.3109/02813432.2012.711190

163 Holman P, Ruud T, Grepperud S. Horizontal equity and mental health care: a study of priority ratings by clinicians and teams at outpatient clinics. BMC Health Services Research 2012;12(1):162. http://dx.doi.org/10.1186/1472-6963-12-162

Chapter 36

164 Major restructuring could jeopardise NHS reform agenda, warns The King's Fund. The King's Fund, 2005. http://v.gd/kingsfund_jeopardise

165 The King's Fund Commission urges politicians to value the role of management in the NHS. The King's Fund, 2011. http://v.gd/kingsfund_rolemanagement

166 Appleby, J. Payment by Results: time for a rethink? The King's Fund, 2012. http://www.kingsfund.org.uk/blog/2012/11/payment-results-time-rethink

167 Hart JT. The Inverse Care Law. Lancet 1971;1:405–12.

168 Gaffney D, Pollock AM, Price D, Shaoul J. The private finance initiative: PFI in the NHS – is there an economic case? British Medical Journal 1999;319:116–9.

     Social Inequalities in Health, New Evidence and Policy Implications. Siegrist J, Marmot M (eds). Oxford University Press, 2006.

169 Principles of Commissioning – Summary. RCGP Centre for Commissioning, 2011. http://www.rcgp.org.uk/revalidation-and-cpd/centre-for-commissioning.aspx

Chapter 37

170 Timmins, N. Never again? The story of the Health and Social Care Act 2012. The King's Fund and the Institute for Government, 2012. http://v.gd/neveragain

171 Managing high value capital equipment in the NHS in England. HC 822, National Audit Office, 2011. http://www.nao.org.uk/publications/1011/nhs_high_value_equipment.aspx

172 Limb M. Half of GPs on clinical commissioning groups have financial links with private providers. BMJ 2012;344:e2431. http://dx.doi.org/10.1136/bmj.e2431

173 Lords financial links to companies involved in private healthcare. Social Investigations, 2012. http://socialinvestigations.blogspot.co.uk/p/lords-financial-links-to-companies.html

174 Changes to public health in England from April 2013. RTPI, 2012. http://www.rtpi.org.uk/media/1570766/changes_in_public_health_for_website.pdf

175 Health reforms will be the end of free care for all, warn experts. BMJ, 2012. http://www.bmj.com/press-releases/2012/03/08/health-reforms-will-be-end-free-care-all-warn-experts

Chapter 38

176 Health at a Glance 2010: OECD Indicators. OECD, 2010. http://dx.doi.org/10.1787/health_glance-2010-en

177 Health at a Glance 2010: OECD Indicators. OECD, 2010. http://dx.doi.org/10.1787/health_glance-2010-en

178 How Does the United States Compare. OECD Health Data 2012. OECD, 2012. http://www.oecd.org/unitedstates/BriefingNoteUSA2012.pdf

179 For example,

   Oishi S, Kesebir S, Diener E. Income inequality and happiness. Psychological Science 2011;22(9):1095–1100. http://dx.doi.org/10.1177/0956797611417262

   Ferrer-i-Carbonell A, Ramos X. Inequality and happiness: a survey. GINI Discussion Paper 38. AIAS, 2012. http://v.gd/inequalityhappiness

180 Wilkinson R, Pickett K. The Spirit Level: Why Greater Equality Makes Societies Stronger. Bloomsbury, 2009.

Appendix

181 Amsterdam JD, Li Y, Soeller I, Rockwell K, Mao JJ, Shults J. A randomized, double-blind, placebo-controlled trial of oral *Matricaria recutita* (chamomile) extract therapy for generalized anxiety disorder. Journal of Clinical Psychopharmacology 2009;29(4):378–382. http://dx.doi.org/10.1097/JCP.0b013e3181ac935c

182 Pittler MH, Ernst E. Kava extract versus placebo for treating anxiety. Cochrane Database of Systematic Reviews, 2010;6:CD003383. http://dx.doi.org/10.1002/14651858.CD003383

183 Pittler MH, Ernst E. Efficacy of kava extract for treating anxiety: systematic review and meta-analysis. Journal of Clinical Psychopharmacology 2000;20(1):84–9.

184 Drug Record: Black Cohosh (*Cimicifuga racemosa*). LiverTox, 2012. http://livertox. nih.gov/BlackCohosh.htm

185 Hawkes N. Herbal medicine might be responsible for high incidence of urinary tract cancer. BMJ 2012;344:e2644. http://dx.doi.org/10.1136/bmj.e2644

186 Wolf M, Tamaschke C, Mayer W, Heger M. [Efficacy of Arnica in varicose vein surgery: results of a randomized, double-blind, placebo-controlled pilot study]. Forschende Komplementärmedizin und klassische Naturheilkunde 2003 Oct;10(5):242–7. [Article in German]

187 Cornu C, Joseph P, Gaillard S, et al. No effect of a homoeopathic combination of *Arnica montana* and *Bryonia alba* on bleeding, inflammation, and ischaemia after aortic valve surgery. British Journal of Clinical Pharmacology 2010;69(2):136–142. http://dx.doi.org/10.1111/j.1365-2125.2009.03574.x

188 Allen-Hall L, Arnason JT, Cano P, Lafrenie RM. *Uncaria tomentosa* acts as a potent TNF-α inhibitor through NF-κB. Journal of Ethnopharmacology 2010;127(3):685–693. http://dx.doi.org/10.1016/j.jep.2009.12.004

189 Brien S, Lewith G, McGregor G. Devil's claw (*Harpagophytum procumbens*) as a treatment for osteoarthritis: a review of efficacy and safety. The Journal of Alternative and Complementary Medicine 2006;12(10):981–993. http://dx.doi. org/10.1089/acm.2006.12.981

190 Kimmatkar N, Thawani V, Hingorani L, Khiyani R. Efficacy and tolerability of *Boswellia serrata* extract in treatment of osteoarthritis of knee – A randomized double blind placebo controlled trial. Phytomedicine 2003;10(1):3–7. http://dx.doi. org/10.1078/094471103321648593

191 Jurenka JS. Anti-inflammatory properties of curcumin, a major constituent of *Curcuma longa*: a review of preclinical and clinical research. Alternative Medicine Review 2009 Jun;14(2):141–53.

192 Kuptniratsaikul V, Thanakhumtorn S, Chinswangwatanakul P, Wattanamongkonsil L, Thamlikitkul V. Efficacy and safety of *Curcuma domestica* extracts in patients with knee osteoarthritis. The Journal of Alternative and Complementary Medicine 2009;15(8):891–897. http://dx.doi.org/10.1089/ acm.2008.0186

193 Altman RD, Marcussen KC. Effects of a ginger extract on knee pain in patients with osteoarthritis. Arthritis & Rheumatism 2001;44:2531–2538. http://dx.doi. org/10.1002/1529-0131(200111)44:11<2531::AID-ART433>3.0.CO;2-J

194 Borrelli F, Capasso R, Aviello G, Pittler MH, Izzo AA. Effectiveness and safety of ginger in the treatment of pregnancy-induced nausea and vomiting. Obstetrics & Gynecology. 2005;105(4):849–856. http://dx.doi.org/10.1097/01. AOG.0000154890.47642.23

195 Rahman K, Lowe GM. Garlic and cardiovascular disease: a critical review. Journal of Nutrition 2006;136(3):736S–740S. http://jn.nutrition.org/content/136/3/736S. short

196 Ried K, Frank OR, Stocks NP, Fakler P, Sullivan T. Effect of garlic on blood pressure: a systematic review and meta-analysis. BMC Cardiovascular Disorders. 2008;8(1):13. http://dx.doi.org/10.1186/1471-2261-8-13

197 Natural Standard Research Collaboration. Omega-3 fatty acids, fish oil, alpha-linolenic acid 2011. http://www.mayoclinic.com/health/fish-oil/NS_patient-fishoil

198 Omega-3 Fatty Acids. University of Maryland Medical Center, 2011. http://www. umm.edu/altmed/articles/omega-3-000316.htm

199 Mori TA, Bao DQ, Burke V, Puddey IB, Beilin LJ. Docosahexaenoic acid but not eicosapentaenoic acid lowers ambulatory blood pressure and heart rate in humans. Hypertension 1999;34:252–60. http://hyper.ahajournals.org/content/34/2/253.long

200 Fish Oil. Medline Plus Supplements. U.S. National Library of Medicine, 2011. http://www.nlm.nih.gov/medlineplus/druginfo/natural/993.html